RADIATION PROTECTION

in Diagnostic X-Ray Imaging

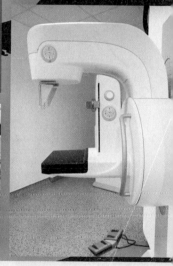

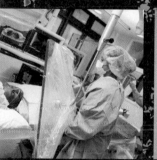

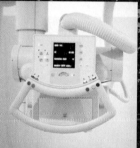

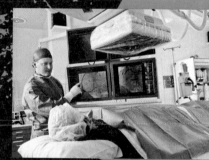

Euclid Seeram, PhD, MSc, BSc, FCAMRT
Honorary Senior Lecturer, Medical Imaging and Radiation Sciences
Medical Image Optimization and Perception Group, Faculty of Health Sciences
University of Sydney
Sydney, Australia

Adjunct Associate Professor, Department of Medical Imaging and Radiation Sciences
Medicine, Nursing and Health Sciences
Monash University
Melbourne, Australia

Adjunct Professor, Faculty of Science
Charles Sturt University
Melbourne, Australia

Patrick C. Brennan, PhD
Professor, Medical Imaging and Radiation Sciences
Medical Image Optimization and Perception Group, Faculty of
Health Sciences
University of Sydney
Sydney, Australia

JONES & BARTLETT
LEARNING

World Headquarters
Jones & Bartlett Learning
5 Wall Street
Burlington, MA 01803
978-443-5000
info@jblearning.com
www.jblearning.com

Jones & Bartlett Learning books and products are available through most bookstores and online booksellers. To contact Jones & Bartlett Learning directly, call 800-832-0034, fax 978-443-8000, or visit our website, www.jblearning.com.

Substantial discounts on bulk quantities of Jones & Bartlett Learning publications are available to corporations, professional associations, and other qualified organizations. For details and specific discount information, contact the special sales department at Jones & Bartlett Learning via the above contact information or send an email to specialsales@jblearning.com.

1453-9

Production Credits
Publisher: Cathy Esperti
Associate Acquisitions Editor: Kayla Dos Santos
Associate Editor: Roxanne McCorry
Production Editor: Leah Corrigan
Marketing Manager: Grace Richards
VP, Manufacturing and Inventory Control: Therese Connell
Composition: Cenveo® Publisher Services
Project Management: Cenveo Publisher Services
Cover Design: Kristin E. Parker
Rights & Media Specialist: Jamey O'Quinn
Cover Image: (radiation symbol) © frees/Shutterstock; (mammogram image) © Serdar Tibet/Shutterstock; (mammogram machine) © zlikovec/Shutterstock; (patient on table) © EPSTOCK/Shutterstock; (x-ray machine) © Tyler Olson/Shutterstock; (surgeon and patient) © Monkey Business Images/Shutterstock
Printing and Binding: RR Donnelley
Cover Printing: RR Donnelley

Library of Congress Cataloging-in-Publication Data
Names: Seeram, Euclid, author. | Brennan, Patrick C. (Patrick Christopher), author.
Title: Radiation protection in diagnostic imaging / by Euclid Seeram and Patrick C. Brennan.
Description: Burlington, MA : Jones & Bartlett Learning, [2017] | Includes bibliographical references and index.
Identifiers: LCCN 2015044232 | ISBN 9781449652814 (paperback : alk. paper)
Subjects: | MESH: Radiation Protection—standards. | Radiometry—methods. | Radiotherapy Dosage.
Classification: LCC RC78.7.R4 | NLM WN 650 | DDC 616.07/575—dc23 LC record available at http://lccn.loc.gov/2015044232

6048

Printed in the United States of America
20 19 18 17 16   10 9 8 7 6 5 4 3 2 1

Dedication

This book is dedicated with love and affection to my son, Dave, and daughter-in-law, Priscilla, two smart and hard-working young people; and to my clever and beautiful granddaughter, Claire. You bring so much joy and happiness to our lives.

Euclid Seeram

To my wonderful little people who keep knocking their heads and to my wonderful big person who keeps knocking my head.

Patrick C. Brennan

Brief Contents

Chapter 1: Radiation Protection Overview   1

Chapter 2: Basic Physics for Radiation Protection: An Overview   17

Chapter 3: Radiation Exposure and Dose Units   45

Chapter 4: The Radiobiology of Low-Dose Radiation   67

Chapter 5: Radiation Protection Practice   99

Chapter 6: Radiation Protection Organizations   135

Chapter 7: Factors Affecting Dose in Radiographic Imaging   147

Chapter 8: Factors Affecting Dose in Fluoroscopy   165

Chapter 9: Dose in Digital Radiography   175

Chapter 10: Radiation Dose in Computed Tomography   199

Chapter 11: Image Quality Assessment Tools for Dose Optimization in Digital Radiography   211

Chapter 12: Diagnostic Reference Levels   221

Chapter 13: Optimization of Radiation Protection: Regulatory and Guidance Recommendations   247

Chapter 14: Protective Shielding in Diagnostic Radiology   261

Chapter 15: Radiation Protection Through Quality Control   279

Appendix A: ARRT Exam Specifications Content Map   285

Appendix B: ASRT Objectives Content Map   287

Index   293

Contents

Preface   xv

Acknowledgments   xxi

About the Authors   xxiii

Reviewers   xxv

1 Radiation Protection Overview   1

Introduction   2

A Rationale for Radiation Protection   3

    Data Sources on Biological Effects   3

    Dose-response Models   3

    Biological Effects   4

The Philosophy of Radiation Protection   4

    The ICRP Framework   5

    Radiation Dose Limits   5

Radiation Protection Concepts   6

    Historical Perspectives   6

    The Four Quartets of Radiation Protection   7

    X-Ray Dosimetry   9

    Dose-Image Quality Optimization   10

    Diagnostic Reference Levels   11

Radiation Protection Organizations and Reports   11

    Organizations   11

    Reports and Publications   11

Radiation Protection and the Technologist   12

    Responsibilities: Four Major Components   12

Discussion Questions   15

References   15

2 Basic Physics for Radiation Protection: An Overview   17

Introduction   18

Atomic Structure   19

    The Element   19

    The Atom   19

    The Nucleus of an Atom   20

    Electrons   21

Types of Radiation   22

    Particulate Radiations   22

    Electromagnetic Radiation   24

    X-Rays and Gamma Rays   27

    Ionizing Radiation   32

X-Ray and Gamma Radiation Interactions   33
    X-Ray Interactions I: Elastic (or Coherent or Rayleigh) Scattering   34
    X-Ray Interactions II: Photoelectric Absorption   35
    X-Ray Interactions III: Compton Scattering   36
    X-Ray Interactions IV: Pair Production   40
Descriptive Terms or Concepts Associated with Radiation   42
    Linear Energy Transfer (LET)   42
    Linear Attenuation Coefficient   42
    Mass Attenuation Coefficient   42
    Inverse Square Law   43
Discussion Questions   44
Reference   44

3   Radiation Exposure and Dose Units   45
Introduction   46
Radiation: A Natural History   46
Sources of Radiation Exposure   47
    Natural Background Sources   47
    Man-Made (Non-Medical) Radiation Sources   50
    Sources of Exposure in Medicine   51
    Diagnostic Exposures   52
    Nuclear Medicine   54
    Radiation Therapy   54
    Footnote to Medical Radiation Doses   56
Basic Dosimetric Quantities and Units   56
    Units of Exposure   57
    Quantities of Radiation Dose   57
    Absorbed Dose   57
    Equivalent Dose   58
    Effective Dose   58
    Collective Effective Dose   61
    Kinetic Energy Released Per Unit Mass (Kerma)   61
Patient Doses in Diagnostic Imaging   63
Staff Doses in Diagnostic Imaging   63
Discussion Questions   65
References   66

4   The Radiobiology of Low-Dose Radiation   67
Introduction   68
Stochastic Effects   68
    Background   68
    Basic Principles and Debate Over Risks with Low-Dose Exposures   68
    Linear No-Threshold (LNT) Model   69
    Do Diagnostic X-Ray Exposures Present Any Risk to Humans?   72
    Mechanisms of Radiation-Induced Change Responsible for
        Stochastic Risks   73

DNA and Cell Repair Mechanisms Following Irradiation   77
How Long Does it Take for Damaged DNA to Manifest Itself in Man?   81
Deterministic Effects   87
Factors Influencing Stochastic Risk or Deterministic Effects
    at Low-Dose Exposures   89
Radiosensitivity of the Cell   89
Kinetics   92
Presence of Oxygen   93
Dose Rate   93
Radioprotectants and Radiosensitizers   93
Changes in Non-Irradiated Cells   94
Genomic Instability   95
Bystander Effect   95
Epigenetics   95
Effects of Radiation on Children, Embryos, and Fetuses   95
Discussion Questions   97
References   97

5 Radiation Protection Practice   99
Introduction   100
Dose Risks in Diagnostic Imaging   100
Justification   104
Optimization   109
Optimization Initiatives   115
Optimization and Cost   116
Optimization: Image Quality Versus Diagnostic Efficacy   116
Radiation Dose Limits   116
Radiation Detection and Measurement   118
Thermoluminescent Dosimetry   118
Dose-Area Product Meters (DAPs)   122
Solid-State Meters   127
Radiochromic Film   129
Discussion Questions   132
References   132

6 Radiation Protection Organizations   135
Introduction   136
International Organizations   136
International Commission on Radiological Protection (ICRP)   136
International Commission on Radiation Unit and Measurement (ICRU)   138
United Nations Scientific Committee on the Effects of Atomic
    Radiation (UNSCEAR)   138
Radiation Effects Research Foundation (RERF)   139
Biological Effects of Ionizing Radiation Committee (BEIR)   139
National Organizations   139
National Council on Radiation Protection and Measurement (NCRP)   140

Center for Devices and Radiological Health (CDRH)   140
Radiation Protection Bureau-Health Canada (RPB-HC)   141
National Radiological Protection Board-United Kingdom
(NRPB-UK)   141
Definition of Terms Used in Reports   141
ICRP's Definitions   142
NCRP's Definitions   142
RPB-HC's Definitions   142
Radiation Protection Recommendations–Common Elements   142
Discussion Questions   145
References   145

7   Factors Affecting Dose in Radiographic Imaging   147
Introduction   148
System Components Affecting Dose: an Overview   148
Radiographic Systems: Exposure Components   148
Clinical Factors   149
Responsibility of Referring Physicians   149
Role of the Technologist   150
Role of the Radiologist   150
Responsibility of the Patient   150
Responsibilities and Radiation Protection   150
Technical Factors in Radiography   151
Exposure Technique Factors   151
Automatic Exposure Control   152
X-Ray Generator Waveform   152
Filtration   153
Collimation and Field Size   154
Beam Alignment   155
Source-to-Image Receptor Distance/Source-to-Skin Distance   155
Patient Thickness and Density   156
Anti-Scatter Grids   156
Sensitivity of the Image Receptor   157
Film Processing   157
Repeat Radiographic Examinations   158
Repeat Rates in Digital Radiography   159
Shielding Radio-Sensitive Organs   159
Discussion Questions   162
References   162

8   Factors Affecting Dose in Fluoroscopy   165
Introduction   166
Radiation Effects From Fluoroscopic X-Ray Exposure   166
Fluoroscopy Systems: Types and Major Components   166
Image Intensifier-Based Fluoroscopic System   167
The Flat-Panel Digital Detector-Based Fluoroscopy System   168

   Major Dose Factors in Fixed Fluoroscopic Imaging Systems ... 169
      Fluoroscopic Exposure Factors ... 170
      Fluoroscopic Instrumentation Factors ... 170
   Major Factors in Mobile Fluoroscopy Systems ... 172
   C-Arm Computed Tomography Fluoroscopy ... 173
   Discussion Questions ... 174
   References ... 174

9   Dose in Digital Radiography ... 175
   Introduction ... 176
   Film-Screen Technology ... 176
   The Digital Imaging Era: A New Paradigm ... 177
      Exposure Creep ... 179
      Highlighting Inappropriate Exposures ... 179
   Principles of Exposure Indices ... 179
      Scientific Criteria for Proposed Exposure Indices ... 179
      Practical Criteria for Proposed Exposure Indices ... 181
   How are Exposure Indices Established? ... 183
      What are the Options? ... 183
      Exposure Indices Represent the Exposure ... 183
      Previous Manufacturer Solutions ... 183
      Aapm Tg 116 Solution ... 185
   Deviation Index ... 190
      Why an Exposure Index? ... 190
      Deviation Index Action Levels ... 190
      IEC Publication ... 191
      What Can Be Gained From Audits of Exposure Index? ... 191
      Other Factors to Consider with the Exposure Index ... 195
   Discussion Questions ... 197
   References ... 197

10 Radiation Dose in Computed Tomography ... 199
   Introduction ... 200
   Early Pioneering Work: Nobel Prize for CT Development ... 200
   The CT Process: Basic Principles and Major Components ... 200
      Data Flow in a CT Scanner ... 202
      Multislice CT Technology: The Pitch ... 202
      CT Image Quality Characteristics: An Overview ... 203
   Risks of CT: A Rationale for Dose Reduction and Optimization ... 203
   CT Dose Descriptors ... 204
      The CTDI ... 204
      The Dose Length Product ... 205
   Factors Affecting Dose in CT ... 206
      Exposure Technique Factors: mAs and kVp ... 206
      Collimation ... 206
      Pitch ... 206
      Patient Centering ... 207

	Automatic Tube Current Modulation	207
	Iterative Image Reconstruction	207
	Dose-Image Quality Optimization Research in CT	208
	An Example of CT Dose Optimization Study	208
	Discussion Questions	210
	References	210

11	Image Quality Assessment Tools for Dose Optimization in Digital Radiography	211
	Introduction	212
	Radiation Dose Quantities	212
	Image Quality in Digital Radiography	212
	What is Image Quality?	213
	Assessment of Image Quality	214
	Visual Grading of Normal Anatomy	215
	Visual Grading Analysis	215
	Dose Optimization Research	216
	Example of a Dose Optimization Study in Computed Radiography	217
	Discussion Questions	219
	References	219

12	Diagnostic Reference Levels	221
	Introduction	222
	Patient Dose Variations	222
	Historical Perspective	222
	Patient Dose Variations Today	222
	What are Diagnostic Reference Levels (DRLs)?	224
	DRLs: An Overview	224
	DRLs: A Definition	224
	What are Diagnostic Reference Levels *Not*?	228
	Why is It Important to Implement DRLs?	229
	Have DRLs Reduced Doses?	230
	Establishment of Diagnostic Reference Values	230
	The Survey to Establish Current Dose Levels	230
	Calculation of DRL Values	237
	Pediatric DRL Values	241
	Diagnostic Reference Levels: A Global Activity	241
	Practical Considerations When Gathering The Data	243
	Discussion Questions	245
	References	245

13	Optimization of Radiation Protection: Regulatory and Guidance Recommendations	247
	Introduction	248
	Radiation Protection Reports	248
	Optimization of Radiation Protection	249
	Education and Training	249

Equipment Specifications   250
Personnel Practices   250
Shielding   250
Equipment Design and Performance Recommendations   250
Radiographic Equipment: General Recommendations   250
Radiographic Equipment: Specific Recommendations   251
Fluoroscopic Equipment   252
Mobile Radiographic Equipment   253
Recommendations for Personnel Practices   254
Protection of Personnel   254
Protection of Patients   255
Recommendations for Radiography in Pregnancy   256
Recommendations for Quality Assurance   259
Discussion Questions   260
References   260

14 Protective Shielding in Diagnostic Radiology   261
Introduction   262
X-Ray Tube Shielding   262
X-Ray Room Shielding   265
Radioprotective Materials   265
General Principles   268
Primary and Secondary Barriers   270
How is the Amount of Shielding Calculated?   272
The Formulae   276
The Planning Process   277
Discussion Questions   278
References   278

15 Radiation Protection Through Quality Control   279
Introduction   280
Definitions of QA and QC   280
Quality Assurance (QA)   280
Quality Control (QC)   280
Dose Optimization   281
Levels of Optimization   281
QC Concepts Leading to Dose Optimization   281
The Tolerance Limit in QC Testing   283
Exceeding the Tolerance Limit   283
Dose Reduction/Optimization as a Consequence of QC   283
Discussion Questions   284
References   284

Appendix A: ARRT Exam Specifications Content Map   285

Appendix B: ASRT Objectives Content Map   287

Index   293

Preface

Radiation protection in diagnostic imaging has evolved through the years, ever since the discovery and use of x-rays to image the human body in 1895. Such evolution has demonstrated several cardinal principles, concepts, procedures, and techniques to reduce the dose to the patient. Such dose-reduction strategies became very important as a result of the evolving knowledge of the biological effects of radiation exposure on both animals and humans, which provides the fundamental basis for radiation protection. The data from human exposure comes from the early instances in which individuals were exposed to high doses, including exposures among radiologists and physicists, individuals working in radiation and nuclear power industries, survivors of the atomic bomb explosions at Hiroshima and Nagasaki, and people living near sites of nuclear reactor accidents, such as the catastrophes at Three Mile Island and Chernobyl. Furthermore, another important source of data on biological effects of radiation exposure has been identified in the Biological Effects of Ionizing Radiation (BEIR) reports. Specifically, Section 7 of BEIR Report VII, presents data on exposure of patients to high doses from medical radiation. It is interesting to note that of the data sources mentioned above, the BEIR VII report puts the maximum emphasis on the data from the Hiroshima and Nagasaki atomic bomb survivors, which has been collected by the Radiation Effects Research Foundation (RERF). Another important concept derived from these studies is that of a dose–risk model, sometimes referred to as a dose–response relationship. The model shows what happens to the risk of radiation injury as the dose increases. Several models have subsequently emerged, and therefore the obvious question in the minds of medical imaging personnel is, which model is best suited when imaging patients? In this regard, Hendee and O'Connor (2012; p. 316) state that while the Linear No Threshold (LNT) model is most widely utilized,

> This model is not chosen because there is solid biologic or epidemiologic data supporting its use. Rather, it is used because of its simplicity and because it is a conservative approach . . . For the purpose of establishing radiation protection standards for occupationally exposed individuals and members of the public, a conservative model that overestimates the risk is preferred over a model that underestimates risk.

With the above ideas in mind, radiation protection is now an integral part of the curriculum in radiologic technology—and more importantly, it provides significant tools to protect not only the patient, but radiology personnel and members of the public as well. For example, a recent and well-established tool in radiation protection is *optimization of the dose-image quality relationship,* in an effort to reduce the dose to as low as reasonably achievable (ALARA) and not compromise the diagnostic quality of the image. This tool has become commonplace in digital radiography (DR) and digital fluoroscopy (DF), and in computed tomography (CT). Yet another popular tool for use in optimization of radiation protection is the diagnostic reference level (DRL) concept. The American College of Radiology (ACR) defines the DRL as "an investigation level to identify unusually high radiation dose or exposure levels for common diagnostic medical x-ray procedures." In 2012, the National Council on Radiation Protection and Measurements (NCRP) developed Report No. 172: *Reference Levels and Achievable Doses in Medical and Dental Imaging: Recommendations for the United States,* "… intended to reach a broad audience of all interested in radiation safety and health protection in medicine."

In addition, several recent developments have been introduced to address the increasing dose to the patient, not only in DR (exposure creep) but also in CT. These include updated knowledge of the exposure indicator and its effect on radiation dose in DR and the use of automatic tube current modulation (ATCM) and iterative image reconstruction algorithms in CT to reduce the noise in the image, and to reduce the dose to the patient. Another significant development that is now receiving attention in North America is that of image quality assessment tools for use in dose optimization studies. These tools include the use of quantitative objective physical measures as well as subjective observer performance when evaluating images in a clinical environment. Observer performance methods fall into two categories depending on the nature of the primary viewing task. If the task of the observer is lesion detection in the image, the method used would be the Receiver Operating Characteristics (ROC) analysis. If the viewing task is the visualization of anatomical structures, the method used would be Visual Grading Analysis (VGA).

Keeping these recent developments in mind, the purpose of this book is to provide a text that brings together a number of the critical issues in radiologic protection and presents these in an understandable way to individuals such as clinicians, radiographers, and other individuals who do not have an in-depth knowledge of medical physics. In particular, it will:

1. Provide a current and detailed overview of the biological effects of radiation exposure, because this topic establishes a firm rationale for radiation protection.

2. Outline the fundamental physical principles and technical aspects of radiation protection, including the essential physics for radiation protection, radiation exposure, dosimetry, dose limits, and the factors affecting dose in DR, DF, and CT.

3. Outline the major components of the DRL and its use in dose optimization.

4. Outline image quality assessment tools for use in dose-image quality optimization studies.

5. Outline the current regulatory and guidance recommendations for radiation protection in diagnostic imaging.

6. Explain the role of quality assurance/quality control in optimization of radiation protection in diagnostic imaging.

With the above objectives in mind, this book can be used as an introduction to radiation protection in diagnostic radiography, as a reference for the professional technologist, and as a supplement for applied fields such as biomedical engineering technology and dental hygiene programs.

Structure of the Book

Radiation Protection Overview

The first three chapters of the text are intended to orient and review the essential background needed for a thorough understanding of the nature and scope of radiation protection. Chapter 1 is a pivotal chapter, and its purpose is to provide a comprehensive overview of the fundamentals of radiation protection and to show a roadmap of topics to be covered in the rest of the book. While Chapter 2 reviews the basic physics necessary for a clear understanding of radiation protection and assumes that the reader has a background in high school-level physics, Chapter 3 outlines the nature of radiation exposure and dosimetry.

Biological Effects of Radiation

Chapter 4 is dedicated to the biological effects of radiation and provides the rationale for radiation protection.

General Radiation Protection Principles and Concepts

The next six chapters are dedicated to explaining general radiation protection principles and concepts. While Chapter 5 presents a detailed description of current radiation protection standards, Chapter 6 examines various international and national radiation protection organizations that are instrumental in developing and promulgating various radiation protection guidelines and recommendations for the safe use of ionizing radiation in medicine. Chapters 7, 8, 9, and 10 should be considered pivotal chapters as well because they deal with the technical factors affecting dose in radiography, fluoroscopy, digital radiography, and CT, respectively.

Tools for Dose Optimization Studies

The following four chapters relate to tools for dose optimization studies. Specifically, Chapter 11 outlines the fundamental tools for image quality assessment for use in dose optimization studies and provides an example of a dose optimization study in computed radiography (CR) imaging. Chapter 12 presents a detailed description of DRLs and how they relate to dose optimization. Chapters 13 and 14 address elements relating to regulatory and guidance recommendations and protective shielding requirements for diagnostic radiology, respectively.

Finally, Chapter 15 discusses the role of quality assurance and quality control in the protection of patients and personnel.

Key Features

A significant challenge in writing this textbook was to meet the wide and varied requirements of its users, both students and instructors alike. In doing so, we have written the materials in a comprehensive manner in order to maintain the student's interest and attention. An important pedagogical feature is the use of detailed chapter outlines and learning objectives at the beginning of each chapter.

- **Outline:** The purpose of the outline is to orient the student to the main topics that will be covered.
- **Learning Objectives:** The use of the learning objectives is to emphasize the importance of each of the topics and subtopics covered through the use of action verbs, such as define, identify, describe, discuss, and outline, for example. Furthermore, the objectives provide criteria for examination.
- **Summary of Key Concepts:** These appear at the end of each chapter and provide readers with a tool to aid in study of the material.
- **Discussion Questions:** These are also provided at the end of each chapter for critical engagement of the material.

The content of this book is intended to meet the educational requirements (for entry to practice) of the following professional radiologic technology associations:

- American Society of Radiologic Technologists (ASRT)
- Canadian Association of Medical Radiation Technologists (CAMRT)
- College of Radiographers in the United Kingdom
- Radiography societies and associations in Asia, Australia, Europe, and Africa

An important consideration to note, however, is that the regulatory and guidance recommendations of all countries could not be included in this textbook, and therefore readers must consult radiation protection reports of their respective national radiation protection organizations and agencies.

Instructor Resources

In addition to the features included in the book, resources have been provided to aid in instruction of the material:

- Lecture outlines in PowerPoint format for each chapter
- A guide for mapping the textbook content to ASRT (American Association of Radiologic Technologists) and the CAMRT (Canadian Association of Medical Radiation Technologists)
- Chapter quizzes and chapter-specific test questions
- Practice activities
- Course syllabi for planning your lessons

Radiation protection in diagnostic imaging is an integral part of the education and skill set of radiologic technologists who play a significant role in the optimization of the radiation dose to the population. This book offers one small step in achieving that goal.

Best wishes in your pursuit of the study of radiation protection of patients, personnel, and members of the public.

Euclid Seeram, PhD, MSc, BSc, FCAMRT
Patrick C. Brennan, PhD

Acknowledgments

The single most important and satisfying task in writing a textbook of this nature is to acknowledge the encouragement of those individuals who perceive the value of the contribution to the literature.

The scope and content of this book are built around the work of several radiation protection organizations made up of expert radiobiologists, medical physicists, and radiologists, who have done the original research. In reality, they are the tacit authors of this text. Each of us, Euclid and Patrick, expresses our gratitude specifically in two parts of this acknowledgments section.

We owe special thanks to the people at Jones & Bartlett Learning. First, thanks are due to David D. Cella (Executive Publisher), who initiated the submission of this text and worked out the contract details for publication. Second, we thank Cathy Esperti (Publisher), Teresa Reilly (Acquisitions Editor), Kayla Dos Santos (Associate Acquisitions Editor), Roxanne McCorry (Associate Editor), Taylor Ferracane (Editorial Assistant), and Leah Corrigan (Production Editor) for their continued support and encouragement to bring this project to fruition.

We must also thank the individuals at Cenveo Publisher Services, especially Moumita Majumdar (Associate Project Manager), for doing a wonderful job on the manuscript to bring it to its final form.

Finally, to all of our students who have passed through our radiation protection classes through the years: Thanks for the questions.

Euclid Seeram

I owe a good deal of thanks to Stewart Bushong, ScD, Perry Sprawls, PhD, Jerrold Bushberg, PhD, Anthony Wolbarst, PhD, Anthony Seibert, PhD, Charles Willis, PhD, Kerry Krug, PhD, Hans Swam, PhD (all medical physicists), and Elizabeth Travis, a radiobiologist at the University of Texas, MD Anderson Cancer Center, from whose research and published works I have learned a great deal. I owe a special thanks to John Aldrich, PhD, for his excellent courses on DR and CT that I have attended and for his instruction on CT and DR quality control. I also thank Francine Anselmo, RTR, MBA, head of the "Medical X-Rays" including the "Diagnostic X-Ray Facility Protection" section of the British Columbia Center for Disease Control, for always inviting me to attend all radiation protection seminars sponsored by her agency.

Hans Swan, PhD, and Rob Davidson, PhD, both from Charles Sturt University in Australia, and Stewart Bushong, ScD, from Baylor College of Medicine in Houston, Texas, have provided me with a good deal of encouragement and explanations of radiation dose optimization in their roles as supervisors of my PhD dissertation, entitled *Optimization of the Exposure Indicator of a Computed Radiography Imaging System as a Radiation Dose Management Strategy.*

I would also like to express my sincere appreciation to two individuals from whom I have learned a great deal on the subject of dose-image quality optimization. These include my coauthor, Patrick C. Brennan, PhD, of the University of Sydney, and Anders Tingberg, PhD, of Lund University, Sweden. Dr. Brennan has taught me the nature and elements of radiation dose-image quality optimization research, which includes several guiding principles, and concepts of radiation protection. Thanks, Patrick, for always providing me with the motivation to specialize in this significant and topical area of radiation protection. Dr. Tingberg, on the other hand, provided me with the bound copies of *Quantifying the Quality of Medical X-Ray Images*—his research focusing on the use of the Visual Grading Analysis (VGA) procedure for evaluating image quality.

I must also thank my family for their continued support and encouragement while I work on writing textbooks. To my charming wife Trish, the cutest Chaplain I know, and overall special person in my life; thanks for your love and encouragement in all my writing activities. To my smart, wise, handsome, and caring son, David, who is the brilliant young editor and publisher of an online digital photography magazine (available at photographybb.com) and of course a wonderful dad. To my beautiful daughter-in-law, Priscilla, a smart, remarkable, and caring young woman, thanks for blessing me with a brilliant, beautiful, and charming granddaughter, Claire. She's the greatest and now considered "number one!"

Last but not least, I would also like to acknowledge here the love, support, and encouragement of both my mother, Betty, and my late father, Samuel, who passed away several years ago (thanks for having me and thanks for the memories, Dad); my father-in-law Edward Penner, and my mother-in-law, Joan (who earned the title "the most well-read person I know" from me, and who passed away several years ago). I love all of you.

Patrick C. Brennan

I am deeply grateful to the University of Sydney for providing me with special study leave to facilitate this text and to all my colleagues for providing much-needed data and expert advice. Thanks are also due to expert agencies such as the Health Protection Agency, UK, (Steve Ebdon-Jackson) and the International Commission on Radiological Protection, whose wealth of superb publications made this task so much easier. I will always be very appreciative of Horace and Michaela at Caffe La Mura, for providing the perfect environment to write. Finally, and very importantly, many many thanks are due to Ms. Phuong Trieu; I am indebted to her for her expertise and huge persistence in helping me provide almost all the figures contained within this text.

I extend my gratitude to my family for their help, love, support, and encouragement. Forever I will be indebted to my parents, my sister, and my wife, each of whom in some way sacrificed something to facilitate my career.

About the Authors

Euclid Seeram, PhD, MSc, BSc, FCAMRT

Dr. Euclid Seeram is currently an honorary senior lecturer, adjunct associate professor, and adjunct professor at the University of Sydney, Australia; Monash University, Australia; and Charles Sturt University, Australia; respectively. He has published over 55 papers in professional and peer review radiologic technology journals and has had 20 textbooks published to date on computed tomography, computers in radiology, radiographic instrumentation, digital radiography, and radiation protection. Presently, he is on the editorial boards for *Radiography, Biomedical Imaging and Intervention Journal, International Journal of Radiology and Medical Imaging*, and the *Journal of Allied Health*. Furthermore, he is currently on the international advisory panel for the *Journal of Medical Radiation Sciences*, and is a founding member and an invited peer reviewer for the *Journal of Medical Imaging and Radiation Sciences*. His current research interests are focused on radiation dose optimization in CT and digital radiography imaging systems and he has published several papers on these two topics.

Patrick C. Brennan, PhD

Patrick C. Brennan is currently Professor of Medical Imaging and Associate Dean, International at the Faculty of Health Sciences, University of Sydney, Australia. In the latter role and within the last 3 years he has forged productive interdisciplinary research and teaching collaborations across health sciences with the leading institutions in China, Southeast Asia, the Middle East, and the Americas. He is also leader of the University of Sydney's Breast Cancer Special Interest Group, consisting of over 100 academic members. Since 2011, he has been (with Professor Warwick Lee) National Co-Director of BREAST. He has won 2 medals of excellence for teaching and has acted as undergraduate, graduate, and PhD examiner in 9 universities across Europe, Asia, and the Americas.

In 2009 he moved from the School of Medicine in University College Dublin, where he was an Associate Professor and Head of Diagnostic Imaging, to the University of Sydney. His new role was to establish an active research group focusing on medical imaging while helping to transform the current teaching program. Since that time he has established a Medical Image Optimization and Perception Group (MIOPeG), which is now leading the world in medical imaging research, with publications in the highest ranking international imaging journals.

Professor Brennan's research involves exploring novel technologies and techniques that enhance the detection of clinical indicators of disease while minimizing risk to the patient. His research has involved most major imaging modalities including x-ray, computerized tomography, ultrasound, and magnetic resonance imaging, with a particular focus on breast and chest imaging. In line with government priorities, his research findings have translated into improved diagnosis and management of important disease states such as cancer, musculoskeletal injury, arthritis, and multiple sclerosis. He is recognized as a leader in clinical translation of medical imaging optimization and radiological perception.

Professor Brennan has presented at the major international imaging meetings, including the annual meetings of the Radiological Society of North America, European Congress, UK Radiological Congress, International Society of Optical Engineering, and Medical Imaging Perception Society. He has published over 180 original papers and these have been accepted by the leading radiological journals such as *Radiology, Radiography, American Journal of Roentgenology, Academic Radiology, European Radiology,* and *British Journal of Radiology.*

Reviewers

Joanne S. Greathouse, EdS, RT(R)(ARRT), FASRT, FAEIRS
Retired
Sun City, AZ

Daniel Snyder, MS, CMLSO
Radiation & Laser Safety Officer, Senior Health Physicist
Geisinger Health System
Danville, PA

Cynthia L. Liotta, MS, RT(R)(CT)
Assistant Professor and Program Director
Gannon University
Radiologic Science Program
Erie, PA

Jera Roberts, EdS, RT(M)
Program Director
Washburn University
Radiography Program
Topeka, KS

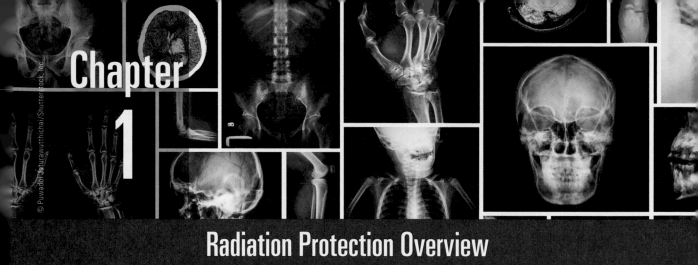

Chapter 1

Radiation Protection Overview

Outline

- Introduction
- A Rationale for Radiation Protection
  - Data sources on biological effects
  - Dose-response models
  - Biological effects
- The Philosophy of Radiation Protection
  - The ICRP framework
  - Radiation dose limits
- Radiation Protection Concepts
  - Historical perspectives
- The four quartets of radiation protection
- X-ray dosimetry
- Dose-image quality optimization
- Diagnostic reference levels
- Radiation Protection Organizations and Reports
  - Organizations
  - Reports and publications
- Radiation Protection and the Technologist
  - Responsibilities: Four major components
- References

Objectives

On completion of this chapter, you should be able to:

1. Discuss the rationale for radiation protection in diagnostic imaging.
2. Describe the philosophy of radiation protection.
3. Explain the four quartets of radiation protection.
4. State the meaning of the terms *x-ray dosimetry*, *dose-image quality optimization*, and *diagnostic reference levels*.
5. Identify several radiation protection organizations and list their respective radiation protection reports.
6. Describe four major responsibilities of the technologist in radiation protection.

Introduction

In their classic textbook, *The Essential Physics of Medical Imaging* (2012), Bushberg et al. state the following:

> Rarely have beneficial applications and hazards to human health followed a major scientific discovery more rapidly than with the discovery of ionizing radiation… Unfortunately, the development and implementation of radiation protection techniques lagged…Within six months of their use, several cases of erythema, dermatitis,…were reported among x-ray operators and their patients…it was not until 1915 that the first radiation protection recommendations were made by the British Roentgen Society, and from the American Roentgen Ray Society in 1922. (p. 751)

The quote above contains several important points that characterize radiation protection in medicine. First, it is clear that the use of ionizing radiation to image humans provides a benefit, but at the same time, such use poses a risk of injury to the living organism. Secondly, the injury is clearly apparent expressed as erythema for example. The third point of significance is that x-rays can cause cancer. This was subsequently proved by experimental confirmation. Finally, as a result of such clearly demonstrated injuries, radiation protection recommendations were introduced as early as 1915. These four major considerations form the bases of this textbook.

Radiation protection in diagnostic imaging is concerned with the physical, technical, and procedural factors involved in protecting both patients and personnel from unnecessary radiation exposure. The physical factors related to the science of the interaction of radiation with matter include physics, chemistry, and biology. While the physics of radiation include topics such as atomic structure, energy deposition in matter, the nature of electromagnetic radiation, interactions of radiation with matter, radiation attenuation, as well as linear energy transfer, and biological effectiveness, chemistry deals with basic chemical reactions that occur when radiation interacts with water and other molecules, such as DNA. The biology associated with radiation protection examines the effects of radiation on biological systems, the study of which is referred to as **radiobiology**. In this regard, the established fact that the biological effects of radiation are real provides a major rationale for radiation protection. Topics such as radiation damage to DNA and chromosomes, cell death and cell survival, total body radiation effects, radiation carcinogenesis, and radiation effects on the embryo and fetus as well as hereditary effects, are fundamental and essential to the study of radiobiology.

Technical factors, on the other hand, deal with the equipment requirements not only for the production of x-rays, but for imaging the patient. Radiographic, fluoroscopic, mammographic, and computed tomography equipment, quality control tools, and protective shielding are fundamental to the technical aspects of radiation protection.

Finally, procedural factors are equally important to the nature of radiation protection. These factors are concerned with radiation dose management; that is, how the dose can be reduced during the imaging of the patient. For example, how can the exposure technique factors (mAs and kVp) be optimized to deliver minimum dose to the patient, without compromising the diagnostic quality of the images? Furthermore, procedural factors take into consideration established formal and official activities of the imaging department that are under the guidance of administrative authorities via regulations, recommendations, laws, licensing, and accreditation.

This chapter introduces the essential elements of radiation protection in diagnostic x-ray imaging, and lays the basic foundation for further study. A rationale for radiation protection is provided based on studies of biological effects of radiation exposure. Current standards of radiation protection are outlined briefly, followed by a short review of patient exposure factors from several diagnostic imaging modalities. Additional concepts of radiation protection, such as radiation quantities and their units, and radiation protection agencies for example will be outlined. The chapter concludes with an overview of radiation dose and image quality optimization, and the responsibilities of the technologist as a radiation worker.

A Rationale for Radiation Protection

Radiation protection deals with the protection of humans from the harmful effects of radiation exposure. These harmful effects (also known as health effects, biological effects, or simply radiation risk) have been studied extensively, and information regarding the kinds of injury stems from several sources of data (Hendee and O'Connor, 2013; Dauer et al. 2010). These kinds of studies are referred to as *epidemiologic studies*.

Data Sources on Biological Effects

As defined by Dr. Elizabeth Travis in her classic textbook *Radiobiology*, epidemiology is the "science that deals with the incidence, distribution, and control of disease in a population" (Travis, 1989). Epidemiologic studies about radiation risk therefore provide data on the health effects of radiation exposure in humans.

Radiation protection guides, standards, and recommendations are based on the knowledge of biological effects of radiation exposure. The data on these effects have been derived from both animal and human studies (Travis, 1989).

The data from human exposure have been placed into four categories (Hendee and O'Connor, 2012), as follows:

1. Early radiation workers who were exposed to high doses, such as radiologists and physicists.

2. Individuals working in radiation and nuclear industries.

3. The survivors of the atomic bomb explosions at Hiroshima and Nagasaki.

4. Workers and local inhabitants exposed to nuclear reactor accidents such as the catastrophes at Three Mile Island and Chernobyl.

In addition to the above four sources, another important source of data on biological effects of radiation exposure has been identified in the Biological Effects of Ionizing Radiation (BEIR) reports. Specifically, Section 7 of BEIR Report VII presents data on exposure of patients to high doses from medical radiation (NRC, 2006). It is interesting to note that of the data sources mentioned above, the BEIR VII report "places by far the greatest emphasis" (Hendee and O'Connor, 2012) on the data from the Hiroshima and Nagasaki atomic bomb survivors. This data has been provided by the Radiation Effects Research Foundation (RERF) (RERF, 2011).

In discussing the *Radiation Risks of Medical Imaging: Separating Fact from Fantasy*, Drs. Hendee and O'Connor (2012) draw attention to the following:

> The RERF studies of the Japanese atomic bomb survivors are the major source of what is known about the health consequences to individuals exposed to ionizing radiation. The RERF data and the models of radiation injury…form the back bone of the BEIR VII report. Hence an analysis of the assumptions and limitations of risk estimates derived from BEIR VII must include a review of the RERF studies from which BEIR VII is derived. (p. 314)

Dose-Response Models

Another important concept derived from these studies is that of a dose-risk model or sometimes referred to as a dose-response relationship. The model shows what happens to the risk of radiation injury as the dose increases. As noted by Hendee and O'Connor (2012):

> RERF data provide statistically significant evidence of increased cancers in Japanese survivors who received doses of 100 mSv and higher with cancer

incidence appearing to increase linearly with dose. At less than 100 mSv, an increase in radiation-induced cancers, if any is too small to be distinguishable from cancer incidence due to all causes. Consequently, a model must be deployed to extrapolate from radiation-induced cancers at doses greater than 100 mSv to a hypothetical and much smaller number of cancers induced by doses of a few millisieverts delivered during medical imaging (p. 316).

Therefore, several dose-response models for extrapolating from a high-dose situation to the low doses used in diagnostic x-ray imaging have been proposed. These models have been placed into two categories: (1) the linear dose-response model without a threshold (LNT model) and (2) the linear dose-response model with a threshold. The LNT model shows that no amount of radiation is considered safe, and that any dose, no matter how small, carries some degree of risk. The linear dose-response model with a threshold proposes that no adverse effect is observed from radiation below a certain level, known as the threshold dose. A biological response occurs only when the threshold dose is reached (Bushong 2013).

Which Model to Use in Medical Imaging?

The obvious question in the minds of medical imaging personnel then is, which model is best suited when imaging patients? To provide a clean answer, it is important to quote the experts—and in this regard, Hendee and O'Connor (2012) state that:

> the model used most widely is the LNT model. This model is not chosen because there is solid biologic or epidemiologic data supporting its use. Rather, it is used because of its simplicity and because it is a conservative approach (i.e., if it is not correct, then it probably overestimates the risk of cancer induction at low dose).

For the purpose of establishing radiation protection standards for occupationally exposed individuals and members of the public, a conservative model that overestimates the risk is preferred over a model that underestimates risk. (p. 316)

Biological Effects

Biological effects can be placed into two categories: (1) *somatic effects*, those effects that appear in the individual exposed to radiation, and (2) *genetic effects*, those effects occurring in future descendants of the exposed individual.

Another system of classification of biological effects is referred to as the *stochastic/non-stochastic* classification system. *Stochastic effects,* which are random in nature, are those in which the probability of the effect occurring depends on the amount of radiation dose. The effect increases as the dose increases. In addition, there is no threshold dose for stochastic effects. Stochastic effects include cancer, leukemia, and genetic effects.

Non-stochastic effects are those effects for which the severity of the effect in the exposed individual increases as the radiation dose increases, and for which there is a threshold dose. Today, these effects are referred to as *deterministic effects* (Bushong 2013). Examples of deterministic effects include radiation-induced skin burns, tissue damage, and organ dysfunction.

The Philosophy of Radiation Protection

The BEIR reports and the RERF studies provide substantial evidence that the biological effects of radiation exposure are real. Both stochastic effects (e.g., cancer and leukemia) and deterministic effects (e.g., skin burns and organ dysfunction) have been observed in human populations exposed to ionizing radiation.

In medical imaging, patients are purposefully exposed to a radiation dose in an effort to restore their health. In this regard, therefore, the International Commission on Radiological Protection (ICRP) provides a radiation protection framework based on three philosophical pillars (Wolbarst et al. 2013) on which the fundamental principles of radiation protection are founded. This framework is subscribed to by various national radiation protection organizations, including the National Council on Radiation Protection and Measurements (NCRP) in the United States (US) (2009); the US Nuclear Regulatory Commission (2007); Health Canada (2008); and the European Medical Exposures Directive (Matthews and Brennan, 2009), to mention only a few.

The ICRP Framework

The framework adopted by ICRP is intended to prevent deterministic effects from occurring by keeping the radiation doses below threshold values and to take all reasonable efforts to minimize the probability of stochastic effects.

The framework encompasses a number of concepts, only two of which will be describe here. The first deals with the types of exposure from which individuals can receive radiation doses: occupational exposure, medical exposure, and public exposure. Whereas occupational exposure refers to exposure due to work activities, medical exposure refers to exposure due to diagnostic examinations and radiation therapy procedures, and does not include occupational exposure of the workers performing the procedures. Public exposure, on the other hand, constitutes all other exposures, such as exposure to natural sources of radiation.

The second concept of the framework, which is of significant importance to radiation workers, including radiology technologists and radiologists, is what the ICRP refers to as "the system of radiological protection." This system is guided by three fundamental principles, namely: justification, optimization of protection, and application of dose limits (ICRP 2007a; ICRP 2007b). While the first two principles deal with individuals

who are exposed to a source of radiation, the third principle examines both occupational and public exposures and does not include medical exposures.

It is not within the scope of this chapter to describe details of each of these three principles; however, the following points are noteworthy:

1. The principle of justification specifically states that any exposure of a patient to radiation should result in more good (benefit) than harm (risk).

2. The principle of optimization of protection implies that "the likelihood of incurring exposures, the number of people exposed and the magnitude of their individual doses should be kept *as low as reasonably achievable (ALARA)* taking into account economic and societal factors" (Moores and Regulla, 2011, p. 23). Furthermore, "this means that the level of protection should be the best under the prevailing circumstances, maximizing the margin of benefit over harm" (ICRP 2007a; ICRP 2007b).

3. The principle of application of dose limits, according to the ICRP, requires that "the total dose to any individual from regulated sources in planned exposure situations other than medical exposure of patients should not exceed the appropriate limits recommended by the Commission" (ICRP 2007a; ICRP 2007b). Note that, as defined by this statement, total dose does not include any medical exposure, but instead accounts for radiation doses from occupational and public sources.

Radiation Dose Limits

Radiation dose limits are based on the linear dose-response relationship without a threshold (LNT model) and are intended to minimize the probability of stochastic effects. These limits are deemed to be acceptable levels of exposure for occupationally exposed individuals.

Radiation dose limits have undergone several reductions throughout the years. In 1990, the BEIR Committee revised its previously documented risk estimates. In Report V, the BEIR estimated the risk of radiation exposure to be four times greater than was previously estimated. This result is based on new risk models, revised dosimetry techniques, and better follow-up of those individuals who were exposed to the atomic bomb explosions at Hiroshima and Nagasaki.

This major revision led the ICRP to change its previously recommended dose limit for occupationally exposed individuals (technologists and radiologists) from 50 mSv (the millisievert [mSv] is a unit of the radiation quantity effective dose which relates exposure to risk) per year to 20 mSv per year (ICRP 1991).

Dose limits have been recommended for occupationally exposed workers and members of the public not only by the ICRP but by national organizations such as the NCRP and the Health Canada Radiation Protection Bureau. A few of these are highlighted in **Table 1-1.**

Radiation Protection Concepts

The development of radiation protection concepts is guided by history; therefore this section takes a cursory glance of what took place after W.C. Roentgen discovered x-rays in 1895.

Historical Perspectives

The need for radiation protection was recognized during the early 1900s, when radiation workers observed skin changes as a result of long exposure to radiation. The history of radiation protection can be broken down into four periods (Brodsky and Kathren, 1989), namely:

1. Era of the protection pioneers (1895–1915).
2. Golden age of radiology (1915–1940).
3. Golden age of radiation protection (1940–1960).
4. Modern era (1960 to present).

Table 1-1 The Exposure Dose Limits in Medicine for Occupationally Exposed Workers and the General Public

Individual	mSv/year		
	NCRP	ICRP	Health Canada
Occupational (Stochastic effects)			
• Whole body	50	20*	20*
Occupational (Deterministic effects)			
• Lens of eye	150	150	150
• Skin	500	500	500
• Extremities	500	500	500
Members of Public			
• Whole body	1	1	1
• Lens of eye	15	15	15
• Skin			
• Extremities			

*Not greater than 20 mSv/year, averaged over 5 years

The interested student should refer to the article by Brodsky and Kathren (1989) for specific details of such history.

During these periods, several concepts emerged that were particularly intended to reduce the amount of radiation exposure to both the patient and radiation worker. These concepts relate to various models of biologic injury, technical aspects of radiation protection, the formation of scientific organizations solely dedicated to the field of radiation protection, and standards of practice for which various guidelines and recommendations for the safe use of radiation in medicine have been established. For example, current radiation protection standards are guided by the philosophy of radiation protection (ICRP 2007a) that includes the principles of justification, optimization, and the application of dose limits.

The development of the principle of dose limits is an interesting topic to explore from a historical perspective. Following early reports of radiation injury, soon after the discovery of x-rays, the idea of limiting the amount of radiation exposure an individual received began to emerge. This was marked by the introduction of the *erythema dose* (a certain amount of radiation need to produce skin reddening), followed by other concepts that have evolved to the present time.

The erythema dose, which was proposed by Mutscheller and Sievert (Brodsky & Kathren, 1989), was followed by the use of the *tolerance dose*, a term used to refer to an acceptable level of radiation exposure. Later, the ICRP replaced the term tolerance dose with the term *maximum permissible dose* (*MPD*), which was subsequently changed around 1977 to a concept referred to as the *dose-equivalent limit*. These changes were attributed to the results of various studies on biological effects of radiation, such as ones identified by the Committee on Biological Effects of Atomic Radiation (BEAR), which provided information on the risks of radiation exposure.

Another change to the concept of dose limits came about in 1990 when the ICRP, in Publication 60 (ICRP 1991), once again made several changes in their radiation protection recommendations. One such change was the replacement of the term dose-equivalent limit with the term *equivalent dose*. This term specifically takes into consideration the fact that different types of radiations (alpha and beta particles and ionizing radiation such as x-rays) have different efficiencies, known as *relative biological effectiveness* (*RBE*), in causing biological effects (Bushberg et al. 2012). This variation is acknowledged using a weighting factor, W_R, that adjusts the total dose based on what type of radiation an individual was exposed to. Furthermore, different tissues have different sensitivity to radiation, and therefore different *tissue weighting factors* (W_T). For example, the W_T for gonadal tissue is 0.20, while for the skin, it is 0.01. The current terminology, effective dose, now takes into consideration both the type of radiation weighting factor (W_R) and the tissue weighting factor (W_T) when calculating the effective dose. Thus, the effective dose relates exposure to risk. For radiation workers, the whole-body effective dose is 20 mSv (ICRP 2007a) and 50 mSv (NCRP 2009) per year.

The biological effects data serve to contribute to the development of radiation protection concepts and procedures. As researchers find out more about the biological effects of radiation, protection guidelines and recommendations will continue to evolve.

The Four Quartets of Radiation Protection

As noted earlier, the overall goal of radiation protection is to prevent deterministic effects and to minimize the probability of stochastic effects. This goal can be accomplished by what Wolbarst et al. (2013) describe as the "four quartets of radiation protection," as illustrated in **Figure 1-1**. These quartets include: (1) personal actions, (2) department activities, (3) administrative structure, and (4) philosophy of radiation protection, including ALARA. It is quite clear that, from the perspective

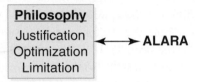

Personal actions	**Activities of department**
Time Distance Shielding (contain)	Control access shield Monitor/survey train

Administrative structure

Recommendations
Laws, regulations,
Licensing
Accreditation

Philosophy

Justification
Optimization   ←——→ **ALARA**
Limitation

Figure 1-1 The four quartets of radiation protection are designed to accomplish the two goals of radiation protection. See text for further explanation.

Reproduced from Figure 5-13, p. 146. Wolbarst, A. B., Patrizio, C., Wyant, A. (2013) *Medical imaging: Essentials for physicians.* Hoboken, NJ: Wiley Blackwell. Reproduced by permission.

of a working technologist, personal actions, some aspects of department activities, and the philosophy of radiation protection are a routine part of their daily practice.

Personal actions include time, shielding, distance, and containment. Department activities "involve the design of new or reconfigured imaging suites; controlling access to radiation areas; routinely monitoring workers and surveying work areas; and training" (Wolbarst et al. 2013). Administrative activities, on the other hand, deal with recommendations, laws, regulations, licensing and enforcement, and accreditation, all of which are intended to ensure effective quality assurance and radiation safety programs (Wolbarst et al. 2013). Finally, the philosophy of radiation protection addresses the principles of justification, optimization, and application of dose limits.

Personal Actions

Anyone who works with radiation or who might be subject to radiation exposure should be familiar with what Bushong (2013) refers to as the "cardinal principles of radiation protection." These principles relate to time, shielding, and distance, and are intended to reduce the radiation exposure an individual may receive. Essentially, radiation exposure can be reduced if:

1. The time of exposure is kept as short as possible, since the exposure is directly proportional to time. In diagnostic x-ray imaging, if the time is doubled, then the dose is doubled.

2. A protective shield is placed between the x-ray tube and the individuals exposed (patient and technologist). The shield is usually made of lead (or bismuth) and can be placed on top of the patient's gonads to absorb unnecessary radiation. A lead apron is generally worn by technologists working in fluoroscopy and mobile radiography by the patient's bedside. Walls of the x-ray rooms are shielded with lead to prevent radiation from exposing individuals outside the x-ray room (e.g., patients waiting for their examination in a waiting room).

3. The distance from the radiation source (an x-ray tube, for example) and the individual exposed is kept as great as possible. As the distance increases, the radiation exposure decreases according to a physical law referred to as the ***inverse square law***. The mathematical expression for this law is:

$$I \alpha \frac{1}{d^2}$$

where I = intensity of the radiation and d = distance. The expression is read as: the intensity of radiation is inversely proportional to the square of the distance.

The Administrative Activity of Quality Assurance

The idea and concepts of ***quality assurance*** (QA) have become mandatory and commonplace in medical imaging departments. QA programs are intended to ensure the production of optimum diagnostic information with minimum dose to the patient and minimum costs to the department. QA involves quality administration and quality control (QC). While quality administration deals with management activities (for example, patient scheduling, policies and procedures, budgets, etc.), QC deals with the technical aspects of equipment performance (Papp 2011).

The technologist plays an important role in QC programs, and with additional education and training, the technologist may even assume the role of a "quality control technologist." The QC technologist is viewed as an individual who comes out to perform QC test procedures, records the results, and, in some cases, interprets and makes recommendations for corrective action if the equipment fails the test.

One of the goals of a QC program is to ensure that diagnostic images are obtained with minimum radiation dose to the patient. In doing so, the QC program is designed to monitor all the appropriate variables in the imaging chain that affect both dose and image quality.

Other terms used to refer to QA are **total quality management (TQM)** and **continuous quality improvement (CQI)**. The TQM system essentially involves the notion that the entire staff of a facility should participate in the activities of QA. CQI, on the other hand, "dictates that every activity in an imaging facility be identified and clear standards (indicators) set and measured to allow development of policies amenable to evaluation and review, with the aim of yet further improvements" (Hynes 1994).

The Philosophy of Radiation Protection

As noted earlier, the philosophy of radiation protection is guided by the three principles of justification, optimization, and the application of dose limits. Of these three principles, the optimization principle is of greatest significance to the daily activities of the technologist. Optimization is concerned with operating under the ALARA philosophy, which means that the radiation worker in medical imaging should always try to use the

minimum radiation dose without compromising the image quality needed to make a diagnosis. In this regard, optimization has often been referred to as **radiation dose-image quality optimization**.

X-Ray Dosimetry

When the x-ray beam falls upon the patient, it is **attenuated**—that is, reduced in intensity as it passes through the patient. This attenuation results in the deposition of the correct radiation dose into the patient. The events surrounding the transmission of the correct dose to the patient (as well as the exposure of the radiation worker to scattered radiation) led to an area of study referred to as **x-ray dosimetry**. Dosimetry includes not only the measurement of the dose to patients and personnel, but also relating the exposure to risk of biologic damage. It is important that technologists understand the essentials of dose metrics in x-ray imaging, in the event that they become engaged in radiation dose optimization research.

It is not within the scope of this chapter to describe dosimetry details; however, the following descriptions are noteworthy. In diagnostic x-ray imaging, several radiation quantities and their units are important to estimating the patient dose and risk to the patient. These include **exposure**, **absorbed dose**, **equivalent dose**, and **effective dose**. Whereas exposure refers to the quantity of radiation falling on the patient (**entrance surface exposure**), absorbed dose is the amount of energy absorbed by the patient per unit mass of tissue. Since it is well known that different types of radiation (particulate and x-rays, for example) have different efficiencies of causing biologic damage, the equivalent dose can be determined using the absorbed dose as follows:

$$H = DW_R$$

where H is the equivalent dose, D is the absorbed dose, and W_R is the radiation weighting factor (W_R for x-rays is 1, while for alpha particles it is 20). This means that for the same absorbed dose, alpha particles will cause more biologic damage than x-rays. Computing the equivalent dose for x-rays "is discouraged in x-ray dosimetry as it can lead to confusion with effective dose…" (Bushberg et al. 2012).

Effective dose relates exposure to risk. In x-ray imaging, only partial body exposures are used (as opposed to whole-body exposure). The beam is always restricted to the anatomy of interest (for example, chest, abdomen, pelvis, etc.,) via **collimation**; in the case of partial body exposure, the stochastic risk is related to the effective dose. Effective dose is based on weighting factors for the various tissues (W_T), since different tissues have different radio sensitivities. W_T for the gonads is 0.08, while it is 0.01 for the skin because the gonads are more radio sensitive (easily damaged by radiation) than the skin. E can be calculated as follows:

$$E = \sum H W_T$$

where E is the effective dose, H is the equivalent dose, and W_T is the tissue weighting factor.

The unit of exposure is the **coulomb per kilogram** (C/kg) which replaced the old unit, the roentgen (R) where $1R = 2.58 \times 10^{-4}$ C/kg. The unit of absorbed dose is the **gray** (Gy) which refers to 1 Joule (J) of energy deposited in 1 kg of material. The unit of equivalent dose is the **sievert** (Sv) which is equal to the absorbed dose multiplied by the quality factor of the particular radiation.

The unit of effective dose is also the sievert (Sv). In diagnostic x-ray imaging, these units are usually very small, so they are often expressed in millisieverts (mSv) or microsieverts (μSv). Similarly, for absorbed dose, it can be milligray (mGy) or microgray (μGy).

Dose-Image Quality Optimization

Optimization refers to using radiation dose within the ALARA philosophy, without compromising image quality. The ICRP (2007) recommends that several iterations be required for optimization, including three options often used by technologists and medical physicists. These include the identification of options for implementing the ALARA principle, selection of the most appropriate option for implementing the ALARA principle, and implementation of this option (Matthews and Brennan, 2009).

Essentially, optimization research involves different methodologies to demonstrate dose reduction without a loss of image quality. In 2005, a special seminal issue of *Radiation Protection Dosimetry* (Mattsson 2005) was dedicated to the topic of optimization strategies in medical x-ray imaging for radiography and fluoroscopy (including digital radiography and fluoroscopy), mammography, and computed tomography (CT). There are three important requirements for optimization research:

1. Ensure that the dose to the patient is safe.

2. Determine the level of image quality required for the particular examination.

3. Reduce the dose in such a manner so as not to compromise the image quality.

To meet the above requirements, various methods are needed to:

1. Determine the level image quality, defined as "the ability to differentiate between images that are normal and abnormal" (Mattsson 2005).

2. Address the perceptions and evaluation of image quality by using human observers, keeping in mind the nature of the detection task. In this regard, various observer performance tests, such as Receiver Operating Characteristics (ROC) and Visual Grading Analysis (VGA), can be used. The task of lesion (pathology) detection would require a different observer performance test than, say, the task of detecting normal anatomical structures.

Several examples of research on optimization during daily operation in x-ray imaging have been described by Matthews and Brenna (2009), and more recently by Seeram et al. (2013), for computed radiography (CR) imaging. The responsibility for optimization of the dose in diagnostic x-ray imaging falls not only on radiologists, technologists, and medical physicists, but also on those who prescribe x-ray examinations for their patients, such as physicians in public emergency departments and private medical care facilities.

Diagnostic Reference Levels

The optimization principle protects patients from unnecessary radiation exposures by using a dose that is as low as reasonably achievable (ALARA). Optimization of a diagnostic imaging procedure can be regarded as the practice of the ALARA philosophy. One tool used in diagnostic x-ray imaging to optimize radiation protection of patients is the *diagnostic reference level* (DRL). DRLs have been used effectively in the United Kingdom (UK) and in Europe for more than a decade (Seeram and Brennan, 2006) and more recently in the US (NCRP, 2012).

There are several definitions of the DRL (Seeram and Brennan, 2006), but only two will be mentioned here. The ICRP Publication 73 (1996) states that DRLs "are a form of investigation level applied to an easily measured quantity, usually absorbed dose in all, or tissue-equivalent material at the surface of a simple standard phantom or a representative patient." The American College of Radiology (ACR), on the other hand, defines the DRL as "an investigation level to identify unusually high radiation dose or exposure levels for common diagnostic medical x-ray procedures."

DRLs are tools that x-ray imaging departments can use to measure and administer radiation doses to patients for a defined set of procedures. If the doses delivered are consistently greater than established DRLs for that facility's country or region, then the department should be concerned about their radiation protection practices and procedures, investigate why exposures are beyond established DRLs, and take corrective action (NCRP 2012).

Radiation Protection Organizations and Reports

In the Introduction, reference was made to an international organization, the ICRP, and two national organizations, the NCRP and Health Canada, that make recommendations about radiation safety. There are a number of other organizations and agencies that play major roles in the development and implementation of radiation protection guides, recommendations, and control procedures, all of which form the content of various reports and publications presented by these organizations.

Organizations

Essentially, organizations can be classified as either international or national. There are several international bodies, including the ICRP, the International Commission on Radiological Units and Measurements (ICRU), the International Atomic Energy Agency (IAEA), the United Nations Scientific Committee on the Effects of Atomic Radiation (UNSCEAR), and the Biological Effects of Ionizing Radiation Committee (BEIR).

The ICRP's recommendations are usually adapted by several countries to meet their own needs. These countries have their own regulatory organizations: the NCRP in the US, the Radiation Protection Bureau (RPB) in Canada, and the National Radiological Protection Board (NRPB) in the United Kingdom are just some of these. The NRPB, for example, has been instrumental in establishing guidelines in magnetic resonance imaging (MRI).

Reports and Publications

Radiation protection standards, guides, recommendations, and control procedures are officially documented in various reports and publications. Several examples that are particularly important to radiologic technologists and radiologists include the following:

1. ICRP Publication 93: *Managing Patient Dose in Digital Radiology.*

2. ICRP Publication 31: *Radiation and Your Patient: A Guide For Medical Practitioners.*

3. ICRP Publication 103: *The 2007 Recommendations of the ICRP.*

4. ICRP Publication 105: *Radiation Protection in Medicine.*

5. NCRP Report 172: *Reference Levels and Achievable Doses in Medical and Dental Imaging—Recommendations for the United States.*

6. NCRP Report 160: *Ionizing Radiation Exposure of the Population of the United States.*

7. Health Canada. *Radiation Protection in Radiology—Large Facilities: Safety Code 35.*

8. NCRP Report 168: *Radiation Dose Management for Fluoroscopically Guided Interventional Medical Procedures.*

9. US Nuclear Regulatory Commission: *Standards for Protection Against Radiation.* US Code of Federal Regulations, 10 CFR 20.

10. US Environmental Protection Agency. *Federal Guidance Report 14: Radiation Protection Guidance for Diagnostic and Interventional X-Ray Procedures.*

Radiation Protection and the Technologist

Ultimately, the radiologist in charge of the department has the responsibility and authority of ensuring radiation protection of patients and personnel. The radiologist must be trained in radiation protection theory and practice and must keep up-to-date with changes in radiation protection recommendations as well as imaging technologies evolve and more information on biological effects continuously becomes available. The radiologist, however, usually assigns this particular responsibility to another individual depending on the size of the radiology facility. In general, this task of radiation safety is assigned to a person specifically trained in health physics, or to a person trained in medical physics. Health physics "is concerned with providing occupational radiation protection and minimizing radiation dose to the public" (Bushong 2013, p. 539). The health physicist, on the other hand "is a radiation scientist, who is concerned with the research, teaching, or operational aspects of radiation safety" (Bushong 2013, p. 539). This person is generally referred to as a *radiation safety officer* (RSO).

In cases where hospitals and/or radiology departments cannot support such officers, other individuals are usually appointed to facilitate radiation protection practices. In this situation, it is essential that these persons be trained in radiation protection.

The radiology technologist receives education and training in radiation protection, including radiographic imaging science (physics), radiographic techniques, and radiation biology. The technologist is therefore prepared to assume a fundamental and significant role as an RSO.

Responsibilities: Four Major Components

There are at least four areas of responsibility in which the technologist must be an active participant in an effort to protect the patient, personnel, and members of the public. These include: responsibility to the patient, responsibility to oneself as a radiation worker, continuing education, and responsibility for dose optimization via the effective application of the ALARA principle.

The technologist conducts the radiographic examination of the patient and is ultimately responsible for the direct radiation protection measures applied to the patient. The first responsibility, therefore, is the required care of the patient during the entire examination, followed by the application of required radiation protection principles that relate to the ALARA philosophy. As a conscientious radiation worker, the technologist plays a significant role in minimizing the radiation risks to the population. In this regard, the technologist must always pay careful attention to the technical and procedural aspects of the examination.

Technical considerations relate to various equipment design intended to minimize and control radiation exposure and the design of the imaging department, to provide a safe environment in which to work (such as the design of protective shielding).

Procedural considerations deal with the ways in which activities are performed to reduce the exposure to the patient. For example, the technologist should always conduct a radiographic examination, keeping the following in mind:

1. Patient positioning must be accurate to avoid repeats due to poor positioning.
2. The technologist should establish and set up correct exposure technique factors for the particular examination.
3. Select the appropriate image receptor for the examination.
4. Perform only the minimum number of images as required.
5. Protect the patient's gonads by using a lead shield.
6. Always collimate the x-ray beam only to the anatomy of interest.
7. Always remain in the protective control booth in the x-ray room during the exposure or wear a lead apron when standing outside the control booth, as in the case of some fluoroscopic examinations.
8. Ensure that the patient understands all instruction with respect to respiration and motion.
9. Always observe the patient during the exposure.
10. Ensure that the patient is free of any foreign objects, such as necklaces, watches, buttons, or hairpins, that may result in a repeat examination, because the objects will appear as image artifacts and interfere with diagnosis.
11. Immobilize the patient if necessary to minimize motion artifacts.

The technologist also has a responsibility to herself/himself and to other personnel who may be subject to radiation exposure where x-ray examinations are conducted. For example, when an examination is conducted with mobile equipment at the patient's bedside or in the emergency department, the x-ray beam orientation does not pose a hazard to other patients and individuals who are present in the room. Furthermore, technologists must always wear personal dosimeters during the course of their work.

A pregnant technologist should inform her department so that appropriate measures can be taken to ensure that the dose limits to her and the fetus are applied (Bushong 2013; Health Canada 2008).

The third area of responsibility falls within the domain of continuing education. It is mandatory that the technologist keeps current with changes and developments not only in radiation protection but also in related topics such as radiation risks.

The fourth area of responsibility is that of dose optimization. This is an area that is becoming increasingly important. As noted in the US Environmental Protection Agency (EPA) *Federal Guidance Report No. 14 on Radiation Protection Guidance for Diagnostic and Interventional X-Ray Procedures* (2012), technologists must play a role to optimize the imaging examination. Furthermore, others have suggested that technologists play an active role in dose-image quality optimization (Matthews and Brenna 2008; Moores and Regulla 2011; Seeram et al. 2013).

Technologists must also get involved and collaborate with radiologists and medical physicists in dose-image quality optimization research. This would require further education and training in image quality assessment tools and dosimetry methods and considerations for close optimization. To meet the above requirement, it is essential that the technologist have a good understanding of:

- Image quality descriptors, such as spatial resolution, contrast resolution and noise
- Methods of image quality assessment that include objective physical methods such as signal-to-noise ratio (SNR) as well as observer performance methods such as the VGA approach mentioned earlier.
- X-ray dosimetry methods, including understanding DRLs.

The significance of radiation protection to the daily activities of the technologist as a medical radiation worker cannot be understated. For this reason, radiation protection and radiobiology are integral parts of the curriculum of radiologic technology programs all over the world.

Summary of Key Concepts

1. The use of ionizing radiation in medicine provides a benefit toward restoring and managing the health of exposed individuals; however, such use poses a risk of injury (harmful effects) to the living organism.

2. Radiation protection deals with the protection of humans from the harmful effects of radiation exposure.

3. The data from human exposure comes from early radiation workers who were exposed to high doses, such as radiologist and physicists; individuals working in radiation and nuclear industries; survivors of the atomic bomb explosions at Hiroshima and Nagasaki; and from nuclear reactor accidents such as the catastrophes at Three Mile Island and Chernobyl.

4. Since the doses from the above four sources of human exposure are high, models have been developed to extrapolate the high doses to the low doses received in medical imaging. These models have been placed into two categories: linear dose-response relationships and non-linear dose-response relationships.

5. The model use in medical imaging is the linear dose-response model

6. The effects of radiation exposure are stochastic effects and deterministic effects.

7. Stochastic effects, which are random in nature, are those in which the probability of the effect occurring depends on the amount of radiation dose. The effect increases as the dose increases. In addition, there is no threshold dose for stochastic effects. Stochastic effects include cancer, leukemia, and genetic effects.

8. Deterministic effects are those effects for which the severity of the effect in the exposed individual increases as the radiation dose increases, and for which there is a threshold dose.

9. Three principles of radiation protection as stated by the ICRP are:

    i. The principle of justification specifically deals with any exposure of a patient should result in more good (benefit) than harm (risk).

    ii. The principle of optimization of protection implies that "the likelihood of incurring exposures, the number of people exposed and the magnitude of their individual doses should be kept as low as reasonably achievable (ALARA) taking into account economic and societal factors" (Moores and Regulla 2011, p. 23).

    iii. The principle of application of dose limits, which according to the ICRP holds that "the total dose to any individual from regulated sources in planned exposure situations other than medical exposure of patients should not exceed the appropriate limits recommended by the Commission" (ICRP 2007a; ICRP 2007b). This statement does not include any medical exposure.

10. The four quartets of radiation protection include: (1) personal actions, (2) department activities, (3) administrative structure, and (4) philosophy of radiation protection, including ALARA. It is quite clear that from the perspective of a working technologist, personal actions, some aspects of department activities, and the philosophy of radiation protection, are a routine part of their daily practice.

11. X-ray dosimetry includes the measurement of the dose to patients and personnel, and relating the exposure to risk of biologic damage. Radiation quantities and their units are important to patient dose and estimating the risk to the patient. These include *exposure*, *absorbed dose*, *equivalent dose*, and *effective dose*. Whereas *exposure* refers to the quantity of radiation falling on the patient (entrance surface exposure), *absorbed dose* is the amount of energy absorbed by the patient per unit mass of tissue. Effective dose (E) relates exposure to risk.

12. While the unit of exposure is the *coulomb per kilogram* (C/kg) the unit of absorbed dose is the *gray* (Gy). The unit of equivalent dose is the *sievert* (Sv) which is equal to the absorbed dose multiplied by the quality factor of the particular radiation. The unit of effective dose is the *sievert* (Sv).

13. Optimization refers to using radiation dose within the ALARA philosophy, without compromising image quality. Essentially optimization research involves different methodologies to demonstrate dose reduction without a loss of image quality.

14. One tool used in diagnostic x-ray imaging to optimize radiation protection of patients is the *diagnostic reference level* (DRL). There are several definitions of the DRL. The American College of Radiology (ACR) defines it as "an investigation level to identify unusually high radiation dose or exposure levels for common diagnostic medical ray procedures" (ACR 2001).

15. Radiation protection organizations can be classified as either international or national, and they issue radiation protection standards, guides, recommendation, and control procedures that are officially documented in various reports and publications.

16. The responsibilities that the technologist must be an active participant in to protect the patient, personnel, and members of the public, include: responsibility to the patient, responsibility to oneself as a radiation worker, continuing education and responsibility in dose optimization in the effective application of the ALARA principle.

Discussion Questions

1. Describe the nature of the data on radiation bioeffects that provide the reasoning for the use of protective measures when imaging patients in diagnostic radiology.

2. Outline the elements involved in what the ICRP refers to as the "philosophy of radiation protection."

3. Discuss the quartets of radiation protection and specifically describe the three guiding principles of radiation protection specified by the ICRP.

References

Brodsky A, Kathren R. Historical development of radiation safety practices in radiology. *Radiographics*. 1989;9:1267–1275.

Bushberg JT, Seibert JA, Leidholdt EM, Boone JM. The Essential Physics of Medical Imaging. 3rd ed. Philadelphia, PA: Lippincott Williams & Wilkins; 2012.

Bushong S. *Radiologic Science for Technologists* (10th ed.). St. Louis, MO: Elsevier-Mosby; 2013.

Committee on the Biological Effects of Ionizing Radiation. *Health effects of low levels of ionizing radiation (BEIR V)*. Washington, DC: National Academies Press; 1990.

Dauer LT, Brooks AL, Hoel DG, Morgan WF, Stram D, Tran P. Review and evaluation of updated research on the health effects associated with low-dose ionizing radiation. *Radiat Prot Dosimetry*. 2010;140(2):103–136.

Health Canada. *Radiation protection in radiology— Large facilities safety code 35*. Ottawa: Ministry of Health; 2008.

Hendee WR, O'Connor MK. Radiation risks of medical imaging: Separating fact from fantasy. *Radiology*. 2013;204(2):312–320.

Hynes DM. Quality management. *J Can Assoc Radiol*. 1994;45:353–354.

International Commission on Radiological Protection (ICRP). *ICRP Publication No 73: Radiological protection and safety in medicine*. Oxford, UK: Pergamon Press; 1996.

International Commission on Radiological Protection (ICRP). *ICRP Publication No. 103: The 2007 recommendations of the international commission on radiological protection. Ann ICRP* 2007a;37(2-4):1–332.

International Commission on Radiological Protection (ICRP). *ICRP Publication No. 105: Radiation protection in medicine. Ann ICRP* 2007b;37(6):1–63.

Matthews K, Brennan P. Optimization of x-ray examinations: General principles and an Irish perspective. *Radiography*. 2009;15:262–268.

Mattsson S (Ed.). Optimization strategies in medical x-ray imaging. *Radiat Prot Dosimetry*. 2005;114(1-3):1–465.

Moores BM, Regulla D. A review of the scientific bases for radiation protection of the patient. *Radiat Prot Dosimetry*. 2011;147(1-2):22–29.

Müller HJ. Artificial transmutation of the gene. *Science*. 1927;66:84–86.

National Research Council. *Health risks from exposure to low levels of ionizing radiation: BEIR VII – phase 2*. Committee to Assess Health Risks from Exposure to Low Levels of Ionizing Radiation. Washington, DC: National Academies Press; 2006.

NCRP. *Report No. 160: Ionizing radiation exposure of the population of the United States*. Bethesda, MD: National Council on Radiation Protection & Measurements; 2009.

NCRP. *Report 172: Reference levels, and achievable doses in medical and dental imaging— Recommendations for the United States*. Bethesda, MD: National Council on Radiation Protection & Measurements; 2012.

Papp J. *Quality Management in the Imaging Sciences* (4th ed.). St. Louis, MO: Mosby-Elsevier; 2011.

Radiation Effects Research Foundation. "Hiroshima, Japan." http://www.rerf.jp/library/archives_e /scids.html (accessed August 11, 2015).

Seeram E, Davidson R, Bushong S, Swan H. Radiation dose optimization research: Exposure technique approached in CR imaging—A literature review. *Radiography*. 2013;19:331–338.

Seeram E, Brennan PC. Diagnostic reference levels in radiology. *Radiol Technol*. 2006;77(5):1–12.

Travis EL. *Primer of Medical Radiobiology* (2nd ed.). Chicago: Year Book; 1989.

U.S. Environmental Protection Agency. *Federal guidance report No. 14: Radiation protection guidance of diagnostic and interventional x-ray procedures*. EPA–402R. Washington, DC: U.S. Environmental Protection Agency; 2012.

U.S. Nuclear Regulatory Commission. *Standards for protection against radiation*. U.S. Code of Federal Regulations 10 CFR 20. Washington, DC: NRC; 2007.

Wolbarst AB, Patrizio C, Wyant A. *Medical Imaging: Essentials for Physicians*. Hoboken, NJ: Wiley Blackwell; 2013.

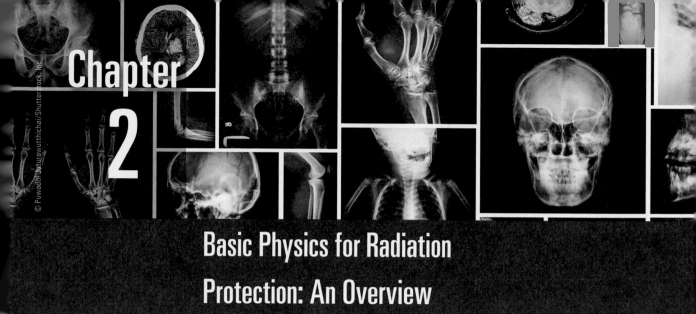

Chapter 2

Basic Physics for Radiation Protection: An Overview

Outline

- Introduction
- Atomic Structure
  - The element
  - The atom
  - The nucleus of an atom
  - Electrons
- Types of Radiation
  - Particulate radiations
  - Electromagnetic radiation
  - X-rays and gamma rays
  - Ionizing radiation
- X-ray and Gamma Radiation Interactions
  - X-ray interactions I: Elastic (or coherent or Rayleigh) scattering
- X-ray interactions II: Photoelectric absorption
- X-ray interactions III: Compton scattering
- X-ray interactions IV: Pair production
- Descriptive Terms or Concepts Associated With Radiation
  - Linear energy transfer (LET)
  - Linear attenuation coefficient
  - Mass attenuation coefficient
  - Inverse Square Law
- References

Objectives

On completion of this chapter, you should be able to:

1. Describe the structure of the atom.
2. Identify two types of radiation and explain the differences between them.
3. State the properties of x-rays.
4. Describe the production of Characteristic and Bremsstrahlung radiations.
5. Outline four characteristics of a diagnostic x-ray beam.
6. Discuss the production of gamma rays.
7. Discuss what is meant by ionizing radiation.
8. Discuss the nature of four interactions of ionizing radiation with matter.
9. Explain the meaning of each of the following terms/concepts regarding the behavior of different radiation types:
   - Linear energy transfer (LET)
   - Linear attenuation coefficient
   - Mass attenuation coefficient
   - Inverse square law

Introduction

Each time a patient is irradiated with x-rays, packets of energy interact with the patient, the image receptor, and anything else that is in the path of the primary beam emitted from the x-ray tube and the subsequently scattered or attenuated radiation (**Figure 2-1**).

It is essential to understand these interaction processes so that we can fully appreciate the events that occur within the patient, the precise risks associated with specific levels of exposure, and how these risks can be kept to a minimal level. A full understanding is also required to make sure that image receptors are being used in an optimal way.

There are two major effects of radiation on human tissue: *stochastic* (also known as non-deterministic) and *deterministic* (also known as non-stochastic). The initial changes that follow irradiation occur at the atomic level, then can build up to the cell and tissue level to manifest

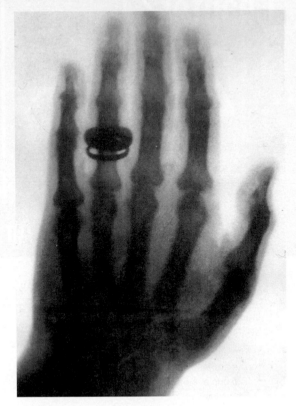

Figure 2-2 The first known x-ray image produced by Roentgen in 1895.

Reproduced from http://clickamericana.com/wp-content/uploads/roentgen-hand-x-ray.jpg.

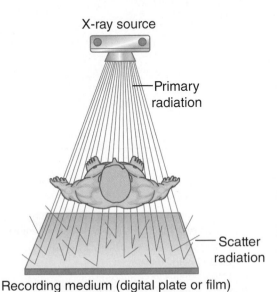

X-ray source

Primary radiation

Scatter radiation

Recording medium (digital plate or film)

Figure 2-1 Diagram demonstrating primary and scattered radiation shown following a patient exposure.

Courtesy of Patrick C. Brennan.

themselves as symptom-like changes. To understand all of these stages in this chain of events, a good grounding in atomic physics is required, along with an appreciation of the unique characteristics of x-radiation that not only dictate the type of events that occur, but also provide the basis for one of the most useful facilities in medicine for well over 100 years (**Figure 2-2**).

This chapter will therefore discuss the atom, x-ray characteristics, and atomic level interactions, so that students will be able to build on this knowledge to explore how these initial events manifest as observable changes in the human organism.

Atomic Structure

The Element

An **element** is the simplest form of matter, consisting of a specific type of atom that cannot be broken down but can undergo chemical reactions with other types of elements. Elements are the basic building blocks of matter, and at this time 118 are known to exist, of which 98 occur naturally. These are listed within the well-known periodic table of elements, which arranges all elements in an order determined by the atomic number of those elements (**Figure 2-3**). Everything we see is composed of elements, but to understand them—as well as the interactions that x-rays have with them—we must first have a good grounding in the anatomy of an atom.

The Atom

An atom simply consists of a nucleus surrounded by orbiting electrons that are positioned at a number of specific distances from the nucleus (**Figure 2-4**).

Originally, the word **atom** originates from the Greek equivalent, *atomos*, which means

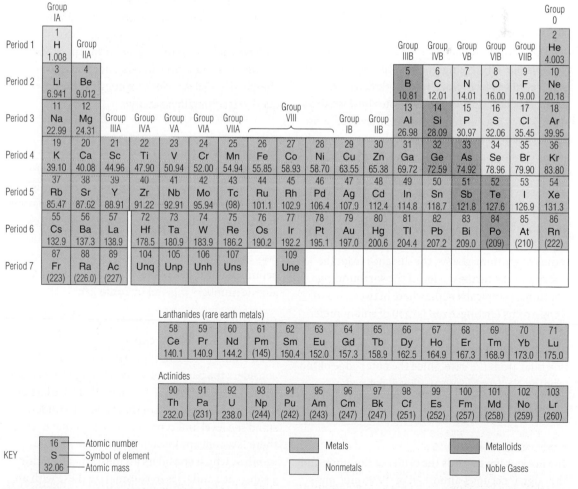

Figure 2-3 The periodic table of the elements.

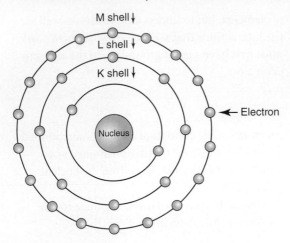

Figure 2-4 A diagram demonstrating the basic structure of an atom (not to scale).
Courtesy of Patrick C. Brennan.

"indivisible"—implying the structure was so small that it couldn't be divided into any smaller parts. While this description demonstrates how small an atom is, it is not entirely accurate, since even most primary school children will now be aware that the atoms contains a number of subatomic particles such as **electrons**, **protons**, and **neutrons**, and scholars with an understanding of more in-depth physics will be familiar with the various forms of **quarks**, which are even smaller, sub-subatomic particles. Nonetheless, the atom is very small; the radius of an atom, that is, the distance from the nucleus to the furthest edge of the surrounding electrons, is typically somewhere between 0.3 to 3 angstroms (an **angstrom** is 1/10 of a nanometer, or 0.00000001 millimeter). It should be stressed that although such measurements imply precision, this is far from the case, since the outer edge of the orbiting electrons is not at all well defined.

The Nucleus of an Atom

Protons and Neutrons
The nucleus lies towards the center of the atom, and although it occupies almost all of the atomic mass (>99.9%), its radius is less than 1/10,000 the length

of the atom—and therefore, its dimensions are tiny. It contains **nucleons**, which are better known as protons and neutrons. These are bound together by a nuclear force that is much stronger than the electrostatic force repelling the positively charged protons from each other, therefore keeping the nucleus together as a unit. The only exception to this arrangement is the most basic element, hydrogen, which does not contain a neutron. Unlike the positive charge of a proton (denoted as e), amounting to approximately 1.6×10^{-19} coulombs, the neutron does not have a charge. The electrical charge of protons and neutrons can be explained by a subatomic unit known as a quark—a fundamental component of matter, which cannot occur singularly, nor is directly observed. There are **up quarks** (each having a charge of $+^2/_3 e$) and **down quarks** (each with a charge of $-^1/_3 e$), and when combined, these form a **hadron**, such as a proton or neutron. The proton has 2 up quarks and 1 down quark, creating a positive charge; the neutron has 1 up quark and 2 down quarks, resulting in no charge.

Atomic Number
The number of protons that exist within the nucleus of an atom determines and is equal to its **atomic number**, and all atoms within a single element have the same number of protons. In other words, the number of protons determine the element type; e.g., an element with nuclei containing one, two, or eight protons will always be hydrogen, helium, and oxygen respectively. A list of some atomic numbers is given in **Table 2-1**.

Effective Atomic Number
The atomic number, as explained above, is specific to an atom or element type. However, when one considers the passage of x-rays through a structure, such as bone within the forearm, there are lots of different elements within that tissue. To understand the level and type of interaction that occurs, there is a concept known as **effective atomic number**, which considers all the elements within a substance and tries to summarize these with an overall atomic number for that structure. Some

Table 2-1 Some examples of atomic numbers.

Element	Atomic number (Z)
Barium	56
Carbon	6
Calicium	20
Iodine	53
Gadolinium	64
Hydrogen	1
Lead	82
Molybdenum	42
Oxygen	8
Nitrogen	7
Phosphorus	15
Sulfur	16
Tungsten	74
Uranum	92

examples of these are summarized in (**Table 2-2**), and while these are helpful to get a grasp of potential x-ray interactions, one should note that the effective atomic numbers listed are dependent on the energy of the x-ray photons.

Table 2-2 Some examples of effective atomic numbers.

Material	Effective atomic number (Z)
Air	7.78
Bone	12.3 - 14.0
Fat	6.46
LiF	8.31
Muscle	7.64
PMMA	6.56
Polystyrene	5.74
Water	7.5

Isotopes

In contrast to the atomic number, the neutron number, which may vary within the same element, determines the *isotope* of the element. If there is a balance between the proton and neutron number, then the nucleus will be relatively stable; however, this stability can be challenged when the neutron number changes, resulting in a process known as *radioactive decay* as the atom attempts to achieve stability. Radioactive decay can involve the release of an *alpha particle* (two protons and two neutrons: equal to a helium nucleus), a *beta particle* following a neutron-to-proton (releasing an electron and antineutrino) or proton-to-neutron (releasing a positron and neutrino) transition, or *gamma radiation* (usually a secondary event after alpha or beta decay). Radioactivity is a science in itself and accounts for its own medical imaging specialty; it is beyond the scope of this text.

Atomic Mass

The total number of neutrons and protons within a nucleus is known as the *atomic mass*. This definition appears to disregard the electrons (which are part of the atom), but as mentioned before, the nucleus accounts for almost all of the atomic mass.

Electrons

At this stage, we know that the proton determines the element type, and the neutron determines the isotope of that element; the electron, on the other hand, is responsible for the element's chemical and magnetic properties. It is a unit with the negative equivalent charge of the proton ($-1.6 ? \times 10^{-19}$ coulombs) that orbits the nucleus in shells at discrete distances from the nucleus (**Figure 2-5**).

The electron is even tinier than a nucleus, with a single electron having approximately 0.05% the mass of a proton. The total number of electrons in a neutral atom will equal the number of protons; however, if there are a greater or lesser number of electrons compared to protons, the atom is known as a negatively or positively charged ion, respectively.

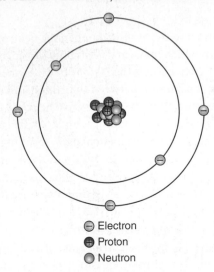

- ⊖ Electron
- ⊕ Proton
- ◯ Neutron

Figure 2-5 A diagram of carbon item demonstrating the electrons orbiting the nucleus.

Table 2-3 Some examples of K-shell binding energies.

Element	K-shell binding energy (eV)
Barium	37.4
Carbon	0.28
Calicium	4
Iodine	33.2
Gadolinium	50.2
Hydrogen	0.01
Lead	88
Molybdenum	20
Oxygen	0.5
Nitrogen	0.4
Phosphorus	2.1
Sulfur	2.5
Tungsten	39.5
Uranium	115.6

Electron Orbits or Shells and Binding Energy

It is fundamentally important to our understanding of the interaction of x-rays with an atom to know that these electrons are held within their orbital positions, otherwise known as *shells*, by an electromagnetic force known as *binding energy*. Electrons can only be released from their shells when a force greater than the binding energy is applied, which may be facilitated by an incoming x-ray, for example. The electromagnetic force results from the positive attractive of the nucleus (protons) on the negatively charged electrons, with the size of the force being proportional to the proximity of the electron to the nucleus. Therefore, the outer-shell electrons, known as *valence electrons*, are most easily removed. In other words, the binding energy of any particular electron is specific to the shell in which that electron is orbiting, and each shell therefore has a letter denoted to it, with the shell closest to the nucleus known as K, the next one L, the next one M, and so on (**Figure 2-4**). The binding energy of an electron in the K shell, for example, is a constant that is unique to each

specific element. K-shell energies for particular elements are listed in **Table 2-3**.

Types of Radiation

Radiation simply describes particles or waves of energy that have the ability to pass through matter or a vacuum. In order to understand the unique properties of x-rays that have made radiologic imaging possible, a short description of the other types of radiation may be useful. In summary, there are five main types: Alpha and beta particles, neutrons, gamma radiation, and x-rays. The first three are known as *particulate radiation* (because they are comprised of physical particles), whereas the latter two are forms of *electromagnetic radiation*. Each of these types of radiation will be considered below.

Particulate Radiations

As mentioned above, there are three main types of particulate radiation, although a number of others are known to exist. All radiation particles have two key features in common: They all have mass, and they all are subatomic entities. Although the amount of mass may vary substantially, each nonetheless has mass, and if one had the right tools, each could be observed as an object in its own right. A number of particulate radiations—but not all—have a negative or positive charge. If the particles are traveling in a single direction, the collection of particles is known as a **particle beam**.

Since particulate radiation has mass and sometimes has a charge as well, this means that when it interacts with matter, there will be substantial interactions between the radiation and matter proportional to the mass or charge of the radiation. This is one reason why particulate radiation is not suitable for radiography, since the ability of the radiation to pass through the patient and still interact with the image detector (in other words, its **penetrating ability**), is critically important. Particulate radiation is limited in this regard, although in nuclear medical imaging, there is a role for some particulate radiation such as positrons; however, x-rays have unique properties that are suited to transmission imaging that will be described later.

Alpha Particles

Alpha particles are high-energy entities released by nuclei of unstable atoms such as uranium-238 or plutonium-236. Each particle is comprised of two protons and two neutrons bound together as a single unit, making them identical to a helium nucleus (**Figure 2-6**).

Since they consist of 2 protons, which are positively charged, and 2 neutrons, which are neutral, the net outcome is a positive charge of 2. They have an atomic mass of 6.6×10^{-27} kg and can have a velocity of approximately 1/20th the speed of light.

Despite their velocity, alpha particles have very little penetrative ability. This is because of their relatively high charge and large weight, particularly when one considers that a single particle has almost 4000 times the mass of an electron. To put it in

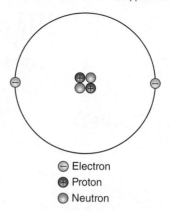

Electron
Proton
Neutron

Figure 2-6 Helium nucleus contained within a helium atom.

perspective, a sheet of paper is capable of completely absorbing an alpha particle (**Figure 2-7**). Put another way, this means that alpha particles have a very high **linear energy transfer** (LET), a measure described below. Alpha particles thus have no clinical relevance to medical imaging.

Beta Particles

There are two types of beta particles, electrons and positrons, both of which originate from an unstable atom and have high energy and speed. In an effort to achieve stability, a neutron can become a proton (when there are excess neutrons) or a proton can convert into a neutron (when there are excess protons). When the former occurs, such as with molybdenum-99, this is known as β^- **decay**, and an electron (along with an antineutrino) is produced. The latter process produces a positron (with a neutrino), and is known as β^+ **decay**. Fluorine 18, a well-known positron emitter within nuclear medicine circles, is the basis for much of the positron emission tomography procedures (**Figure 2-8**). β^- decay is rarely used in imaging.

The electron, as discussed above, and its positron counterpart have a very low atomic mass compared with a proton. They also have charge, this being negative (–1) or positive (+1) for the electron and positron respectively. Due to this lower mass

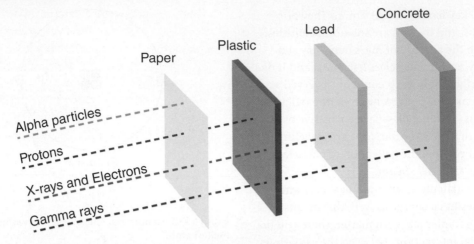

Figure 2-7 Types of attenuators that will absorb different types of radiation.
Courtesy of Patrick C. Brennan.

and charge when compared with an alpha particle, beta particles have a lower LET and therefore can penetrate further, being stopped by a few millimeters of aluminum.

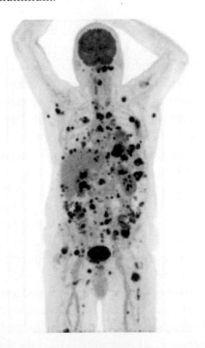

Figure 2-8 PET scan obtained with gallium-68.
Courtesy of Patrick C. Brennan.

Neutrons

Neutron radiation is a byproduct of nuclear fission (the splitting of an atomic nucleus) or nuclear fusion (the collision of two highly energetic nuclei to form a new nucleus). The properties of neutrons are given above. They have a similar mass to a proton, but no charge, which is different from the other particulate types of radiation described earlier. Their mass means that they have high LET properties; depending on their energy, they can be highly penetrating, sometimes even more so than x-rays or gamma rays.

Other Types of Particulate Radiation

The key particulate radiations are described above, but it should be noted that there are many others, including protons, neutrinos (tiny mass; charge-less), mesons (mass around two-thirds of a proton; some have either positive or negative charge) and muons (mass between an electron and proton; positively charged).

Electromagnetic Radiation

X-rays and gamma radiation belong to a family of radiation types known as ***electromagnetic radiation***. These are distinct from particulate radiation in that they do not exist as a particle with mass and do not have charge. Rather, they are packets of pure energy.

The Electromagnetic Spectrum

The electromagnetic spectrum consists of a very broad array of radiation types (**Figure 2-9**). At the left side of **Figure 2-9**, we can see radio waves, which can be as long as a kilometer or mile; however, they have a frequency that is relatively low at 10,000 cycles per second. On the other end of the spectrum are gamma rays, which have a wavelength around 1 picometer (or 0.000001 micrometer, which in itself is 0.000001 meter), but have a frequency of 1×10^{20} waves per second.

Properties of Electromagnetic Radiation

Even though the radiation types contained within the electromagnetic spectrum seem completely diverse, they do share the following properties:

- They can travel through empty space or a vacuum in a straight line.
- They are transmitted by electric and magnetic fields oscillating at right angles to each other (**Figure 2-10**).
- In a vacuum, they all travel at the speed of light: 300,000 km/s or 180,000 miles/s;

- They can be described in terms of their wavelength or frequency, which can vary hugely depending on the radiation type.
- They are unaffected by external magnetic or electric fields.
- They exhibit exponential absorption through a homogeneous type of material. This means that for *additional equal thicknesses* of material, there are *equal fractional reductions* in radiation intensity (**Figure 2-11**).
- They exhibit wave and photon (particle) behavioral characteristics.

Particles of Electromagnetic Radiation?

As one will see from the last point above, sometimes there is reference to particles when talking about the behavior of electromagnetic radiation such as x-rays. It is important to remember, however, that this does not mean particles in the sense described within the particulate radiation section where mass and sometimes charge is involved. Rather, it means packets of energy, which are otherwise known as photons.

Dual Characteristics of Electromagnetic Radiation

The dual characteristics of electromagnetic radiation mean that when one is describing its

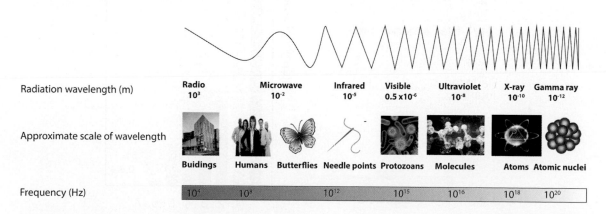

Figure 2-9 The electromagnetic spectrum.
Courtesy of Patrick C. Brennan.

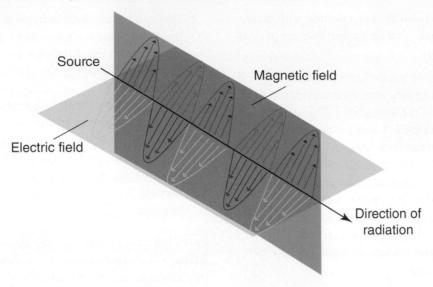

Figure 2-10 Electric and magnetic field oscillating at right angles to each other and to the direction of radiation.

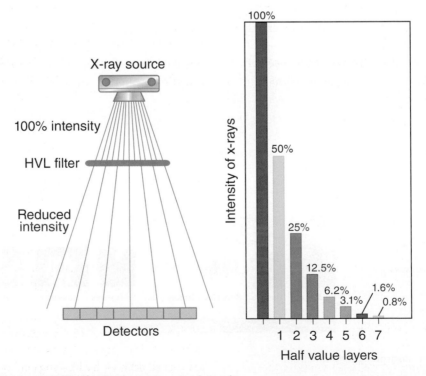

Figure 2-11 The impact of half-value layers on x-ray intensity.

behavioral properties, we often think of waves in terms of interference when passing through matter and photons (particles) when we think of energy and momentum. Certainly, when describing the interaction of x-rays with matter (human or otherwise), we will use the concept of photon energies much more than waves, but if we were discussing the interaction of light with filters, the use of wave characteristics may be more useful. With the help of Max Planck, the German theoretical physicist responsible for proposing quantum theory, these concepts can be combined in the simple formula:

$$E = hf$$

where E is the energy of the photon, h is Planck's constant (6.626×10^{-34}), and f is cycles per second (Hz).

X-Rays and Gamma Rays

Within the electromagnetic spectrum, we can see that both x-rays and gamma rays are positioned towards the right. They share the properties of having a very short wavelengths and a very high frequency. Nonetheless, they are distinct from each other—sufficiently so that only x-rays can be used in radiographic imaging.

X-Ray Properties

X-rays have no mass or charge; they are invisible photons of energy. From the simple formula above we can see that energy is proportional to frequency, and therefore as the frequency of electromagnetic radiation goes up, so does its energy. X-rays, which are at the upper end of the frequency range in Figure 2-9, therefore have higher energies than, say, light, but lower energies than gamma rays. In medical imaging, the energy of photons within a single x-ray beam can range from 0–150 kiloelectron-volts (keV). Some of these energies are too low to be useful and only add to the radiation dose received by an individual, but others are higher and can easily penetrate through the patient, yet still interact with the detector and produce an image.

Types of X-Rays

To understand the type of x-ray energies that are contained within a diagnostic exposure, it is necessary to understand how x-rays are produced. This is too big a subject to describe in detail here, but a brief description is in order.

As a result of the interactions of electrons with a target such as tungsten, we have two types of x-rays: *characteristic radiation* and *bremsstrahlung radiation*. Characteristic x-rays are named as such because the energy of these x-rays remains constant for a specific element, such as tungsten, within the x-ray tube target. Bremsstrahlung x-rays take their name from the German word that means "braking radiation" or "deceleration radiation"—and the name describes the x-ray radiation in that it is produced by deceleration of a charged particle deflected by the target.

Production of Characteristic Radiation

Characteristic radiation is produced when an electron emitted from the x-ray tube filament interacts with an inner shell electron (such as a K shell) (**Figure 2-12 [1]**) of the tungsten target; ionization takes place and the electron is removed from its orbiting shell (**Figure 2-12 [2]**). The atom cannot continue in the state of having a missing electron on its inner shell, and therefore an outer-shell electron (e.g., from the L shell) moves into the vacant place (**Figure 2-12 [3]**). In turn, the resultant vacancy on the L shell is filled by another outer-shell electron from the M shell or beyond, and so on (**Figure 2-12 [4]**). However, since the binding energies of electrons differ between the orbiting shells, when the L-shell electron (for example) moves into the K shell, it now has excessive energy that must be released. This energy is released in the form of characteristic x-rays.

Even though the example given above refers to an L–K interaction, this could happen between any shell pairing; however, the released characteristic x-ray specific to certain shell-to-shell transitions may not be of sufficient energy to even leave the target, never mind reach the patient.

Characteristic Radiation Energies

With tungsten, for example, when an L-shell electron with a binding energy of ~11.5 keV moves into the K-shell orbit with a binding energy of ~69.5 keV, there is a difference in energies of ~58 keV. This is

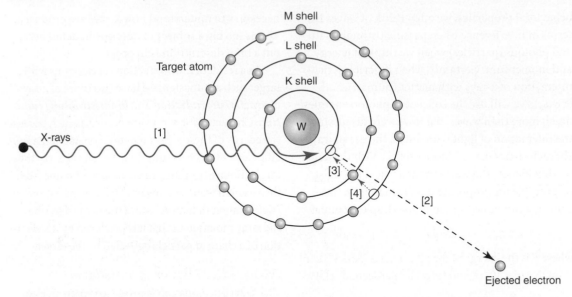

Figure 2-12 Events happening within a tungsten atom following the interaction between x-rays and the inner-shell electron.

released in the form of x-rays, and since the binding energies of these two shells within tungsten always remain at the values stated above, the x-ray energy released with this L–K transition remains constant and can be seen from the vertical spike on the left shown in **Figure 2-13**.

To the right of this spike in Figure 2-13 is another one, which represents the transition of an M-shell electron to a K-shell vacancy. Because the binding energy of an M shell is approximately 2.5 keV, the M–K binding energy difference (and x-ray energy released) is greater compared to the L–K difference. The reader will note that there will be other shell transitions such as an M–L or N–L transition following an L-shell electron ejection but the energy of resultant x-rays will be small. It also should be

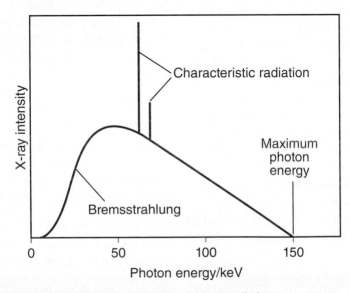

Figure 2-13 Demonstration of characteristic and bremsstrahlung radiation.

noted that for any of these transitions to occur, the electron interacting with the tungsten target must exceed the relevant binding energies, and if, for example, one has set a kilovoltage peak (kVp) of 50, then there will be no K ejections (Figure 2-13).

Finally, to reiterate, the energies described for tungsten are specific to tungsten. If the target consisted of molybdenum or rhenium, the energies of the characteristic radiation would be very different due to the different K-shell (**Table 2-3**) and other binding energies.

Bremsstrahlung Radiation Production

With characteristic radiation, the incoming electrons emitted from the filament of the x-ray tube interact with electrons within the x-ray tube's target (**Figure 2-14**). Simplistically, an alternative to the target's electrons with which the filament's electrons could interact at the target is the nucleus. While a direct interaction is not going to occur at x-ray tube voltages, the electron can pass close to the positively charged nucleus. When this happens, the positive force of the nucleus can cause a change in the negative electrons' direction, resulting in a release of bremsstrahlung x-ray radiation.

Bremsstrahlung Radiation Energies

Unlike characteristic radiation, where very specific energies are produced, the bremsstrahlung process results in a much wider range of energy levels. The basis for this is straightforward: When incoming electrons pass close to the nucleus, they can undergo a whole range of direction changes, from a very small amount where the electron only very marginally changes its path, to a huge level where the electron is traveling almost in the reverse of its original direction. The **kinetic energy** of the electron is lost as direction changes and is converted into x-ray energy, with the amount of energy released proportional to the level of direction change. Therefore, if the electron direction can vary by a large range, there will be a large range of energies, and this results in the well-known continuous spectrum of energies as shown in Figure 2-13. In practice, rarely does an

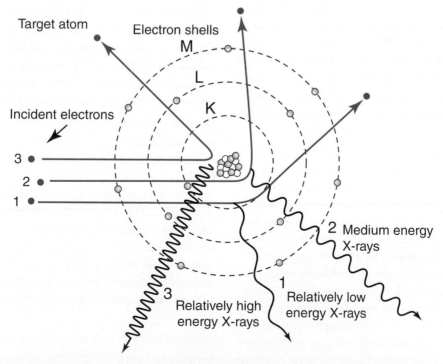

Figure 2-14 Image demonstrating a Bremsstrahlung radiation: [1] on the figure demonstrates a smaller angle of electron deflection and lower energy of x-rays produced, compared with [2] and [3].

electron give up all its energy as an x-ray, but instead undergoes various direction changes resulting in a variety of x-ray energies being released.

Close examination of Figure 2-13 describing bremsstrahlung radiation and including the characteristic radiation, both of which are typical of the energies contained within a diagnostic x-ray beam, leads one to the following conclusions:

1. A range of energies exist from just above zero to close to the kVp set for the exposure. The *potential energy* and subsequent kinetic energy (as it is moving) of the incoming electron within the x-ray tube is determined by the potential difference applied across the cathode and anode. Since the kVp set by the radiographer determines the maximum energy an electron can have, this in turn determines the maximum energy that can be lost when this electron passes close to a target nucleus.

2. The highest intensity of x-rays is situated at an energy somewhere close to around one-third the maximum energy. This emphasizes the importance of not using simple descriptors such as kVp to represent the x-ray beam's energy. Even *average beam energy* may be inappropriate once one considers the non-Gaussian appearance of the energy distribution, and more appropriate descriptors such as *effective beam energy* should be used instead.

3. A number of x-rays are at a very low energy, which would contribute little to the image-making process but would instead increase patient dose (if indeed these x-rays actually escaped from the x-ray tube). This highlights the need for filtration to be inserted into the x-ray tube housing so that as many of these lower energy x-rays as possible are removed, and indeed such filters are legally required in most countries. In practice, inherent filtration resulting from materials simply existing in the x-ray tube by nature of its construction (glass envelope, oil within the housing, etc.) removes about 50% of the x-rays generated at the anode,

and the added filtration such as aluminum removes 80% of the remainder.

4. The insertion of the characteristic radiation vertical peaks highlights that when an x-ray exposure takes place, both types of x-ray radiation will be produced as long as the energy levels described on the X axis exceed the energy required to remove a target electron from its orbiting shell.

Efficiency of X-Ray Production

If asked whether the production of characteristic and bremsstrahlung radiation is efficient, the answer must be *No*. If one uses the intensity of electrons as the baseline value at 100%, then about 1% of this turns into x-rays, and the other 99% results in heat and light, highlighting the importance of effective heat dispersion systems. As mentioned above, of this 1%, perhaps 0.5% gets through the inherent filters and a further 0.1% passes through the added filtration. While the level of efficiency remains low, whatever the conditions, it does vary depending on the kVp selected and the atomic number of the anode material, with efficiency being directly proportional to both these factors. Other factors restrict the use of anode materials with a very high atomic number, limiting the ability to improve efficiency by altering the anode.

Gamma Radiation

Gamma radiation has some similar properties to x-rays in that it is a form of electromagnetic radiation and therefore has neither mass nor charge. Since gamma radiation is positioned immediately to the right of the x-rays within the electromagnetic spectrum (Figure 2-9), gamma photons generally have energies that are higher than x-rays, and therefore are highly penetrating. One other noticeable difference between gamma and x-rays is the production processes, which will be discussed below.

Gamma Ray Production and Energies

Gamma rays are produced from unstable, radioactive isotopes, and therefore have energies that are specific and characteristic to the mother isotope (the original unstable element). These specific energies are known as *line spectra*, and those that are useful in medical imaging vary from 100 to 511 keV.

The main method of gamma ray emission is known as *isomeric transition*. Here, the unstable mother nucleus is trying to achieve stability, and its first step is to release alpha or beta particles as described above. In this transition, the nucleus achieves a *metastable state*, which requires the further release of a gamma photon of energy.

Gamma Ray Production: An Example

A typical example of this process that is relevant to nuclear medicine imaging techniques is when the unstable isotope molybdenum-99 converts to technetium-99^m (the superscript m represents a metastable state) with a release of a negative beta particle and a gamma particle of 740 keV. However, technetium-99^m is still unstable and therefore undergoes a further decay to technetium-99 with a release of gamma radiation at the specific energy of 140 keV. Incidentally, the latter then goes on to become ruthenium-99—but only after more than 200,000 years of further decay! A diagrammatic summary of all this is given in **Figure 2-15**.

The transition from technetium-99^m to technetium-99 is widely used within nuclear medicine. It is introduced into the patient as a pharmaceutical while being attached to another agent that leads the technetium-99^m to a specific part of the body; subsequently, gamma radiation is released from that part of the body and captured by imaging equipment, revealing functional and morphological indicators of disease. An example of this is when sestamibi is attached to technetium-99^m and administered intravenously; imaging subsequently indicates how well the blood is flowing through the heart (**Figure 2-16**). Since the specific technetium-99^m to technetium-99 transition does not involve the release of alpha or beta particles (pure gamma radiation) and has a short half-life of just over 6 hours (meaning the intensity of radiation is reduced to 50% in 6 hours and to ~6% in 24 hours), the radiation dose to the patient is relatively low. Also, the energy of the gamma ray at 140 keV means that the radiation can easily escape from the patient and can be captured by the external gamma ray detectors.

Internal Conversion

It should be acknowledged that there is a competing process to the above gamma-release transition, which is known as *internal conversion*. In order to achieve ground state (stability), the excited nucleus may not release the excess energy as gamma

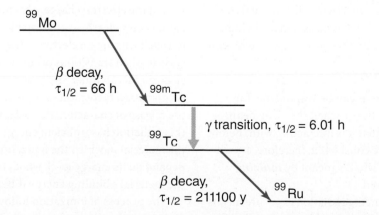

Figure 2-15 Production of gamma rays following the transition of technetium-99^m to technetium-99 as part of molybdenum-99 to ruthenium-99 series of events.

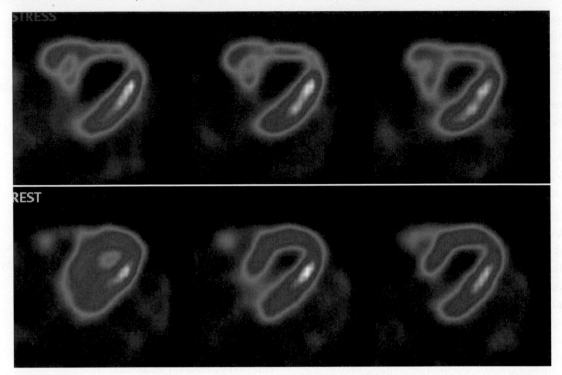

Figure 2-16 An image generated from combination of sestamibi and technetium-99^m.
Courtesy of Patrick C. Brennan.

radiation, but instead transfers the energy to an electron, usually within the K shell, and the electron is emitted from the atom with an energy equal to the original energy minus the binding energy of the specific electron. This process can reduce the gamma release transitions by approximately 9%. The level of reduction can be summarized by the internal conversion coefficient, which is measured by dividing the internal conversion rate by the gamma emission.

Ionizing Radiation

The interactions that can be responsible for biological change occur when the x-ray beam *ionizes* the atoms that it is interacting with. Before the interactions are considered, therefore, a good understanding of what is meant by *ionizing radiation* is required.

Ionization following radiation exposure means that an interaction has taken place between an orbiting electron and another agent—x-rays, gamma rays, or alpha particles—leading to the complete removal of the electron from its atom. This results in an *ion pair*—the electron that has been emitted, which obviously carries a negative charge, and the remaining atom, which is now positively charged since it has lost an electron and the positive nucleus is no longer balanced by the sum of the electron charge. This positively charged atom is now clearly in an unstable state, since there is a shell without an electron; therefore, a series of shell-to-shell transitions occur in which an outer electron fills an inner-shell vacancy (**Figure 2-17**). As discussed before, these transitions will result in the release of characteristic radiation, but whether this radiation has sufficient energy to escape from the material in which the ionization took place will depend on its energy level, which in turn relies on the material's binding energy differences.

The process of ionization following x-ray interactions can be direct or indirect. *Direct ionization* occurs when the x-ray enters the atom and interacts directly with the electron, which is removed

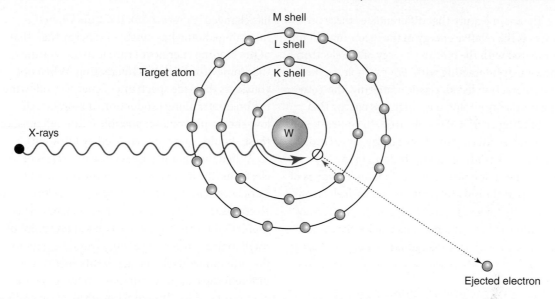

Figure 2-17 X-rays interacting and ejecting an inner-shell electron. One can see the outer-shell electron from the L shell moving into the subsequent vacancy.

from the atom (Figure 2-17). ***Indirect ionization*** occurs when the x-ray removes the electron; that electron, which then goes on to be a beta particle, is responsible for removing another electron. X-rays, gamma rays, and neutron particles are both directly and indirectly ionizing radiation types, whereas alpha and beta particles would mainly be directly ionizing.

Alternatively, ***excitation*** may occur. This is where the electron is not removed from the atom, but instead it has received just the right amount of energy to transfer it to an outer orbiting shell. This remains in this higher orbit for a short period of time before returning to its original shell, releasing some form of electromagnetic radiation such as visible light. This is the basis for processes of luminescence, such as fluorescence and phosphorescence.

Finally, ionizations can be damaging to the organism and indeed can be the first step towards many biological changes. It is important to note that some electromagnetic radiation is nonionizing, such as light and radio waves; x-rays, however, are ionizing, as are gamma rays and alpha, beta, and neutron particles. For this reason, each exposure presents a potential risk to the individual being exposed.

X-Ray and Gamma Radiation Interactions

The properties of x-rays and gamma radiation should now be clear. They are mass-less, charge-less, and therefore at higher energies have the ability to penetrate through human tissue. That penetration, however, does not mean that x-rays or gamma rays do not have critical interactions within the body; they do, and the focus of this section is to explore and detail those interactions. As a result of those interactions, human tissue can undergo change that can manifest itself in cancer (although the risk is normally very low for diagnostic x-ray exposures) or in direct change to the body such as reddening of the skin.

There are four main interaction processes that may occur when x-ray or gamma radiation interacts with matter such as human tissue. These are listed below, but two of these (in boldface) are of much greater importance for x-ray interactions than the others:

- Elastic or coherent scattering
- **Photoelectric absorption**
- **Compton scattering**
- **Pair production**

The main feature that differentiates these processes is the relative energy of the incoming photon compared with the binding energy of the electron the x-ray is interacting with. For example, in the first interaction listed, elastic scattering, the x-ray or gamma ray photon has much less energy that the binding energy of the electron. In contrast, in Compton scattering the x-ray energy far exceeds the relevant binding energy. Indeed, in the first three interaction processes, the photon energy is of a level that the only interactions are with electrons; the fourth, however, involves energies >1.022 meV that allow nuclear interactions to take place and only occurs with gamma radiation. Each of these interaction processes will be considered in turn.

X-Ray Interactions I: Elastic (or Coherent or Rayleigh) Scattering

Elastic scattering, also called coherent or Rayleigh scattering, is the only process of the four in which no change in energy occurs. It accounts for only 10% of all x-ray interactions. The term *elastic scattering* means that the energy of the incoming photon, in this case an x-ray, is completely conserved; however, the direction of the photon has changed (**Figure 2-18**). It occurs when the incoming photon has much less energy than that of the binding energies of the electrons within the atom with which it is interacting. When one considers the wide spectrum of energies following the bremsstrahlung production of x-rays, such low-energy photons are possible (although most of these should have been removed by filtration).

When the photon passes close to a series of electrons, the oscillating electromagnetic field associated with the photon (Figure 2-10) forces the electrons to oscillate at the same frequency. This oscillation means that as electrons at one point of oscillation are receiving energy from the photon, they are immediately replacing this energy at a different stage of the oscillation, so there is no net loss of energy. This constant absorption and replacement of the photon's energy is the basis for the term *elastic* scattering. The probability of elastic scattering happening is directly proportional to the atomic number squared and inversely proportional to the energy, so as the photons increase in energy, elastic scattering is less likely to occur.

The vast majority of elastic scattering interactions are of the Rayleigh type as described above; however,

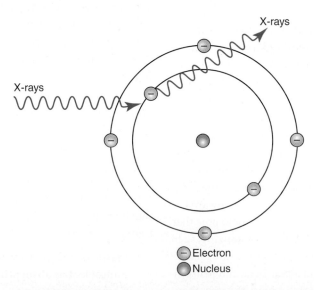

Figure 2-18 Diagram of elastic scattering. Note the electron has not been ejected and the energy of the x-ray has remained the same, even after the interaction within the electron.

there is another type called Thomson elastic scattering, which occurs when the photon passes close to only a single electron. This is much rarer than even the Rayleigh type. Again, no loss of energy occurs.

X-Ray Interactions II: Photoelectric Absorption

Photoelectric absorption is an important interaction that occurs between the photon and electrons. In photoelectric absorption, the incoming photon has an energy very close to or slightly exceeding that of the binding energy of the electron with which the photon is interacting. When the interaction takes place, all of the photon's energy is transferred to the electron, resulting in complete absorption (as the name would suggest). The electron is ejected from the atom as a photoelectron, with an energy that equals the original photon energy minus the binding energy (**Figure 2-19**), with this energy being absorbed close to where the interaction took place. In addition, the atom in which the interaction took place will *recoil* to satisfy the Law of Conservation of Momentum, which tells us that the total momentum of two objects

before a collision is equal to the total momentum of the two objects after the collision.

The removal of the electron from the shell will result in an outer-shell electron filling the vacated space and characteristic radiation (as described above) being given off; alternatively, this excess energy is transferred to an outer-shell electron, which is ejected from its shell and becomes what is known as an ***Auger electron***. With regard to human exposure, since the atomic numbers of elements in biological tissue are low, so too is the difference in binding energies, and therefore the characteristic radiation released will be unable to move very far from its site of origin.

There are a number of key points relating to photoelectric absorption:

1. Photoelectric absorption cannot occur if the photon energy is less than the binding energy of the electron with which it is interacting.

2. All the photon energy is given up to the electron and is therefore completely absorbed.

3. The photon energy must be close to or slightly greater than the electron's binding energy.

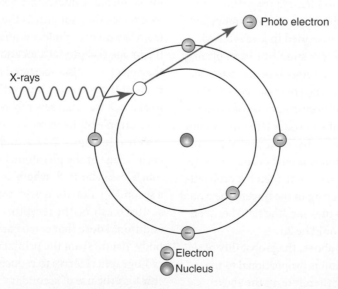

Figure 2-19 Diagram of photoelectric absorption. With this interaction process, the x-ray has ejected the electron and has been totally or almost totally absorbed.

4. For binding energies to be close to the photon energies typically used in diagnostic imaging, the energy of the x-ray photon should not be excessive. Therefore, the probability of photoelectric absorption is reduced as photon energy is increased, the relationship being:

Photoelectric absorption is inversely proportional to the photon energy cubed (E^3);

However, as the photon energy increases above 200 keV and beyond, E^3 becomes E^2 and eventually E.

5. To ensure that photon energies match binding energies, the interaction usually only happens with inner-shell electrons, mainly the K shell; otherwise, the energy differences between the photon and electron would be too great. Since binding energies increase with atomic numbers, the probability of photoelectric absorption occurring is higher with higher atomic numbers, the relationship being:

Photoelectric absorption is proportional to the atomic number cubed (Z^3).

As the photon energy increases, the probability of absorption changes from Z^3 to Z.

This last point—that is, the probability of photoelectric absorption being proportional to the atomic number cubed—is critically important to the image contrast obtained in x-ray–based diagnostic imaging. A very simplistic example may help demonstrate why: A finger is being examined, and we wish to enhance the contrast between the bone (with an effective atomic number of 14) compared with the adjacent soft tissue (effective atomic number of 7). Hypothetically, if the probability of photoelectric absorption was only proportional to the atomic number (not cubed), then the probability of absorption occurring in the fingerbone would be twice that of soft tissue—i.e., the ratio between the two tissue types would be 2:1.

However, as stated above, the probability of photoelectric absorption is proportional to the atomic number *cubed*; therefore, in the above (simplistic) finger example, the probability of the photoelectron being absorbed in the bone compared to in the soft tissue is 2744 ($14 \times 14 \times 14$) to 343 ($7 \times 7 \times 7$), or 8:1. This means that the probability of absorption of x-rays in bone is 8 times rather than 2 times that of soft tissue, ensuring that the contrast between the two tissue types is significantly enhanced.

This is why every radiographer is taught that if contrast is to be enhanced within the image, the energy of the x-rays (kVp) must be kept as low as possible so that the probability of photoelectric absorption is enhanced. Of course, there are dose implications with lower beam energies, but these will be discussed elsewhere.

X-Ray Interactions III: Compton Scattering

Photoelectric absorption is considered in favorable terms in terms of image contrast; however, Compton scattering challenges quality. From **Figure 2-20**, we see that when photoelectric absorption predominates, the object is reasonably accurately represented and discriminable from the background (**Figure 2-21**).

On the other hand, when Compton scattering is the main interactive process (**Figure 2-22**), we can see that not only is the radiation scattered from the object of interest no longer arriving at the image receptor at a location that represents the object, but also, scattered radiation from other parts of the subject is interacting with the object's image in a way that severely reduces the contrast. An example of the impact of scattered radiation is shown in **Figure 2-23 A** and **B**: In A, we have a clear image of the phantom, but the spine becomes much less clear in B, where due to the absence of a secondary radiation grid, we have much more scatter reaching the receptor. This, as well as the additional dose that can be achieved in parts of the body distant from the primary radiation, is why radiographers strive to reduce scattered radiation through the use of secondary radiation grids and accurate levels of collimation.

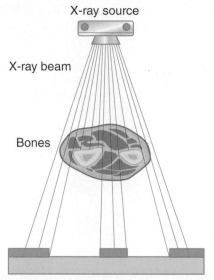

Figure 2-20 A diagrammatic representation of pure absorption, where all the x-rays are absorbed by the two bones.

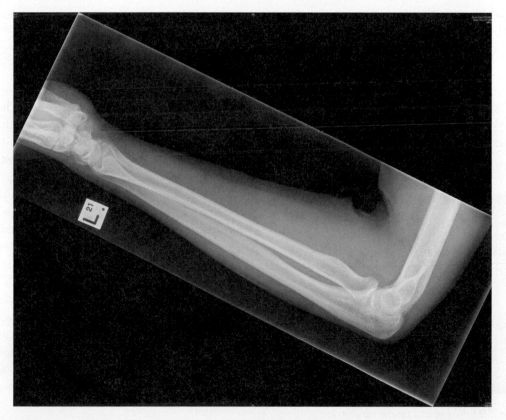

Figure 2-21 Image of a forearm, where photoelectric absorption is the main interaction process.
Courtesy of Patrick C. Brennan.

X-ray source

X-ray beam

Bones

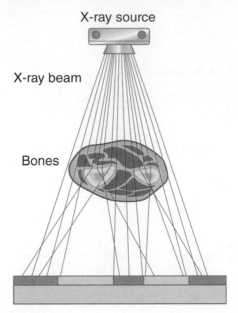

Recording medium (digital plate or film)

Figure 2-22 A diagrammatic representation of Compton scatter, where all the x-rays are no longer absorbed by the bone, and radiation representing a certain part of the attenuating structure is arriving at inappropriate locations on the image receptor.

Compton scattering occurs when the incoming x-ray photon has much more energy than the binding energy of the electron with which it is interacting. When the interaction takes place, the x-ray is no longer fully absorbed; rather, it loses only some of its energy to a recoil electron. The x-ray then continues in a direction that is different from its original one—that is, it has been scattered (**Figure 2-24**)—and since energy has been lost, Compton scattering can be referred to as "inelastic scattering." The recoil electron, known as a Compton electron, is ejected from the atom and can go on to cause further ionizations. Since the binding energy of the electron must be considerably less than the x-ray photon's energy, the interaction often takes place with electrons positioned in shells other than the K shell (i.e., the vast majority of electrons).

So if the x-ray energy is reduced following a Compton-type interaction, the question becomes, by how much is it reduced? The answer is dependent on a few factors, including the conservation of energy and momentum, and is summarized by this formula:

$$\lambda_2 - \lambda_1 = h \, / \, mc(1 - \cos\theta)$$

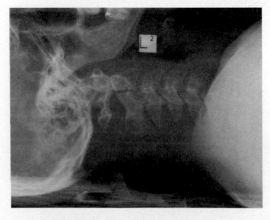

Figure 2-23 Image of a lateral cervical spine using a horizontal beam technique.
Courtesy of Patrick C. Brennan.

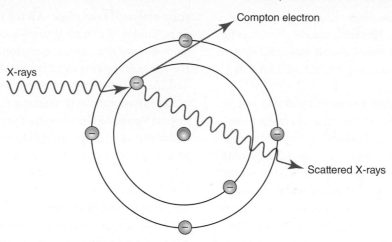

Figure 2-24 Compton scattering. Note the x-rays have continued after the interaction, albeit in a changed direction.

where λ_2 is the wavelength of the scattered x-ray photon, λ_1 is the wavelength of the incident x-ray photon, h is Planck's constant (see above), m is the mass of the electron, c is the velocity of light, and $cos\ \theta$ is the cosine of the angle of the scattered x-ray photon. You will remember from our discussion above on electromagnetic radiation that as frequency or energy increases, wavelength decreases. So wavelength is an inverse representation of energy.

The bottom line of all of this is that since **h**, **m**, and **c** are constants, the amount of energy lost by the x-ray photon (or the level of wavelength increase) is highly dependent on the angle of the scattered x-ray. As this angle increases, the level of photon energy loss is greater; as the angle decreases, the energy lost is less. Two consequents of this formula should be apparent: first, **h, m, c**, and **cos θ** are the *only* determinants of the lost energy, so the characteristics of the attenuator are not relevant; second, since a given scattered photon angle will give a very specific wavelength change, this means that if the wavelength of the photons are small (high energy), it leads to a large fractional change in the wavelength and a lot of energy loss. If the photon wavelength is large

(low energy) for a specific scattered photon angle, a given wavelength reduction leads to a small fractional change and therefore low energy loss. In other words, *if the incident photon energy is high, much energy can be lost and transferred to the Compton electron; this is not the case if the incident photon energy is relatively low.*

Unlike photoelectric absorption, which generally occurs with only a very limited number of inner-shell electrons (e.g., K shell has two electrons), Compton scattering can occur with a much greater number of electrons. Therefore, the probability of Compton scattering occurring is closely related to the number of electrons that are present within the atom. The electron number can be calculated by estimating the number of electrons existing within a gram of tissue using the formula:

$$\text{Electrons / gram} = \frac{\text{Avogadro's number } (6.023 \times 10^{23}) \times \text{atomic number}}{\text{Atomic mass}}$$

A practical example of this is to calculate the electron numbers for bone and adjacent muscle. For bone, the effective atomic number is 13.8, the atomic mass is 27.7, and therefore the electron density is approximately 3×10^{23}; with muscle, the values for effective atomic number, atomic mass, and electron density are approximately 7.5, 14.5, and 3.4×10^{23}, respectively.

From these approximate calculations, one can see two key facts: First, that there is a huge number of electrons available for x-rays to interact with (and remember, this is simply electrons/gram). Second and more important, even though the atomic numbers of these two human tissues are different by almost factor of two, the number of electrons is very similar. In other words, the number of electrons, and hence the probability of Compton scattering, is independent of the atomic number.[1] This is very unlike photoelectric absorption, as discussed above.

The key issues regarding Compton scattering are therefore:

1. The incoming x-ray photon has an energy that is considerably greater than the binding energy of the electron it is interacting with.

2. Following the x-ray/electron collision, the x-ray loses some of its energy and changes direction—that is, it scatters.

3. The electron is ejected from the atom and is known as a Compton electron.

4. The interaction generally involves outer-shell electrons.

5. The probability of Compton scattering occurring is directly related to the electron number and independent of the atomic number of the attenuator.

Finally, one further issue from **Figure 2-25**: One can see that when a diagnostic exposure is made, one cannot eliminate Compton scattering. Both photoelectric absorption and Compton scattering will take place. All the radiographer or technologist can do is to choose a kVp that helps answer the clinical question. While from the above it appears to be reasonable to suggest that photoelectric absorption should be the predominant interaction process (and therefore a lower kVp should be chosen), every experienced technologist or clinician will know that imaging forces lots of compromises. From an image quality perspective, a lower kVp may be preferable; however, this can increase radiation dose levels, due to more radiation being absorbed within the body. Also, in terms of penetrating larger patients, and sometimes deliberately reducing image contrast to enhance image quality such as with chest radiography (**Figure 2-26 A and B**), higher kVps maybe preferable. The challenge to the radiographer, technologist, and radiologic clinician is clear.

X-Ray Interactions IV: Pair Production

Pair production involves energies beyond those used with diagnostic x-rays, so it will only be treated briefly here. Unlike the other three interaction processes, pair production involves the incoming photon interacting with the nucleus of the atom. To be able to achieve this, it needs an energy of at least 1.02 meV to overcome the nuclear electrostatic forces. This type of energy is far beyond that used with x-rays, but would be relevant to gamma radiation and therefore nuclear medicine.

When the incoming photon does have at least an energy of at least 1.02 meV and interacts with the nucleus, two particles are produced (hence the term *pair production*): an electron and a positron. Excess photon energy above 1.02 meV will be given to the two particles in the form of kinetic energy. This process is a very clear example of the very

---

[1]For a more comprehensive listing of electron numbers per gram, and also electron densities, which multiplies the electrons/gram by the densities of atoms in an attenuator (g/cm³), please see Chapter 5 of the excellent textbook by Dowsett, Kenny and Johnston: *The Physics of Diagnostic Imaging* (2006).

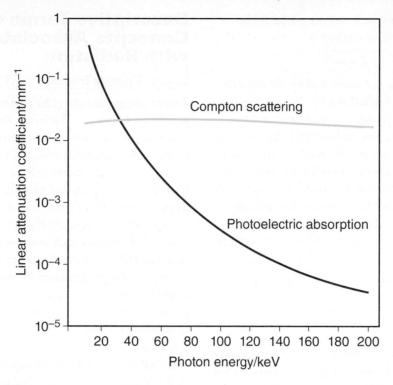

Figure 2-25 Diagram showing the relative contributions of photoelectric absorption and Compton scattering to the attenuation processes at x-ray energies relevant to diagnostic imaging.

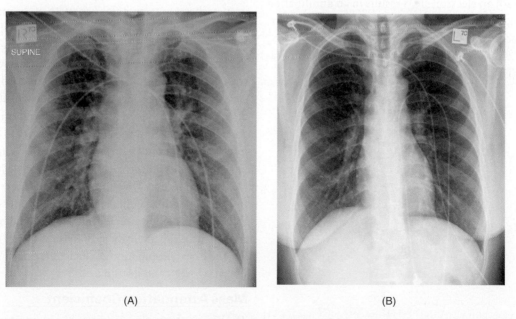

(A)   (B)

Figure 2-26 (A) Low kVp chest x-ray. (B) High kVp chest x-ray. Note the reduced contrast using the high energy.
Courtesy of Patrick C. Brennan.

well- known formula from Einstein for the law of conservation of mass-energy:

$$E = mc^2$$

where e = energy, m = mass, and c is the constant velocity of light. From this it can be seen that the energy is proportional to its mass or vice versa. With pair production, we have the original energy of the photon that is transformed into the electron and positron following its nuclear interaction. If the original energy was 1.02 meV exactly, then the two particles would be stationary; however, any spare energy, i.e., above 1.02 meV, is given off as kinetic energy to the two particles. All this can be summarized in the following formula:

$$\text{Energy of the Photon E} = \text{total energy}$$
$$\text{of the electron } (m_s c^2 + k_e)$$
$$+ \text{ total energy of the positron } (m_s c^2 + k_p)$$

where $m_s c^2$ is the stationary mass of a particle, and k_e and k_p are the kinetic energy of the electron and positron, respectively.

As the positron reduces its momentum to a low level, within a mm or less it can then go on to interact with an electron. This results in an annihilation event, which produces two gamma rays moving in opposite directions, each having an energy of 511 keV. This is the basis of positron emission tomography (**Figure 2-27**).

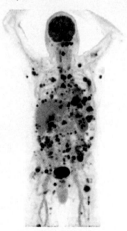

Figure 2-27 Positron emission tomography.
Courtesy of Patrick C. Brennan.

Descriptive Terms or Concepts Associated with Radiation

Linear Energy Transfer (LET)

Linear energy transfer (LET) is a measure of the density of ionizations that occur along the path of a beam of radiation. If radiation such as alpha particles deposits all its energy within something as thin as a piece of paper, this means that all the ionizations have occurred within a distance of only a few microns (Figure 2-7). This would be known as high LET radiation. On the other hand, electromagnetic radiations such as x-rays or gamma rays have low LET, since they are much more penetrating than alpha particles and the ionizations occur in low densities over a much greater thickness of matter. Beta and neutron particles would be somewhere in between. Radiation with high LET is much more damaging to biological tissue and this feature determines dosimetric quantities.

Linear Attenuation Coefficient

Linear attenuation coefficient describes the level of x-ray (or other radiation types) attenuation that occurs when x-rays pass along the path of the material with which it is interacting. It is defined as the level of fractional reduction in x-ray intensity per unit thickness of the material. Since we are dealing with fractional reductions in x-ray intensity, the coefficient clearly obeys the exponential law. The level of attenuation is obviously due to absorption and scattering, and therefore sometimes one hears reference to the *total linear attenuation coefficient* being made up of *linear absorption coefficient + linear scatter coefficient*.

Half-value layer (HVL) is closely related to the linear attenuation coefficient and simply refers to the thickness of the attenuating material that will reduce the x-ray intensity by 50% (Figure 2-11).

The linear attenuation coefficient is often referred to as *u* and its unit is m⁻¹.

Mass Attenuation Coefficient

The linear attenuation coefficient concentrates on unit thickness of an attenuator; however, the level of attenuation that occurs is also dependent on the density (p) of the attenuator. Mass attenuation coefficient therefore is defined as the fractional reduction in x-ray intensity that occurs in a unit cross-sectional area in an attenuator of unit mass. To convert from linear to mass attenuation coefficient, we simply divide the former by the density of the attenuator (p):

$$\text{Mass attenuation coefficient} = \text{linear attenuation coefficient} / p$$

The advantage of the mass attenuation coefficient is that one does not need to elaborate upon the attenuator type, since this is taken into consideration when it is being calculated, and therefore the number provided is independent of the attenuator. This is unlike the linear attenuation coefficient, where the final value is only specific to a particular attenuator and thus without specifying the attenuating material the value is meaningless.

Inverse Square Law

The Inverse Square Law applies to electromagnetic radiation only and is summarized as follows:

$$I = 1 / d^2$$

where I is the intensity of radiation and d is the distance from the source of the radiation.

In **Figure 2-28**, we can see that the radiation is being emitted from a point source (which in reality with x-rays is impossible, as the focal spot is of a finite size, but let us put this to one side for the moment). As we move from distance X1, which is positioned at a distance of 100 cm from the source, and then to distance X2, which is 200 cm from the source (a doubling of the distance), two key changes occur *as long as there is no attenuation of the radiation*: First, the area of the exposure area is increased by a factor of 4, but second and more important, since the area has quadrupled, the intensity per unit area must have *decreased* by a factor of 4 as well. We can see a similar change as one moves from X2 to X3.

As shown in Figure 2-28, if the exposure at distance X1 was 16 mSv, at distance X2 (a doubling of the distance from the source) there would be a reduction in radiation dose to 4 mSv, further reducing to 1 mSv at X3.

The definition of the Inverse Square Law therefore is as follows: *The intensity of radiation emitted from a point source is proportional to the inverse square law of the distance from the source as long as the radiation has not been attenuated.*

It can be seen that in x-ray practice, there are some practical difficulties with the Inverse Square Law, namely: (1) we do not have a point source of x-rays, (2) there will be some attenuation since

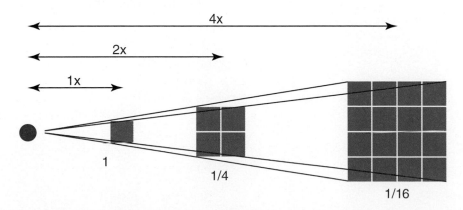

Figure 2-28 Diagrammatic presentation of the Inverse Square Law, where the radiation is reduced per unit area to one-fourth the original exposure when the distance is doubled.

Summary of Key Concepts

1. **Overall structure of the atom**. An atom consists of a nucleus surrounded by orbiting electrons that are positioned at a number of specific distances from the nucleus.

2. **Subatomic entities**. Atoms contain a number of subatomic particles, such as electrons, and a nucleus (the latter containing protons and neutrons), while physics scholars will be familiar with the various forms of quarks.

3. **Differences between particulate and electromagnetic radiation**. There are five main types: alpha and beta particles, neutrons, gamma and x-rays. The first three are known as particulate radiation (they are comprised of physical particles), whereas the latter two are forms of electromagnetic radiation.

4. **Properties of x-rays**. X-rays are mass-less, charge-less, invisible photons of energy. The energy of x-rays is proportional to frequency, and therefore as the frequency of electromagnetic radiation goes up, so does its energy. X-rays, being at the upper end of the frequency range, have higher energies than light, but lower energies than gamma rays.

5. **X-ray interactions with biological tissue**. At higher energies, x-rays have the ability to penetrate through human tissue. That penetration, however, does not mean that x-rays or gamma rays are not having critical interactions within the body; they do. These interactions form the basis of biological injuries that radiation technologists must understand for correct dosimetry.

imaging departments do not operate in a vacuum, and (3) the intensity of radiation at a given distance from the source is not equal in all directions (due to the anode heel effect). Nonetheless, this is a hugely important law and is arguably the most important principle when trying to offer staff effective measures of x-ray radiation protection.

Discussion Questions

1. Discuss the constituents and characteristics of the atom.

2. Discuss how certain types of electromagnetic radiation are more suited to medical imaging compared with particulate radiation.

3. Discuss the two key processes that occur when x-rays interacts with human tissues.

Reference

Dowsett DJ, Kenny PA, Johnston RE. *The Physics of Diagnostic Imaging*, 2nd edition. London: Hodder Arnold; 2006.

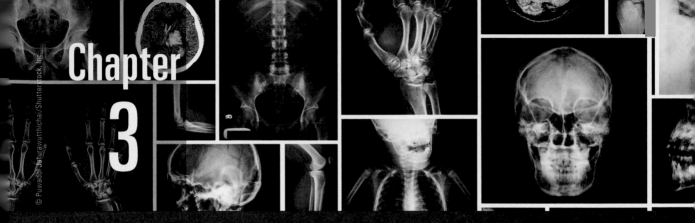

Chapter 3

Radiation Exposure and Dose Units

Outline

- Introduction
- Radiation: A Natural History
- Sources of Radiation Exposure
  - Natural background sources
  - Man-made (non-medical) radiation sources
  - Sources of exposure in medicine
  - Diagnostic Exposures
  - Nuclear Medicine
  - Radiation Therapy
  - Footnote to Medical Radiation Doses
- Basic Dosimetric Quantities and Units
  - Absorbed dose
  - Equivalent dose
  - Effective dose
  - Collective effective dose
  - Kinetic energy released per unit mass (kerma)
- Patient Doses in Diagnostic Imaging
- Staff Doses in Diagnostic Imaging
- References

Objectives

On successful completion of this chapter, you should be able to:

1. State briefly the history of radiation exposure to humans.
2. Identify and describe briefly the sources of radiation exposure to humans.
3. Identify three categories of medical radiation exposure and briefly explain exposures from diagnostic radiology.
4. Discuss essential features of the following radiation quantities and state the units associated with each:
   - Exposure
   - Absorbed dose
   - Equivalent dose
   - Effective dose
5. Discuss the stages in the calculation of the effective dose.
6. State typical patient and personnel doses from diagnostic imaging examinations.

Introduction

This chapter will introduce the reader to the sources and levels of radiation to which we as humans are exposed on a daily basis. It will include a discussion regarding the contribution of medical, and particularly diagnostic, radiation to these radiation levels, as well as examine different dose units used to describe these radiation exposures.

Since radiation has been omnipresent since life began, a brief history of radiation and a summary of how exposure levels have changed since our earliest predecessors will be our starting point.

Radiation: A Natural History

Our species, *Homo sapiens*, and its evolutionary predecessors have been exposed to ionizing radiation since life began around 4 billion years ago. At that time, radiation was between 5 to 10 times higher than it is now (**Figure 3-1**), yet organisms were able to evolve and develop while being exposed to such high doses. While the current sources of radiation are considered below, it is interesting to consider, albeit briefly, the reasons why radiation levels have decreased since prokaryotic life began.

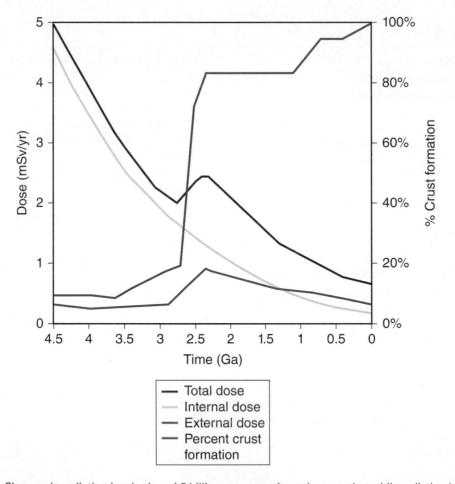

Figure 3-1 Changes in radiation levels since 4.5 billion years ago. It can be seen that while radiation levels have decreased by between a factor of 5 and 10, there was a brief increase that coincides with the formation of the Earth's crust.

Courtesy of Patrick C. Brennan.

Radioactive decay accounts for a lot of this change. Each nuclide has a *half-life*, wherein after a particular period of time, the intensity of radiation is reduced by half. Even though the half-life of some of these earlier products is very long—for example, ^{232}thorium has a half-life of 14×10^9 years, ^{238}uranium has a half-life of 4.5×10^9 years, and ^{235}uranium has a half-life of 7×10^6 years—enough time has passed over the last 4.5 billion years to see these radioactive levels fall by a significant amount. There was a competing factor, however, and that was the formation of the earth's crust. Large ion *lithophiles* (elements having an affinity to rock), while present in molten magma, tended to congregate in the earth's crust as it developed, a process that mainly occurred about 2.6 billion years ago, although some early formation was evident 1 billion years earlier. Since the amount of radiation (gamma) released was proportional to the concentration of these products, it is reasonable to assume that radiation levels went up at the time of Earth's crust formation. These temporal changes in both direction can be seen in Figure 3-1, which has been adapted from the text by P. Andrew Karam and Stephen A. Leslie (Karam & Leslie, 1996), who summarize this topic extremely well.

Ultraviolet (UV) radiation levels have changed through time. Four billion years ago, there was a paucity of free oxygen and hence ozone, and ultraviolet levels of radiation were higher than now. Even so, two factors helped mitigate (to a limited extent) against this effect. First, earth's atmosphere was much thicker: It consisted of substances such as nitrogen, water vapor and CO_2 held at a higher pressure, e.g., 10 bars, which is about 10 times the current atmospheric pressure. This led to greater surface temperatures and extra cloud cover—an extreme example of greenhouse effect. In addition, greater volcanic activity led to higher levels of sulphur compounds in the atmosphere, which were particularly efficient at absorbing UV radiation. Second, when life was beginning, lower sun surface temperatures gave off UV levels that were approximately 50% of current levels.

In summary, it is clear that billions of years ago, the earth was a much more hostile environment than now from a radiation perspective. Nonetheless, perhaps it is due to these early challenges that early life, and subsequently man, developed sophisticated mechanisms for adapting to and repairing damage inflicted by exposure to ionizing radiation.

Sources of Radiation Exposure

Each year, we are exposed to ionizing radiation from a variety of sources. It is interesting to observe that while at least half of the radiation dose we receive comes from background sources such as cosmic rays and radon, we tend to get much more concerned about the risks associated with medicine, mobile phones, or nuclear power plants. Perhaps this biased weighting of risk is associated with whether the radiation is man-made (e.g., nuclear power plants) or whether we can choose to be exposed (e.g., medicine), but regardless, it is useful to remember that cosmic radiation and radon have ionizing properties as well as x-rays.

The sources of radiation to which we are exposed are summarized in **Figure 3-2**, and medicine makes up just less than 50% of the total amount of radiation received. It is interesting to consider, however, a similar pie graph from 20 years ago (**Figure 3-3**). Here, one can see that medical radiation is making up a much smaller part of the pie, and this substantial change over the last 20 years is due to the large increase in the use of computed tomography (CT) scanners along with the proliferation of radiation doses associated with certain interventional procedures and nuclear medicine. This will be discussed in more detail below, but for now, let us consider the other radiation sources.

Natural Background Sources

Table 3-1 further details exposures that can occur in different world regions. The first four items here are from natural radiation background sources collectively accounting for annual doses of anywhere between 1.5 and 3 millisieverts (mSv), with up to

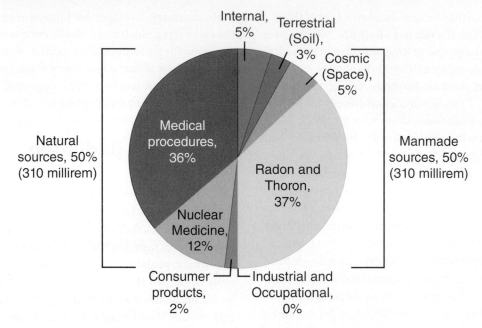

Figure 3-2 Sources of radiation exposure within the United States (2009). 310 millirem = 3.1 millisieverts (mSv).
Courtesy of Patrick C. Brennan.

70–80% of this being from inhalation of radon. **Radon** is an odorless and colorless radioactive gas and an indirect daughter product of uranium-238 (via radium-226), which is commonly distributed within the earth's crust. Radon itself has a short

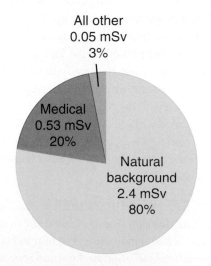

Figure 3-3 Sources of radiation exposure, including medical detail, within the United States of America in 1980.

half-life of about 4 days; however, its daughter products, which include polonium-218, lead-214, and bismuth-214, can be inhaled in particulate form and lodge within the lungs, continuing exposing the individual. In the United States, it is estimated that radon accounts for up to 20,000 deaths annually, being the second biggest causal agent of lung cancer after smoking.

Radon and its daughter products have always been exposing humans to radiation, but recently this has become a much greater problem because homes are much better insulated to reduce air flow through walls and windows. The unintended consequence is that radon gas and its daughter products can seep into the house's basement (which is often much less insulated) and then become trapped within the living areas by the insulation. There is a large geographic variation in the concentration of radon due to the distribution of uranium and, to a lesser extent, thorium, which produces the radon-220 isotope (there are 39 varieties) in the crust. An example of this can be seen from **Table 3-1**, which shows the contribution of radiation exposure from radon in the United States is approximately 6 times

Table 3-1 Levels of annual doses in millisieverts from three locations for a variety of radiation sources

Radiation source	World	USA	Japan	Remark
Inhalation of air	1.26	2.28	0.4	Mainly from radon, depends on indoor accumulation
Ingestion of food & water	0.29	0.28	0.4	K-40, C-14, etc.
Terrestrial radiation from ground	0.48	0.21	0.4	Depends on soil and building material
Cosmic radiation from space	0.39	0.33	0.3	Depends on altitude
Sub total (natural)	2.4	3.1	1.5	Sizeable population groups receive 10-20 mSv
Medical	0.6	3	2.3	World-wide figure excludes radiotherapy; US figure is mostly CT scans and nuclear medicine.
Consumer items	-	0.13		Cigarettes, air travel, building materials, etc.
Atmospheric nuclear testing	0.005	-	0.01	Peak of 0.11 mSv in 1963 and declining since; higher near sites
Occupational exposure	0.005	0.005	0.01	World-wide average to all workers is 0.7 mSv, mostly due to radon in mines. US is mostly due to medical and aviation workers.
Chernobyl accident	0.002	-	0.01	Peak of 0.04 mSv in 1986 and declining since; higher near site
Nuclear fuel cycle	0.0002		0.001	Up to 0.02 mSv near sites; excludes occupational exposure
Other	-	0.003		Industrial, security, medical, educational, and research
Sub total (artificial)	0.61	3.14	2.33	
Total (mSv per year)	3.01	6.24	3.83	

greater than in Japan. In particular, high levels of radon have been reported in the United States, Iran, Scandinavian countries, Italy, and Ireland. The level of variation that can be seen is amply illustrated by the fact that within an average house there will be approximately 50–100 Becquerels/m³ (Bq/m³), in contrast to the well-reported incident in 1984 of a Pennsylvania home in which levels of around 100,000 Bq/m³ were reported. Exposure in mines can be up to 10 times this value.

While the other types of natural radiation collectively represent a low dose (and hence relatively low risk) compared to the challenge presented by radon in variation locations, it is important to briefly consider internal exposure from ingestion of food and water, terrestrial radiation, and cosmic radiation. Humans have always had radioactive products within our body that we have ingested—and they are critically important to our survival. The doses are low, at around 0.3–0.4 mSv per year, and include such products as potassium-40 (^{40}K) and carbon-14 (^{14}C), which present with 4000 and 1200 disintegrations per second respectively. ^{40}K is an essential element for all cells, being particularly being necessary for optimum nerve, cardiac, and renal function, among others. ^{14}C is an essential ingredient of DNA (and provides a good postmortem indication of the age of an individual).

In addition to the radioactive sources within the ground, soil, and air, which can be part of the food we eat, water we drink, and air we breathe, radiation arises from the earth itself and affects us externally. This is known as **terrestrial radiation** and accounts for between 0.2 and 0.5 mSv per year. A number of these we have encountered before, such as uranium-238 and thorium. Compared with the earliest life on the earth 4 billion years ago, these products currently have about 50% of their original activity; however, their impact upon modern humans, who have only been around for ~150,000 years, has remained largely unchanged.

Cosmic radiation comes from the skies. We are constantly being irradiated by charged ions and nuclei that primarily arise from outside our solar system. When these particles interact with our atmosphere, a cocktail of other radiation entities are generated, including particulate radiation such as electrons, neutrons, and alpha particles and electromagnetic radiation such as x-rays. The most intense amount of radiation comes from about the **troposphere**, 7 miles above the earth's surface, which has special relevance to those who undergo supra-terrestrial travel, such as astronauts or even the crew of ordinary aircraft. In addition, the level of cosmic radiation can vary depending on where we live, with people at higher altitudes receiving more radiation than those at sea level.

Man-Made (Non-Medical) Radiation Sources

Up to 99% of man-made radiation is derived from medical exposures; however, a small level of exposure is received from nuclear power generators. In particular, when there is an accident at a nuclear power plant such as Chernobyl or Fukushima, radiation levels affecting workers and those living in the vicinity can be considerable. For example, following the Chernobyl accident in the Ukraine

in 1986 that resulted from a fire at the plant, it is estimated that around 237 individuals experienced the acute radiation syndrome, with 30 workers or fireman dying from this within 3 months. On the first day of the disaster, doses of up to 20,000 mSv (the equivalent to about 4000 years of living!) were experienced. In addition, radiation exposures, particularly from iodine-131 and cesium-137, to the surrounding areas were significantly higher than normal; approximately 220,000 individuals in the immediate, strictly controlled zones and between 6 and 7 million people in the more widespread contaminated regions were exposed to excessive levels of radiation. However, it is important to note that in the 20 years since the accident, the *average* excessive exposure in the controlled zones and contaminated regions amounted to an additional ~31 and ~9 mSv, respectively, which is not that significant an increase over the radiation levels (between 50 and 100 mSv) that individuals would have received if the incident never occurred.

At the time of this writing (2013), it is much harder to accurately describe the implications of the Fukushima Daiichi nuclear disaster following the Tōhoku earthquake and tsunami in Japan in 2011. Once again, iodine-131 and cesium-137, along with cesium-134, were responsible for the released radioactivity. To date, there have been no reported incidents of death directly attributable to radiation exposure, although some estimates have been proposed and debated regarding future increased death as a result of stochastic effects. The doses appear to be much lower than the Chernobyl incident, with 111 workers (of the 8300 workers) receiving doses in excess of 100 mSv, with 6 of these receiving more than 250 mSv. It has been estimated that of 132,011 residents of the Fukushima Prefecture surveyed between July 2011 and May 2013, 99.9% received internal doses of less than 1 mSv, with 14, 10, and 2 individuals receiving doses of 1, 2, and 3 mSv respectively. However, for this incident at Fukushima, it is still early days and all these figures will require revisiting once more scientifically validated data are published.

Finally, there is another radioactive particle strontium-90, which is released from nuclear power plants. It is interesting to note that while this is a relatively new, man-made product, it is present within all humans.

In summary, while there is much fear around nuclear power plant accidents, the two best-known incidents of recent years would suggest that while the potential radiation levels to workers and rescue personnel immediately following the incident can be very high, the overall increased radiation dose and risk to individuals living within the surrounding areas may not be catastrophic. Interestingly, there appears to be less concern with the doses that may be administered from medical radiation, even though the average person will receive much higher radiation levels from this source compared with nuclear power plant incidents.

Sources of Exposure in Medicine

Medical exposures are increasingly making a more important contribution to the overall radiation levels received by mankind. When one considers data relevant to the US population (**Figures** 3-3 and **3-4**), it can be seen that from 1980 to 2006 there has been a dramatic shift in terms of contributing factors, with the relative amount of medical exposures increasing from approximately 20% to 50% at the expense of natural background levels (see above). Since we can safely assume that natural levels have not changed in absolute terms in those 30 years, it follows that medical sources have increased. The reader is directed to the excellent United Nations Scientific Committee on the Effects of Atomic Radiation (UNSCEAR) report to the UN General Assembly: *Sources and Effects of Ionising Radiation* (UNSCEAR 2008). Within this document is much valuable data, and these have been used extensively to support this section.

It should be noted that the level of contribution is very much dependent on geographic regions. While Figure 3-4 suggests that medical radiation accounts for about 50% of the total effective radiation dose given per capita, it should be noted that

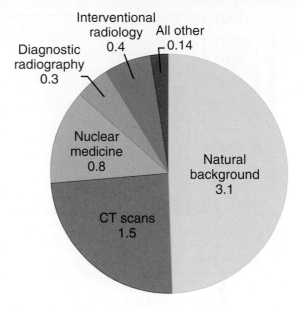

Figure 3-4 Annual per capita effective dose (mSv) for the United States population in 2006.
Data from: UNSCEAR Report/United Nations.

this is for the US population, and one shouldn't assume that this graph represents countries from other world regions such as those located in South east Asia or Africa. Indeed, if instead of looking at a country-specific situation, the global situation is investigated, we can see that over the period 1997–2007 the contribution of medical exposures to the overall collective effective dose remains close to 20% (Table 3-1). Clearly, the rapid rise in recent years of medical radiation doses is within the domain of the wealthy nations.

To unravel this geographic variation a little, UNSCEAR has divided countries into four main groupings based on the number of physicians per capita: healthcare levels I, II, III, and IV representing the presence of at least 1 physician per a population of 1000, 1000–2999, 3000–10,000, and ≥10,000 persons respectively. Once we categorize countries this way, it can be seen that almost 70% of diagnostic examinations take place in health-care level I countries, where 24% of the population

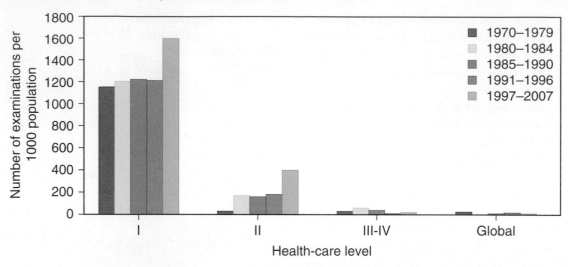

Figure 3-5 Annual frequency of diagnostic radiologic investigations in the varying healthcare level countries from 1970–2007.

(*Source*: UNSCEAR report © 2008 United Nations. Reprinted with the permission of the United Nations.)

Data from: UNSCEAR Report/United Nations.

reside and the frequency of examinations per 1000 individuals has risen from 820 in 1970s to 1332 between 1997 and 2007. In level II countries, the increase in the frequency of the examinations is even more marked, with the numbers rising for the same period from 26 to 332; however, the numbers in level III and level IV countries have remained consistently low. All these data are summarized in **Figure 3-5**.

The delivery of medical radiation can be categorized into the following three groupings: (1) diagnostic exposures, (2) nuclear medicine, and (3) radiation therapy. Each of these will be considered below.

Diagnostic Exposures

It is estimated that there are approximately 3.6 billion diagnostic x-ray examinations performed each year. These are responsible (with nuclear medicine examinations) for a collective dose of around 4,000,000 man-sieverts (manSv), or 0.62 mSv individual effective doses annually, keeping in mind that this annual figure for effective dose is highly variable and the number presented simply represents a global mean (**Table 3-2**). So which are the big contributors when it comes to radiation dose?

CT is currently the largest contributor to diagnostic radiation doses. In UNSCEAR's 2008 report, it is noted that CT was responsible for 47% of the

Table 3-2 Annual per capita and collective effective doses from medical x-ray investigations across the four healthcare levels

Health-care level	Population (millions)	Annual per caput dose (mSv)	Annual collective effective dose (manSv)
I	1540	1.91	2,900,000
II	3153	0.32	1,000,000
III	1009	0.03	330,00
IV	744	0.03	24,000
World	446	0.62	4,000,000

(*Source:* UNSCEAR report © 2008 United Nations. Reprinted with the permission of the United Nations.)

radiation dose while only accounting for ~8% of the number of examinations. The picture was similar in the National Radiological Protection Board (NRPB) publication *Radiation Exposure of the UK Population from Medical and Dental Examinations* (2002), with CT examinations having a frequency of just over 3% of all examinations but resulting in ~40% of the collective dose (**Table 3-3**).

If we look at the publication from Hall and Brenner (2008), we can see that the number of CT examinations has increased by a factor of 20 and 12 in the United States and the United Kingdom (UK), respectively, over the last two decades. While the number of examinations and the dose produced is likely to increase due to more CT examinations being performed, wider availability of CT units, quicker examination times due to advanced helical and multi-slice technologies, more elaborate and complex examinations, and better evidence on the utility of CT, there may be some initial signs that the rate of increase is starting to slow

down, but this will need to be monitored. It should be acknowledged, however, that the frequencies described earlier in this paragraph are specific to healthcare level I countries; if we look at the UNSCEAR data on other levels, an interesting trend is emerging where CT accounts for 15% of the collective dose in level II countries but 65% in level III and IV countries. Globally, the figure sits at ~43%.

While CT is a big contributor to medical diagnostic exposures, there are other major players including angiographic, interventional, dental, and general exposures. If one considers **Table 3-4,** adapted from the NRPB 4 report (2002), it can be seen that the number of angiographic studies account for slightly less than 1% of diagnostic examinations, but 10% of collective dose with angiocardiography, peripheral and abdominal angiography being responsible for 75% of this dose. The data available for interventional procedures are not dissimilar to the angiographic

Table 3-3 Sources of radiation exposure, including medical details, within the United States in 1980

Computed tomography	Number of examinations	Percentage frequency	Collective dose (manSv)	Percentage collective dose
CT abdomen	297,244	0.72	2972.4	15.4
CT angiography	5129	0.01	31	0.16
CT chest	192,885	0.46	1543.1	8
CT bone mineral densitometry	1594	0	2	0.01
CT extremety	18,401	0.04	9.2	0.05
CT head	618,391	1.49	1237	6.41
CT interventional	13,184	0.03	131.8	0.68
CT neck	24,332	0.06	60.8	0.32
CT pelvis	139,722	0.34	1397.2	7.24
CT spine	63,183	0.15	253	1.31
CT pelvimetry	8200	0.02	2	0.01
CT other	4771	0.01	24	0.12
Subtotal	1,387,036	3.33	7662	39.71
Overall X-ray radiation	41,541,000	100	19,298	100

Data from: UNSCEAR report © 2008 United Nations. Reprinted with the permission of the United Nations.

Table 3-4 The number of examinations and the associated collective dose from angiographic examinations in the UK (2002)

Angiography	Number of examinations	Percentage frequency	Collective dose (man Sv)	Percentage collective dose
Abdominal angiography	12,711	0.03	285	1.48
Aortography	11,161	0.03	122.6	0.64
Angiocardiography	162,871	0.39	1076.4	5.58
Cerebral angiography	11,999	0.03	48	0.25
Peripheral angiography	116,903	0.28	361.5	1.87
Pulmonary angiography	5529	0.01	29.9	1.16
Subtotal	321,174	0.8	1923	10
Overall X-ray radiation	41,541,000	100	19,298	100

Data from: NRBP 2002 © Crown copyright. Reproduced with permission of Public Health England.

figures, with these examinations accounting for again just less than 1% of examination number but 6% of dose, with cardiac, biliary, and urinary interventions accounting for over 90% of this latter value.

Dental examinations, according to the UK data (NRPB W5 2002), interestingly show the opposite trend, with numbers of examinations being responsible for approximately 30% of diagnostic examinations but less than 0.5% of the total dose. Again, frequency variations between countries are evident for all these figures (with the dental values) as shown by UNSCEAR (2008) shown in (**Figure 3-5**).

Finally, one should not forget that in a typical healthcare level I country, general radiographic examinations account for almost 95% and 41% of the number of examinations and collective dose, respectively, and therefore still deserve major attention when directing resources towards optimization of diagnostic x-ray examinations. The top 20 examinations in terms of frequency and dose are shown in **Tables 3-5** and **3-6,** respectively.

One should note that the numbers presented above are only relevant at the time of the relevant publications. It is quite likely that the values will have changed between the time of writing and the publication of this text.

Nuclear Medicine

While the focus of this book is radiography, it is important to briefly consider the impa ct of nuclear medicine on collective dose, since from the diagram above it can be seen that within the United States, nuclear medicine contributes to approximately 12% of the total collective dose received and about 25% of medical exposures. UNSCEAR (2008) estimates that about 33 million nuclear medicine investigations take place globally; however, 90% of these are only with healthcare level I countries. There has been an approximate doubling in the number of diagnostic nuclear medicine procedures between the 1970s and 1997–2007, accompanied by an increase in dose per examination from an average value of 4.6 mSv to 6.0 mSv within the last decade. In terms of collective dose globally (**Table 3-7**), at approximately 200,000 manSv per year, nuclear medicine makes up about 5% of medical investigative procedures (4,000,000 manSv/year).

Radiation Therapy

Radiation therapy is definitely outside the scope of this text, but very briefly, it is worth considering the amount of individuals exposed for cancer treatment. Treatment consists of either external radiation (teletherapy) using x-ray machines, cobalt units, and especially linear accelerators;

Table 3-5 Examinations within the UK ordered according to the frequency of examinations

Type of Examination	Number of Examinations
XRAY	
Teeth(Intraoral)	9,562,500
Chest	8,286,520
Mammography	1,726,303
Abdomen (plain film)	1,217,192
Pelvis	919,740
Hip	885,489
Cervical spine	858,547
Lumbar spine	824,763
Colon	359,436
Lumbar sacral joint	338,901
Thoracic spine	281,215
Angiocardiography	162,871
Intravaneous urogram	162,502
Esophagus	123,751
Cardiovascular interventional	121,810
Peripheral angiography	116,903
Stomach and duodeum	98,581
Bladder and urethra	82,941
Biliary system	67,627
Billary and urinary interventional	47,968
Small intestine	41,089
Abdominal angiography	12,711
Cerebral angiography	11,999
Aortography	11,161
COMPUTED TOMOGRAPHY	
CT head	618,391
CT abdomen	297,244
CT chest	192,885
CT pelvis	139,722
CT spine	63,183
CT neck	24,332
CT interventional	13,184

NRBP 2002 © Crown copyright. Reproduced with permission of Public Health England.

Table 3-6 Examinations within the UK ordered according to the level of collective dose being delivered

Examinations	Collective Dose (SV/person)
XRAY	
Colon	2587.9
Angiocardiography	1076.4
Cardiovascular interventional	903.9
Abdomen (plain film)	852.0
Lumbar spine	824.8
Pelvis	643.8
Mammography	466.3
Intravaneous urogram	390.0
Peripheral angiography	361.5
Hip	321.2
Abdominal angiography	285.0
Biliary system	270.3
Stomach and duodeum	256.3
Billary and urinary interventional	235.1
Thoracic spine	196.9
Esophagus	185.6
Chest	165.8
Small intestine	154.2
Aortography	122.6
Bladder and urethra	102.5
Lumbar sacral joint	92.2
Cervical spine	60.1
Cerebral angiography	48.0
Teeth(intraoral)	47.8
COMPUTED TOMOGRAPHY	
CT abdomen	2972.4
CT chest	1543.1
CT pelvis	1397.2
CT head	1236.8
CT spine	252.7
CT interventional	131.8
CT neck	60.8

NRRP 2002 © Crown copyright. Reproduced with permission of Public Health England.

Table 3-7 Examinations within the UK ordered according to the to the level of collective dose being delivered

Health-care level	Population (millions)	Annual collective effective dose (manSv)			
		Medical	Dental	Nuclear medicine	Total
I	1,540	2,900,000	9,900	186,000	3,100,000
II	3,153	1,000,000	1,300	16,000	1,000,000
III	1,009	33,000	51	82*	33,000
IV	744	24,000	38		24,000
World	446	4,000,000	11,000	202,000	4,200,000

Data from: UNSCEAR Report/United Nations.

the latter machine is 10 times more available compared with each of the other two. In addition, brachytherapy is a form of treatment in which the radioactive source is placed in the body close to the tumor site. Approximately 5.1 million radiotherapy treatments are performed each year, with 90% of these being of the external radiation type, the remaining resulting from brachytherapy exposures. Approximately 75% of exposures occur in the healthcare level I countries. The total amount of radiation being delivered *specifically to the treatment site* can vary from between 20 to 80 Gy, but this is delivered in many daily fractions over a period of weeks that can be tolerated by the patient.

Footnote to Medical Radiation Doses

Finally, while it is important to be aware that the contribution of medical radiation to collective doses is considerable and likely to increase, this must be balanced against benefit to the patient. While nuclear power accidents confer no human advantage, medical radiation has both diagnostically and therapeutically transformed medical care, resulting in much improved prevention, identification, and management of disease. One should therefore be very careful at simply thinking that high medical radiation doses automatically need to be reduced. While justification and optimization of medical exposure are critical features that need to be employed each time the patient is exposed, this should not be at the detriment of diagnostic and treatment efficacy.

Basic Dosimetric Quantities and Units

There are a plethora of dosimetric quantities and units that present ample opportunity to confuse students and individuals unfamiliar with the topic. For example, what are the differences between (and need for) all of the following (and these are not all of them): gray, sievert, roentgen, rad, rem, kerma, effective dose, dose equivalent, and absorbed dose? Some belong to the International System of Units (SI system) and some are specific for different countries. Nonetheless, each is distinct and each can be recognized and remembered for having a specific function. The aim of this section is to steer students through these units in a way that facilitates understanding and recall.

Before we get into the units, it is important to be aware that they fall into two main categories: Some measure **radiation exposure** and some measure *radiation dose*. What is the difference between exposure and dose?

- Radiation exposure refers to *radiation traveling through air*. It is the amount of ionization-induced *charge produced in a unit mass of air* at a particular part of the x-ray or gamma beam. Its precise definition is: The sum of all electric charges *of one sign* (either negative or positive) when all the radiation-induced released electrons in a specific volume of air are completely stopped, divided by the mass of that volume of air.
- Radiation dose refers to *radiation traveling though a medium*. It is the amount of *energy absorbed within an object*, such as a person. Its definition is: The total amount of ionizing radiation absorbed by a medium.

While the distinction should be clear, exposure and dose are related to each other, and this will be specified below.

Units of Exposure

The SI unit of exposure is the ***coulomb per kilogram*** (C/kg). This should come as no surprise, since coulomb is the SI unit of charge and kilogram the SI unit of mass. However, there is an older (non-SI) unit that may still used: the ***roentgen*** (R) where $1 R = 2.58 \times 10^{-4}$ C/kg.

One can ask why one would bother with a unit that deals with radiation traveling through air, when one should deal primarily with radiation interactions with media such as human tissue. However, it is interesting to note that the effective atomic number of air, at 7.8, is very similar to that of muscle (7.6) and water (7.5). This means that the attenuation processes for air and a lot of human soft tissue is very similar, meaning that a number of dosimetric experiments and measurements can take place quite easily in air to represent what might be happening in the human body.

Quantities of Radiation Dose

One of the reasons why there is such a variety of dose quantities is that different quantities represent different aspects of dose. In particular, we have three key categories: ***absorbed dose***, which simply measures the radiation level imparted within tissue; ***dose equivalent***, which takes into consideration the type of radiation involved with the exposure; and ***effective dose***, which takes dose equivalent and applies a weighting factor depending on the radio sensitivities of the organs that are being exposed. Each of these has an SI unit along with at least one other more traditional unit, and each will be considered in greater depth below. All of these have been defined and discussed in the essential reference text, *ICRP 103: The 2007 Recommendations of the International Commission on Radiological Protection* (ICRP 2007).

Absorbed Dose

Absorbed dose is a baseline quantity used in radiological protection and from which many other dose units we will consider below are derived. Absorbed dose simply measures the amount of energy that is imparted to media and is defined as the mean energy deposited to a medium by ionizing radiation divided by the mass of that medium. Since the SI units for energy and mass are the ***joule*** (J) and kilogram (kg), respectively, it should be no surprise that the SI unit for absorbed dose is J/kg. In practice, this is less commonly used than the ***gray*** (Gy); however, since 1 Gy = 1 J/kg, conversion could not be easier. However, there is another unit commonly used in the United States called the ***rad***—which is simply 0.01 Gy.

So to summarize all this, the unit of absorbed dose is:

$$1\,J/kg = 1\,Gy = 100\,rads$$

At this stage, one should be able to clearly distinguish between the gray (absorbed dose) and the roentgen (exposure, abbreviated as R). However, based on the above, it is reasonable to assume that some level of proportionality should exist between the two, and indeed there is a fixed relationship based on the fact that $1\,R = 2.58 \times 10^{-4}$ C/kg (see above) and that 1 Gy (in air) would equal 2.95×10^{-2} C/kg. Relatively simple arithmetic will tell us that:

$$1 \text{ Gy} = 115 \text{ R } or \text{ 1 R } = 8.7 \text{ mGy}$$

Equivalent Dose

The problem with absorbed dose is that it does not differentiate between different types of radiation, and the damage that occurs following radiation does not only depend on the absorbed dose, but also on the radiation type. For example, 1 Gy of alpha particles equals 1 Gy of x-rays, even though the alpha particles have a much higher linear energy transfer than x-rays and therefore can inflict much more damage. The dose equivalent is used to make this distinction between types of radiation. It does this by applying a radiation weighting factor to each type of radiation (and energy, where relevant). A list of some of the latest ICRP weighting factors is given in **Table 3-8**.

Equivalent dose is defined as the average absorbed dose multiplied by a radiation weighting factor (the latter being determined by the type and energy of the radiation) such that the effect of the radiation exposure can be better characterized. It therefore takes into consideration the absorbed dose *and* the radiation weighting factors.

The SI unit of equivalent dose is the J/kg; however, the *sievert* (Sv) is commonly used, and particularly in diagnostic radiology, the *millisievert* (mSv) is used. In the United States, however, one will hear reference to the *rem*, which is simply 0.01 sievert. So, in summary:

$$1 \text{ J/kg} = 1 \text{ } sievert = 100 \text{ } rems$$

Once we have the absorbed dose value (in grays), we can then convert this to equivalent dose (in Sv) by simply multiplying the absorbed dose by the radiation weighting factor. From Table 3-8, we can see that the weighting factor for alpha particles is 20; therefore, 1 Gy of alpha particles will equal 20 Sv, which offers a much better indication of the damage that an alpha particle will cause. Interestingly, the reader will note that the weighting factor for x-rays and gamma rays is 1, meaning that 1 Gy of x-rays equals 1 Sv, making our life in diagnostic radiology much more simple than some of our physics colleagues dealing with other radiation types.

Finally, one should be careful with terminology: The *equivalent dose* (see definition above), which considers the *average* absorbed dose, should not be confused with an earlier version of this weighted absorbed dose, the *dose equivalent*, which considered the absorbed radiation dose at one particular location within the beam.

Effective Dose

At this stage, based on the above definitions, we have now a dose measure—equivalent dose—that takes into consideration not only the patient's absorbed dose, but also the type of radiation that has been delivered by using a specific radiation weighting factor based on the damage that that radiation type might inflict on the patient. There is still a problem, however: For example, if we have a single dose of 1 Sv (which would be very high for diagnostic purposes), but we deliver that dose in a highly collimated way, first to the shoulder and then to the breast, the biological response in the breast will be much higher than that in the shoulder. This is due to the *radio sensitivities* of the tissues within the breast being higher than

Table 3-8 List of radiation types with radiation weighting factors

Radiation type	Radiation weighting factor (wR)
Photons	1
Electrons and muons	1
Proton and charged pions	2
Alpha particles, fission fragments, heavy ions	20
Neutrons	A continuous function of neutron energy

Data from: ICRP, 2007.

those in the shoulder. There is a need, therefore, for a further measure that takes into consideration the differing sensitivities of exposed tissue to radiation. This measure is the *effective dose* and is summarized as the weighted sum of tissue equivalent doses (ICRP 2007) as described by the following formula:

$$E = \Sigma W_T H_T$$

where E is the effective dose; W_T is the weighting factor for a specific tissue, where the sum of all the weighting factors for all tissues is 1 (see explanation in the following section); and H_T is the equivalent dose delivered to a particular tissue.

The SI unit for effective dose is again J/kg; however, the sievert is most widely used. Since the sievert is used for both the equivalent dose and effective dose, it is essential when reporting dose quantities that the specific dose measure being used is made clear.

To arrive at this very useful quantity, two things are then needed: The equivalent dose delivered to the various tissues along with weighting factors for each tissue that somehow summarizes their radio sensitivities. How these values are derived is very well described within the ICRP document and summarized below.

Deriving the Equivalent Dose

With regard to equivalent doses to specific organs, this clearly cannot be measured for each patient exposure, so calculations have been made to establish conversion factors that can be applied to an external dose unit such as *entrance surface dose* in radiography (the equivalent dose to the patient's entrance surface—meaning, the first tissue to encounter the x-ray beam, often the skin) or activity intake in nuclear medicine. This has been achieved using mathematical phantoms, such as the adult Reference Male and Reference Female often used by the ICRP.

The relative radiation risk to specific tissues is defined using the latest knowledge derived from epidemiological studies of cancer and hereditary risks following radiation exposures. Weighting factors are given to all individual organs and tissues that are known to demonstrate cancer or hereditary effects in such a way that all weighting factors, when combined, result in a value of 1. In this way, by multiplying all exposed tissue by their respective weighing factors and adding all the final products together, we arrive at a figure that represents the total detriment resulting from a specific exposure. This figure is the *equivalent dose*. The most recent tissue weighting factors published by the ICRP are given in **Table 3-9**. It should be noted that these have changed from the previous recommendations of the ICRP (ICRP 60: 1990): for example, the weighting factor for breast tissue increased from 0.05 to 0.12, arguably one of the biggest changes between ICRP 60 and ICRP 103.

There is the issue of gender and age variations when it comes to establishing tissue and organ weighting factors; however, to simplify

Table 3-9 List of radiation weighting factors for various organ and tissue types

Tissue	w_T	Σw_T
Bone marrow (red), colon, lung, stomach, breast, remainder tissues*	0.12	0.72
Gonads	0.08	0.08
Bladder, oesophagus, liver, thyroid	0.04	0.16
Bone surface, brain, salivary glands, skin	0.01	0.04
	Total:	1.00

* Remainder tissue: Adrenals, extrathoracic (ET) region, gall bladder, heart, kidneys, lymphatic nodes, muscle, oral mucosa, pancreas, prostate, small intestine, spleen, thymus, uterus/cervix.

Data from: ICRP, 2007.

calculations, the ICRP has averaged these weighting factors across genders and ages. This has the advantage of simplifying considerably the calculation of effective dose for the end user (the clinician or radiologic technologist), described further below—but it does mean that *one should not use effective dose to calculate an absolute risk to the individual*. Once we know a quantifiable risk associated with a particular effective dose, and we have a typical effective dose for a specific projection or examination, we can give to our patient population—which is increasingly concerned and likely to inquire—a reasonable estimate of the relative risk. This, of course, relies on a linear, non-threshold model and the extrapolation of high-dose risks to the (generally) low doses that exist in diagnostic radiology—a subject discussed elsewhere.

Calculation of Effective Dose

The overall calculation of effective dose is best summarized in **Figure 3-6**, which has been adapted from ICRP 103 (2007). The calculation of effective dose has been considerably simplified by the availability of specific software tools such as PCXMC, a user-friendly tool issued by the Finnish Radiation and Nuclear Safety Authority (STUK).

In this diagram we can see the following stages:

- **Stage 1**: There is an initial exposure representing a specific examination.
- **Stage 2**: The measurement of the absorbed dose to a male or female phantom is performed following the exposure in stage 1.
- **Stage 3**: These absorbed doses are multiplied by relevant radiation weighting factors (which for x-rays is 1) and equivalent dose values are established.
- **Stage 4**: These equivalent doses are averaged across genders.
- **Stage 5**: Age- and gender-specific tissue weighting factors are applied to this gender-averaged equivalent dose, and an effective dose is derived.

While one now has a measure of the effective dose that is immensely valuable for assessing risk or detriment from exposures and has been widely employed, it is important to acknowledge that there are some

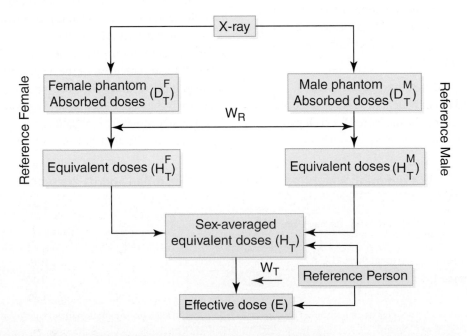

Figure 3-6 Method for calculating effective dose according to the ICRP 103.

Data from: ICRP 103 (ICRP, 2007). The 2007 Recommendations of the International Commission on Radiological Protection. ICRP Publication 103. Ann. ICRP 37 (2-4).

dissenters. One of these dissenters, Brenner (2008), best summarizes the potential disadvantages of effective dose making the following points:

1. The weighting factors are subject to the opinions of the specific ICRP committee at the time of publication. Brenner cites the change in the breast weighting factor between ICRP 60 and ICRP 103 as an example of this subjectivity, which he argues was not a result of additional data suggesting greater risk, but rather that the committee placed a greater emphasis on cancer *incidence* rather than cancer *mortality* in making the determination.

2. The age- and gender-specific averaging described above has led to much misuse of effective dose; in cases, for example, where it has been used inappropriately in children and other individuals for whom the average dose might be considerably higher or lower than the optimal dose for that individual's situation.

3. The description itself has led to much confusion. It could be argued that really the calculation represents an expression of *detriment* rather than *dose*, yet "dose" is maintained in the descriptive phrase. Brenner suggests that "effective dose" could be replaced with "effective risk" using epidemiologically proven cancer risks, and therefore changing the formula above from

$$\text{Effective dose } (E) = \Sigma W_T H_T$$

To

$$\text{Effective risk } (R) = \Sigma r_T H_T$$

where r_T is defined as lifetime organ-specific, radiation-attributable cancer risk estimates. This would then be expressed in risk of say 1:100,000 of inducing a cancer, which is arguably more readily understood than representing risk in terms of a dose value. The reader will note that hereditary factors have been removed from Brenner's proposal, but this may be justified based on the significant downgrading of, hereditary effects from radiation described in ICRP 103.

Nonetheless, effective dose is still the prefered option for presenting an assessment of radiation detriment and certainly the one currently proposed by the ICRP.

Collective Effective Dose

Collective effective dose takes into account the amount of radiation being delivered to a specific geographic population. Its usefulness is shown earlier in this chapter, where the amount of radiation delivered to a country, for example, allows the average dose to an individual to be calculated (collective effective dose divided by the population) which facilitates comparisons of doses to populations (or individuals) living in different geographic regions. It also facilitates an overall evaluation of the benefits of a new radiologic technique or technology on a whole population, including a complete health economics assessment.

The collective effective dose is therefore *the sum of all individual effective doses* within a certain population within a particular time frame. The unit is the man-sievert (manSv). Examples of collective doses are given in Table 3-6, adapted from data published in the UK by the NRPB in 2002.

Kinetic Energy Released Per Unit Mass (Kerma)

There is one more very important quantity that should be considered: The *kinetic energy released per unit mass*, more commonly known as the *kerma*. The kerma is the unit currently used for most dosimetric devices used in clinical departments. The good news is that for x-ray radiation used in medical imaging, its units (J/kg or Gy) and its numerical values (e.g., 10.5 mGy) are the same as absorbed dose, and only for higher energies do differences start to emerge. To understand what is meant by kerma, we should step back and reconsider absorbed dose.

As stated above, the absorbed dose is the energy deposited to a medium divided by the mass of that medium. Let us consider more closely what is meant by *energy deposited to a medium*. From the

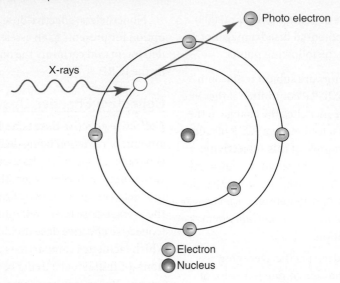

Figure 3-7 Diagram of photoelectric absorption. With this interaction process, the x-ray has ejected the electron and has been totally or almost totally absorbed.

physics surrounding interaction processes— specifically, photoelectric absorption and Compton scattering (described elsewhere)—we know that when an x-ray interacts with an electron, the energy deposited is expressed by the energy lost by the photon, but also the energy contained within released electrons (**Figure 3-7**).

However, for a specific unit of mass, some of those released electrons will be contained within that mass, but others—if they have enough energy— will escape from that mass and deposit their energy at some distance away from the original interaction process. This means that *absorbed dose equals the energy deposited in a particular mass (i.e. the energy given up by the photons in the original interactions) + the energy of electrons entering the mass – the energy of electrons escaping from that mass.*

If the energy of the electrons is high enough— or, in other words, if sufficient energy has been given to the electrons by the photons—the amount of energy absorbed along the axis of a material would look like the solid-line curve in **Figure 3-8**, unlike when the photon energies remain in the realm of diagnostic x-rays (dashed line). The main difference between the curves in **Figure 3-8** is

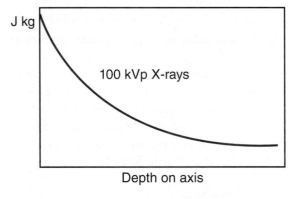

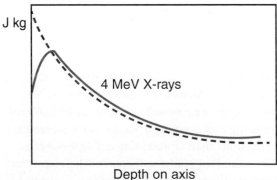

Figure 3-8 Comparing the energy absorbed in an attenuator for low and high energy electrons emitted following radiation interaction.

contained in the first few microns of tissue: For the higher-energy x-rays, the absorbed dose (J/kg) starts to increase over distance, since the higher-energy electrons have escaped from the original interaction site and are being deposited further into the depth of the tissue. In contrast, the lower-energy electrons are absorbed much closer to their site of origin. This clearly becomes a complication for small tissue volumes, where some of the energy will not be contained within that volume and therefore will not be accounted for, even though the initial attenuation took place there.

Kerma addresses this problem of the small volume: Focusing, as it does, on *kinetic energy released per unit mass*, and on the production of the electrons, rather than their absorption, by using kerma, we do not see this initial discrepancy in the absorption within the initial few microns for higher-energy electrons (**Figure 3-8** [blue line]), but rather a more continuous line. As stated previously, for the energy of electrons used in diagnostic radiology, the kerma and absorbed dose remain the same.

Patient Doses in Diagnostic Imaging

If we accept the linear no-threshold model, which is generally advocated by most radiobiologists, then we must also accept that there is a risk associated with each x-ray exposure that is administered. When such a risk is evident, then clinicians and radiographers need to be prepared for questions from an increasingly inquisitive public, which is becoming much more aware of radiation issues following incidents such as the recent episode at the Fukushima Daiichi power plant. Thus, if a parent arrives at an x-ray department with a 7-year-old requiring lumbar spine exposures, it is perfectly possible (and reasonable) for questions to be raised about the radiation dose and associated risks. X-ray personnel need to be prepared for this type of scenario. The first step is to have a good grasp of the radiation doses that are being delivered for typical examinations, and then we can make a very rough estimate of potential risk,

acknowledging of course all the caveats associated with such estimations.

Table 3-10 therefore summarizes typical effective doses delivered for an array of x-ray examinations. These data have come from the NRPB in the UK. In no way do the values suggest that this dose is what has been delivered for a particular examination, since dose variations can be substantial between and within medical centers, even for standard-sized patients. Instead, the values may serve simply as rough indicators as to the type of radiation levels that are being delivered.

Staff Doses in Diagnostic Imaging

The focus of most of this discussion is on patients following medical exposures, but it is important to note that radiologic staff can also be exposed following patient examinations, mainly from scattered radiation and primarily from fluoroscopic examinations. The level of radiation that staff may receive depends on the size of the radiation field, the angle of the scattered radiation, and very importantly, the distance of the operator from exposures (as described by the Inverse Square Law). Typically, doses to staff have been very low, often immeasurable on personnel dosimeters; however, the advent of increasingly complex interventional procedures present the potential of higher staff doses. Methods of monitoring and protecting staff are considered elsewhere; however, we will present some data here on staff dose levels.

A recent publication by Chida et al. (2013) measured staff doses in a hospital where almost 7000 cardiac catheterization procedures were being performed each year (about 30 per day). The staff were divided into three groups: Physicians ($n = 18$), nurses ($n = 7$) and radiologic technologists ($n = 8$), and the mean annual effective doses for each of these groups were 3.0 mSv, 1.34 mSv, and 0.6 mSv, respectively—with large variations around these mean values. For example, some physicians received doses as low as 0.8 mSv, while others had dose levels as high as 6.2 mSv—almost 8 times

Table 3-10 Patient radiation doses for various examinations. The values give some indication of radiation doses being delivered for specific procedures; however, they do not describe what will be delivered for future examinations

Type	Room mean DAP distribution $(Gy.cm^2)$
Radiograph	
Adomen AP	2
Cervical spine AP	0.23
Cervical spine LAT	0.2
Chest AP	0.18
Chest PA	0.09
Lumbar spine AP	1.3
Lumbar spine LAT	2.1
Pelvis AP	1.8
Thoracic spine AP	0.8
Thoracic spine LAT	1.3
Complete Examination	
Barium Enema	16
Barium Meal	9
Barium Small Bowel Enema	18
Barium Swallow	7
Coronary Angiography	25
Coronary Graft Angiography	40
Femoral Angiography	46
Fistulography	7
IVU	11.5
Proctography	15
T-tube Cholangiography	4
Water Soluble Swallow	14
Interventional Procedure	
Biliary Intervention	33
Nephrostomy	8
Oesophageal Stent	13
Pacemaker(permanent)	7
PTCA 1 stent	34

Data from: NRBP 2002 © Crown copyright. Reproduced with permission of Public Health England.

Summary of Key Concepts

1. **Radiation has affected humankind, and indeed all life, from the dawn of time**. Our species, **Homo sapiens**, and its evolutionary predecessors have been exposed to ionizing radiation since life began around 4 billion years ago. At that time, radiation exposure was 5 to 10 times higher than it is now, yet organisms were able to evolve and develop while being exposed to such high-dose levels. While the current sources of radiation are considered below, it is interesting to consider the reasons why radiation levels have decreased since prokaryotic life first developed on Earth.

2. **Radiation emits from a variety of sources**. Each year, humans are exposed to ionizing radiation from a variety of sources. While at least half of radiation that we receive comes from background sources, such as cosmic rays and radon, we tend to get much more concerned about the risks associated with medicine, mobile phones, or nuclear power plants. Perhaps this biased weighting of risk is associated with whether the radiation is man-made (e.g., nuclear power plants) or whether we can choose to be exposed (e.g., medicine), but regardless, we must remember that cosmic radiation and radon has ionizing properties as well as x-rays.

3. **A variety of radiation measures currently exist**. There are multiple dosimetric quantities and units that present great opportunity to confuse students and individuals unfamiliar with the topic. We must understand the differences between (and need for) all of the following: gray (Gy), sievert (Sv), roentgen (R), rad, rem, kerma, effective dose, dose equivalent, and absorbed dose (and these are just a sampling). It is important to be aware that these measurements fall into two main categories: Some measure **radiation exposure** and others measure **radiation dose**. We look at the differences between exposure and dose.

4. **Patients and staff in diagnostic imaging departments need to be advised of radiation dose levels**. Due to increased awareness of the issues surrounding radiation exposure, many patients will want to know the risk presented by radiation exposure. Means of calculating such risks are discussed, and calculations for the typical effective doses delivered for an array of x-ray examinations are described. Moreover, occupational exposures among physicians, nurses, and technologists should be considered. Traditionally, doses to staff have been very low, often immeasurable on personnel dosimeters; however, the advent of increasingly complex interventional procedures present the potential of higher staff doses. We present some data on staff dose levels.

higher. The fact that physicians generally received the highest doses is well reported elsewhere, but it is interesting to note that the level of radiation that they received could potentially be as high as the radiation they would have received without any occupational exposures. Even so, this exposure still remains well below the average 20 mSv/year (over 5 years) recommended by the ICRP for radiation workers. While other researchers have similarly reported effective doses below permissible limits, it has been noted that individual organ doses may exceed recommended limits—such as the dose delivered to the eye lens, as reported by Koukorava et al. (2011) and Sanchez et al. (2012), as well as doses to the extremities (Koukorava et al. 2011). The need for protective devices, clothing, and practices, along with regular monitoring, is emphasized.

Discussion Questions

1. Discuss the constituents and characteristics of the atom.

2. Discuss why certain types of electromagnetic radiation are more suited to medical imaging compared to particulate radiation.

3. Discuss the two key processes that occur when x-rays interacts with human tissue.

References

Brenner DJ. Effective dose: a flawed concept that could and should be replaced. *Br J Radiol.* 2008;81(967):521–523.

Chida K, Kaga Y, Haga Y, Kataoka N, Kumasaka E, Meguro T, Zuguchi M. Occupational dose in interventional radiology procedures. *AJR Am J Roentgenol.* 2013;200(1):138–141.

Dowsett DJ, Kenny PA, Johnston RE. *The Physics of Diagnostic Imaging,* 2nd edition. London: Hodder Arnold; 2006.

Hall EJ, Brenner DJ. Cancer risks from diagnostic radiology. *Br J Radiol.* 2008;81:362–378.

Hart D, Wall BF. *Radiation Exposure of the UK Population from Medical and Dental X-ray Examinations.* NRPB W4 publication. Oxford, UK: National Radiological Protection Board; 2002.

International Commission on Radiological Protection. 1990 Recommendations of the International Commission on Radiological Protection. ICRP Publication 60. *Ann ICRP.* 1991;21(1–3). (Available at http://www.icrp.org/publication.asp?id=ICRP%20Publication%2060; Retrieved August 15, 2015.)

International Commission on Radiological Protection. 2007 Recommendations of the International Commission on Radiological Protection (Users Edition). ICRP Publication 103 (Users Edition). *Ann ICRP.* 2007;37(2-4).

Karam PA, Leslie LA. The evolution of the earth's background radiation level over geological time. *International Radiation Protection Association.* 1996;2(69). (Available at http://www.irpa.net/irpa9/cdrom/VOL.2/V2_69.PDF; Retrieved August 15, 2015).

Koukorava C, Carinou E, Simantirakis G, Vrachliotis TG, Archontakis E, Tierris C, Dimitriou P. Doses to operators during interventional radiology procedures: focus on eye lens and extremity dosimetry. *Radiat Prot Dosimetry.* 2011;144:482–486.

Ministry of Education, Culture, Sports, Science, and Technology of Japan. *Environmental Radioactivity and Radiation in Japan.* (n.d.) (Available at http://www.kankyo-hoshano.go.jp/en/; Retrieved August 17, 2015.)

National Council on Radiation Protection and Measurements. *Ionizing radiation exposure of the population of the United States.* NCRP No. 160. Bethesda, MD: NCRP; 2009. (Available at http://www.ncrponline.org/Publications/Press_Releases/160press.html; Retrieved August 17, 2015.)

[No author] Schoolgirl in Fukushima exposed to high level of radiation in September. 2 November 2011, *The Mainichi Daily News.*

[No author] Fukushima city says radiation dose level unlikely to harm health. 13 January 2012, *The Mainichi Daily News.*

Sánchez RM, Vano E, Fernández JM, Rosales F, Sotil J, Carrera F, García MA, Soler MM, Hernández-Armas J, Martínez LC, Verdú JF. Staff doses in interventional radiology: a national survey. *J Vasc Interv Radiol.* 2012;23:1496–1501.

United Nations Scientific Committee on the Effects of Atomic Radiation. (2010). Sources and effects of ionizing radiation. New York: United Nations. p. 4. (Available at www.unscear.org/docs/reports/.../09-86753_Report_2008_Annex_A.pdf; Retrieved August 17, 2015.)

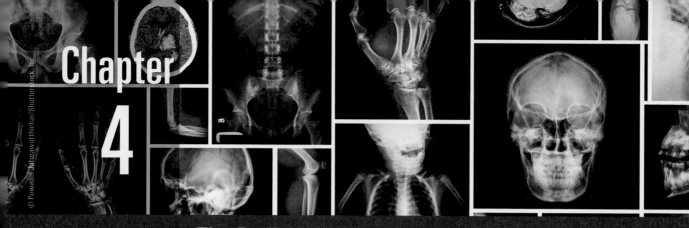

Chapter 4

The Radiobiology of Low-Dose Radiation

Outline

- Introduction
- Stochastic Effects
  - Background
  - Basic principles and debate over risks with low-dose exposures
  - Linear No-Threshold (LNT) Model
  - Do diagnostic x-ray exposures present any risk to humans
  - Mechanisms of radiation-induced change responsible for stochastic risks
  - DNA and cell repair mechanisms following irradiation
  - How long does it take for damaged DNA to manifest itself in man?
- Deterministic Effects
- Factors Influencing Stochastic Risk or Deterministic Effects at Low-Dose Exposures
  - Radio sensitivity of the cell
  - Kinetics
  - Presence of oxygen
  - Dose rate
  - Radioprotectants and radio sensitizers
- Changes Within Non-Irradiated Cells
  - Genomic instability
  - Bystander effect
- Epigenetics
- Effects of Radiation on Children, Embryos, and Fetuses
- References

Objectives

On completion of this chapter, you should be able to:

1. Identify and describe the essential characteristics of the following two categories of biological effects of radiation exposure:
   - Stochastic effects
   - Deterministic effects
2. Discuss the essential features of the Linear No-Threshold (LNT) Dose Response Model.
3. Discuss the mechanisms of radiation-induced change responsible for stochastic risks.
4. Describe the reactions involved in the radiolysis of water.
5. Describe the structure of DNA and explain the mechanisms of the effects of radiation exposure on the DNA molecule.
6. Outline the repair mechanisms of DNA following irradiation.
7. Describe briefly each of the stages of the cell cycle.
8. Discuss the manifestations of DNA damage in man in terms of:
   - Chromosomal aberrations
   - Hereditary effects

9. Identify and describe briefly the three main stages of changes that occur in an irradiated cell that changes it in to a cancerous cell.

10. Discuss the characteristics of deterministic effects.

11. State the law of Bergonie & Tribondeau, and explain practical examples of this law.

12. Discuss the radio sensitivity of immature and mature cells.

13. Explain briefly what is meant by each of the following:
    * Oxygen enhancement ratio
    * Dose rate
    * Radioprotectants
    * Radiosensitizers
    * Epigenetics

14. Discuss the bioeffects of radiation on children, the embryo and the fetus.

Introduction

The first thing to note when one considers the impact of radiation on biological tissue is that the effects can be divided into two main categories: *stochastic effects*, which are focused on the risks associated with inducing certain long-term outcomes—including cancer within the exposed individual and hereditary changes apparent in the exposed individual's future offspring—and *deterministic effects*, which are direct effects on the cells that are irradiated, resulting in symptoms such as skin reddening or ulceration. While both of these effects will be dealt with here, it is around the stochastic effects that the greatest debate remains.

The effects of low-dose radiation will be considered in some detail here, from the earliest molecular changes to the actual symptoms apparent in man.

Stochastic Effects

Background

As mentioned above, the stochastic effects[1] are concerned with the risks associated with radiation exposure, such as cancer within the exposed individual or hereditary changes passed on to an individual's offspring. *There is no guarantee whatsoever that these changes will occur following irradiation.* In the recent publication of the International Commission on Radiological Protection (ICRP 2007), it was reported that cancer remains the largest risk following exposure, with the risk of radiation-associated hereditary effects being substantially downgraded. Nonetheless, both will be considered here.

Basic Principles and Debate Over Risks with Low-Dose Exposures

Throughout this chapter, one must keep in mind the following three key principles relevant to stochastic effects:

1. It is generally accepted that there is *no safe threshold dose* below which radiation exposure has no effect (although the debate around this is detailed below). This means that, however low the exposure, there is always the risk of inducing a mutation leading to a cancer or hereditary change.

2. The *risk is proportional to the dose*, highlighting the importance of consistently applying the "as low as reasonably achievable" (ALARA) concept.

3. The eventual effect (cancer or hereditary change) can result from mutations occurring within a single cell following radiation exposure.

There is much controversy around the stochastic risks associated with low-dose exposures; however, the knowledge surrounding the risks of radiation levels close to those we deliver to patients in x-ray departments is growing, with new data constantly arriving. These data are forcing scientists to adjust their understanding of the effects of radiation and reconfigure associated risk models. While a great deal of the information gathered originates from laboratory investigation, the data that is possibly (and paradoxically) the most useful and relevant to man comes from catastrophic events involving humans: The atomic bomb blasts in August 1945 in Hiroshima

---

[1]Stochastic effects are sometimes referred to as "non-deterministic effects." These terms can be used interchangeably.

and Nagasaki, Japan, and the nuclear power plant accidents that occurred in Chernobyl, Ukraine in 1986 and the more recent disaster at the Fukushima Daichii power plant in Japan in 2011 (**Figures 4-1** and **4-2**). In particular, the data arising from the Life Span Study, undertaken from 1950–2000 by the Radiation Effects Research Foundation (RERF), has provided a wealth of knowledge regarding the effects of ionizing radiation to man from large doses. By extrapolating from these higher exposures to lower doses, similar to those we might encounter in medical imaging departments, we get a sense of the long-term effects of therapeutic radiation.

At the outset of this chapter, one must be clear that extrapolating risks associated with low-dose exposures, say 1–100 mSv, from high-dose data is fraught with difficulties. We rely on having accurate data on the original high doses (which is difficult to verify), acceptance of the value of effective dose concept—something very much under debate—and assessment of risks based on this measure. The relationship between the effects of

high and low levels of radiation, particularly in the absence or paucity of good data supporting calculated risks associated with low doses, and related conclusions about treatment are highly reliant on the *Linear No-Threshold Model*, which in radiobiology circles is generally accepted, but far from universally accepted. The next section will explore the concept of the Linear No-Threshold Model.

Linear No-Threshold (LNT) Model

So if the Linear No-Threshold Model (LNT) is a critical ingredient of the current consensus on low-dose risk, what is it? Simply put, it describes the risks of inducing cancer at varying doses of radiation; by definition, this description takes the position that risk is *linear* and has *no threshold*.

The "Linear" Part

The "linear" part of the model is based upon the premise that we have evidence for risks associated with high-dose levels of radiation, and based upon that evidence, we try and calculate risks associated with lower doses (**Figure 4-3**). For example,

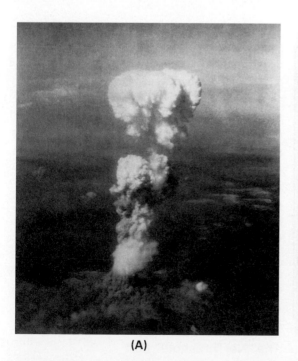

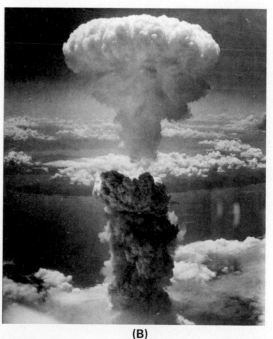

(A)   (B)

Figure 4-1 Nuclear explosions in Hiroshima (A) and Nagasaki (B) in 1945.
U.S. Army Photo.

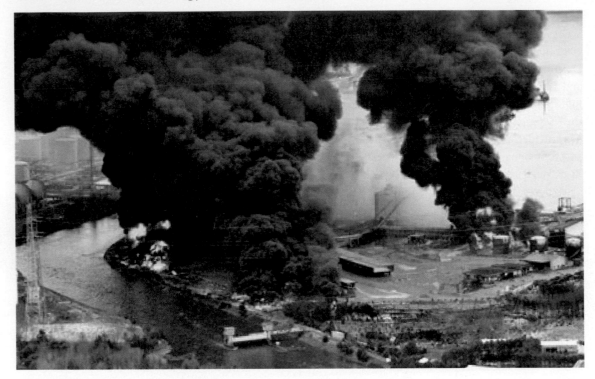

Figure 4-2 Nuclear power plant accident at Fukushima Daichii in 2011.
Courtesy of Reuters.

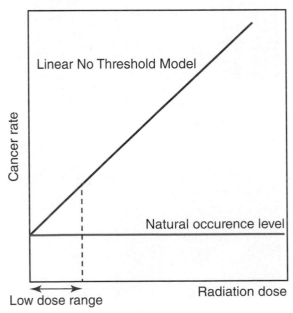

Figure 4-3 The Linear No-Threshold (LNT) Model. Note that the risk increases as the radiation dose increases.

suppose there is evidence that a 5-Sv effective dose delivered to each of 1000 individuals will result in a fatal cancer being induced in 250 of those individuals, and also evidence that 1 Sv effective dose of radiation will similarly produce a fatal cancer in 50 of the 1000 individuals; in both situations, we see a strikingly constant, or linear, relationship between the number of affected persons in the population compared to the effective dose of radiation given. The natural inclination is to extrapolate downwards to doses more relevant to diagnostic exposures. Using a diagnostic imaging example, if we have dose data that show that 1,000,000 individuals each received an effective dose of 5 mSv from x-ray examinations, then, in theory, based on the above numbers, a fatal cancer will be induced in approximately 250 of those individuals.

The "No-Threshold" Part

The no-threshold means that the model assumes there is no "safe" level of radiation; in other words, however low the dose might be, there will always be a risk associated with an x-ray exposure. Together with the linear part of the model, this forms the basis of the *as low as reasonably achievable (ALARA) principle*, which is well known by all personnel working with x-rays. Since there is no safe threshold and the risk is directly associated with dose in a linear fashion, ALARA means that, every time a patient is x-rayed, the dose must be kept as low as possible (consistent with acceptable image quality).

The Debate Over the LNT Model

The LNT model is, however, open to much debate, particularly since there is very little evidence to support radiation effects below 100 mSv. Certain bodies such as the French Académie des Sciences and the Health Physics Society in the United States present opposing views. In fact, three potential

alternatives to this model have been proposed, as illustrated in **Figure 4-4** and summarized here:

1. A threshold exists (purple line), and the risks below 100 mSv are proportionally lower than those above 100 mSv. This is shown by the green line in Figure 4-4.

2. A threshold exists, but below the threshold dose, radiation doses incur a benefit to the exposed individual—a concept known as *hormesis*—as shown by the red line in Figure 4-4.

3. A threshold does not exist; however, the effects of radiation below 100 mSv are proportionally higher than those above 100 mSv (indicated by the blue line in Figure 4-4).

In addition to these alternative approaches, the United Nations Scientific Committee on the Effects

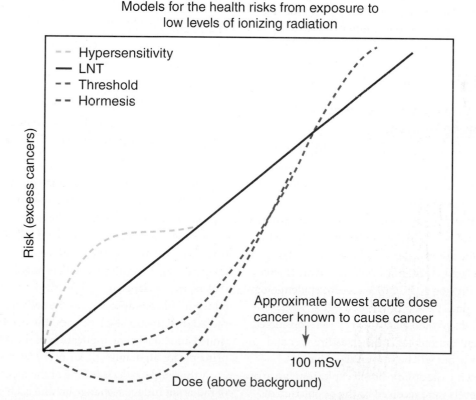

Figure 4-4 The LNT model and three alternative models.

of Atomic Radiation (UNSCEAR), in contrast to its previous stance, has recently issued recommendations to the UN General Assembly stating that they no longer recommend attempting to calculate radiation-induced health detriment by multiplying low doses of radiation (at or below background levels) by the number of individuals exposed. Adherence to this recommendation presents certain challenges when attempting to establish potential risks to specific population from low diagnostic x-ray exposures (e.g., 5 mSv and below).

Application of the LNT: A Prudent Approach

Despite all the debate, and accepting that there is no certainty, the LNT Model remains the most accepted model by radiation agencies across the world when attempting to understand the risks from various doses of radiation. It is most likely prudent for medical imaging clinicians and radiographers to continue to employ this model until the ICRP states otherwise. This stance is supported by continued endorsement of the LNT model by the US National Research Council of the National Academy of Science (BEIR 2006), UNSCEAR, the US Environmental Protection Agency, and a collection of other radiation protection bodies.

Do Diagnostic X-Ray Exposures Present Any Risk to Humans?

Despite these recommendations, at this stage the reader may have some serious doubts about whether the levels of radiation encountered in x-ray departments have any radiobiological implications or present any risk to humans. This will be explored further in the sections below, but it may be useful to consider evidence provided by two sources of data: the Japanese atomic bomb survivors (Pierce et al. 1996; Preston et al. 2007); a recent epidemiological study on CT exposures (Pearce et al. 2012). The implications of these data are very well considered by eminent radiobiologists such as Brenner and Hall (2012), but will be summarized here.

Following the atomic bomb explosions, an array of dose levels were received by the population of exposed individuals, which numbered well over 100,000; however, a subpopulation ($n = 30,000$) received organ doses that were not dissimilar from doses received from a few sequential CT scans (Pierce et al. 1996; Preston et al. 2007). This group of individuals demonstrated an increased risk of cancer in long-term follow up.

The epidemiological work of Pearce and colleagues (2012) considered 180,000 individuals who had received 280,000 CT scans between 1985 and 2002. All individuals were younger than 22 at the time of exposure and thus would have had higher radio sensitivity than older patients. The authors focused on leukemia and brain tumors—cancers that have a shorter latency period and would appear in the study's 10-year follow-up period. The work showed that there was a positive significant relationship between the dose to the bone marrow and brain and the risk of leukemia and brain tumors, respectively, at the rate of 1 excessive case of each cancer per 10,000 patients undergoing CT examinations in the first year of life. The results from this work provides some powerful conclusions:

1. There is a risk of cancer from diagnostic x-ray exposures.

2. This risk is very low.

3. The risk, although low, is detectable, so statements that radiation risks associated with diagnostic exposures are simply undetectable must be questioned.

While this study by Pearce and coworkers has effectively demonstrated the risk with diagnostic exposures, the age of patients, the limited cancer types considered, and the restricted follow-up periods insists that further work be done to further clarify the risks—and this work is ongoing. Nonetheless, the evidence highlights the importance of taking a cautious approach to the delivery of x-ray radiation at diagnostic levels and the need for continued and consistent application of the ALARA principle for all diagnostic x-ray exposures.

A thorough understanding of the mechanisms of radiation induced-change behind each exposure is now required.

Mechanisms of Radiation-Induced Change Responsible for Stochastic Risks

This part of the chapter will consider the changes that immediately occur within cells that have been exposed to radiation, looking first at the impact on DNA and the presentation of the chromosomal mutations and associated genetic mutations. These changes within the exposed cell occur at very early time-points compared with the manifestation of eventual symptoms; for example, the initial ionizations occur in less than one-billionth of a second (**Figure 4-5**).

It should be stressed here, as elsewhere, that a highly informative and detailed discussion of the processes that occur are presented in the full version of the ICRP 99 and 103 publications (ICRP 2005; ICRP 2007). Much of the material described here is drawn from those documents and associated publications.

DNA

Prior to 1970, there was much uncertainty regarding the most sensitive component with the cell; however, following the elegant work of Munro (1970), it was shown that the cell was much more likely to express effects of radiation exposure when the nucleus was exposed compared with other organelles. Munro established this by inserting a polonium radioactive source, a producer of alpha particles, at the end of a tungsten needle at a variety of sites within the cell. His work showed that cell death occurred at ~26 cGy when the source was placed within the nucleus, compared with 50,000 cGy when the polonium was positioned at other parts of the cell such as the cytoplasm. While this showed that the location of the radio-sensitive component of the cell was at the nucleus, or within at least 2 microns of the nucleus, it wasn't until further radiolabeling work was done that the DNA was shown to be more radio sensitive than mRNA, which in turn was more sensitive than rRNA, tRNA, and amino acids.

How Does Radiation Cause Change Within the DNA?

It should be emphasized that x-rays can be directly or indirectly ionizing. With the direct route, the x-ray simply causes the ionization, whereas with the indirect route, the x-ray produces a secondary

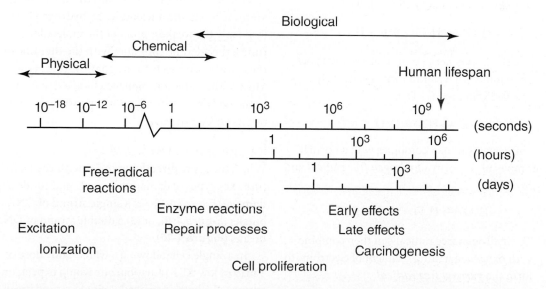

Figure 4-5 A summary of the time taken for post-irradiation effects to manifest from the earliest ionization events through effects manifesting in the whole organism.

particle, such as an ejected electron, that causes subsequent ionizations.

The x-ray or its secondary particle can then go on to cause direct or indirect effects on biologic tissue. The direct option involves the x-ray (or its secondary particle) directly interacting with the DNA, causing ionizations potentially leading to subsequent morphological change (see below). However, DNA only makes up about 1% of the human body, unlike water, which comprises up to 80% of the body. Therefore, it is highly likely that instead of interacting with DNA, the x-ray (or the secondary particle) will interact with and ionize water, leading to radiolysis of water and the formation of *free radicals*. Free radicals are highly reactive agents with an unpaired electron in their outer shell. The process for the formation of these free radicals, according to Holahan (1987), is as follows:

1. X-ray interacts with water (H_2O) to form ionized water molecule (H_2O^+) and an ejected electron (e^-):

$$x\text{-ray} \rightarrow H_2O = H_2O^+ + e^-$$

2. The ionized water then combines with a normal water molecule to form the *hydroxy free radical* (OH·) and a hydrogen ion (H^+):

$$H_2O^+ \rightarrow H_2O = OH\cdot + H^+$$

3. The electron generated in [1] above then goes on to join with water to form a negatively charged water ion (H_2O^-):

$$e^- \rightarrow H_2O = H_2O^-$$

This water ion then combines with a normal water molecule to form a *hydrogen free radical* and a hydroxyl ion:

$$H_2O^- \rightarrow H_2O = H\cdot + OH^-$$

4. The hydrogen free radical can then combine with oxygen, a willing recipient of electrons, to form the *peroxyl free radical*.

$$H\cdot + O_2 = HO_2.$$

All of these free radical species are highly reactive molecules with an unpaired electron on the outer shell and the potential to do much damage, such as breaking chemical bonds within DNA. The peroxyl free radical, while less oxidizing than the other two, has a longer life and therefore can do damage at sites further from its origin. Also, the hydroxyl and hydrogen free radicals can combine to form hydrogen peroxide, another oxidizing agent (something that can accept electrons and cause subsequent biological damage). The combined consequence of the free radicals acting on DNA is responsible for approximately 70% of radiation damage following low-dose x-rays, whereas for high-LET radiation exposures, most damage occurs following the direct impact of the radiation on the DNA.

What is DNA?

A little reflection on the structure of DNA may help understand the effects of radiation or free radicals on this molecule. DNA is a nucleic acid that is shaped as a double helix or a spiral ladder (**Figure 4-6**). The sides of the ladder are made up of nucleotide (sugar-phosphate) chains, while the rungs comprise four types of nitrogen bases: Adenine, cytosine, guanine, and thymine, which are attached to the nucleotides by hydrogen bonds (arguably the weakest point of the molecule). At the rungs, the adenine combines with the thymine *or* the cytosine connects to the guanine (**Figure 4-7**). Most of the radiation-induced change that occurs in the body results from a post-exposure disruption of this DNA structure.

X-Ray Interaction with DNA

When the x-ray directly interacts with the DNA, three key types of damage occur: (1) nucleotide base damage (**Figure 4-8**), (2) a single strand of DNA breaks (**Figure 4-9**), or (3) a double strand of DNA breaks (**Figure 4-10**).

In a single cell following a whole-body dose of 1 mSv of low-LET radiation, one would expect, on average, 2.5 bases damaged, 1 single-strand break, and 0.04 double-strand breaks. The bottom line is

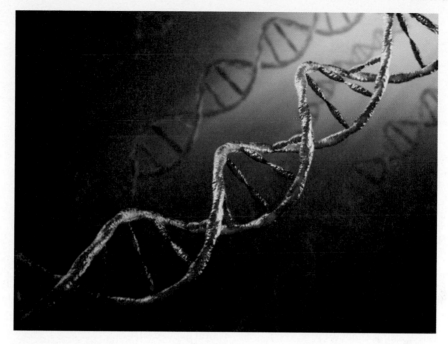

Figure 4-6 Double stranded DNA.
© The Astrophysics and Astrochemistry Laboratory/NASA.

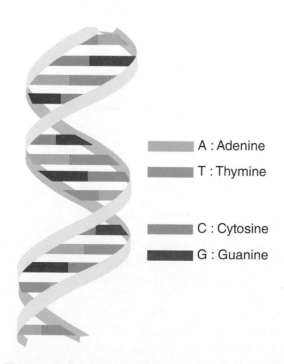

A : Adenine

T : Thymine

C : Cytosine

G : Guanine

Figure 4-7 Nitrogen bases.

that DNA change following x-ray damage can subsequently lead to a variety of mutations and chromosomal aberrations, resulting in variety of signaling pathways that may protect or cause damage and may contribute to the pathogenesis of cancer.

With regard to the specific type of post-radiation lesion, while some specific base damage may cause significant health impact—for example, damage to 8-hydroxydeoxyguanosine and thymine glycols (ICRP 2007)—isolated base damage that would generally occur with low-dose x-rays has limited effects. The main source of radiation mutagenesis is double-strand breaks. These are harder to repair than single-strand breaks, since there is no intact strand from which repair to the other strand can be modeled. Double-strand breaks occur when damage to the DNA occurs at several sites within close proximity to each other that may result from the initial ionization complimented by the production of secondary particles (collectively known as a cluster). It is estimated that with x-rays, 30% of the

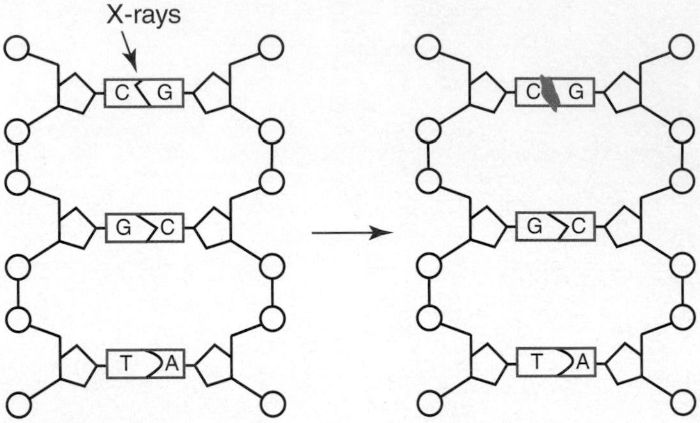

X-rays

Figure 4-8 Nucleotide base damage.

double-strand breaks occur following this clustering effect where two or more double-strand breaks are evident, compared with 70% with higher-LET radiation. This clustering effect (**Figure 4-11**) following direct x-ray damage actually provides a distinction between this type of DNA damage and damage that occurs spontaneously (without radiation exposure).

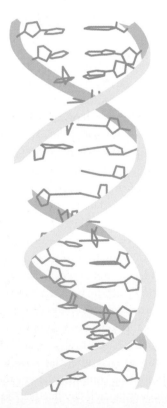

Figure 4-9 Single-strand breaks.

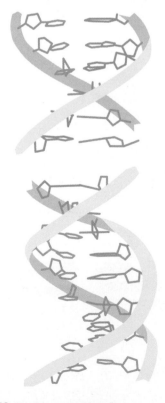

Figure 4-10 Double-strand breaks.

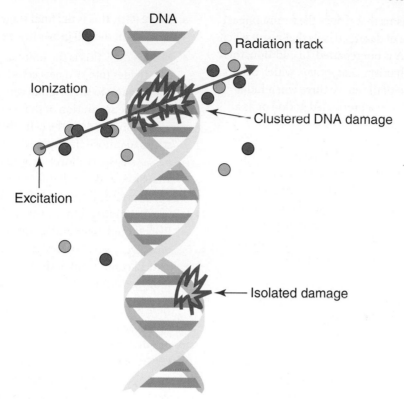

Figure 4-11 Clusters of damage and an isolated incident following a radiation interaction with DNA.

Free-Radical Damage on DNA

Radiation damage following free-radical damage is similar to that described for direct x-ray damage above, with certain distinctions. The predominant types of DNA lesions are again base damages and single-strand breaks, however, the double-strand breaks are usually spread more evenly throughout the DNA.

More Than Just DNA Interactions

Finally, while the focus here has been on DNA interactions, damage, and repair, one must note that radiation directly or mediated by free radicals can cause effects in other structures, such as RNA, proteins, mitochondria, and cell membranes. These can all cause damage to the cells' structure or function, either in an isolated way or comple-menting other post-radiation changes. However, the evidence to date on these other changes has generally relied on high doses of radiation, so at present it is difficult to know the relevance of these other changes to the x-ray doses delivered during diagnostic x-ray exposures.

DNA and Cell Repair Mechanisms Following Irradiation

Producing single- or double-strand DNA breaks or base damage does not automatically mean detrimental effects on the cell, organ, or organism. There are three highly effective repair mechanisms of which one needs to be aware, including *cell cycle arrest*, *DNA repair*, and *apoptosis*. Via these three mechanisms working together and interdependently, the majority of the damage that occurs following radiation is repaired. The defense against damage is not just about fixing the majority of broken DNA strands, there must also be mechanisms that reduce the future impact and propagation of damaged cells that result when some of the DNA is not repaired. In addition, there is a further mechanism, *adaptation*, which occurs as a combination of the above three when radiation is delivered over a protracted period or as a fractionated regime.

Repair Mechanism 1: Cell Cycle Arrest

Before we consider the arrest of the cell cycle, a review of what happens during the cell cycle may be useful. The cell cycle is a sequence of events relevant to dividing cells that facilitate the production of the next generation of cells. There are four main stages, as shown in **Figure 4-12**):

1. Gap 1 (G_1): During this phase, the cell is producing a lot of proteins and enzymes, increasing the number of organelles present and growing in size.

2. Synthesis (S): DNA replication occurs, in which all chromosomes are duplicated by producing two sister chromatids. At the end of this phase, the DNA present within the cell has doubled.

3. Gap 2 (G_2): This is the final stage before mitosis; here, again the cell grows in size.

4. Mitosis (M): This is the point at which the cell divides into two new cells identical to one another and to the original cell. The key event here is the separation of the two chromatids to opposing ends of the cell. There are five stages to mitosis: interphase (which encompasses steps 1–3 above), prophase, metaphase, anaphase, and telophase. At the end of mitosis, cytokinesis is responsible for the cell's cytoplasm dividing into the two separate cells. Even though temporally, mitosis makes up only a very small part of the cell cycle, it is a critical component of the cell with regard to radio sensitivity.

There is a further stage, quiescence, which is simply when a cell has left the cycle and has stopped dividing.

If DNA has received insult from an external (or internal) agent such as ionizing radiation, rather than let the cell cycle continue as normal, resulting in cell progenies with mutations and hence

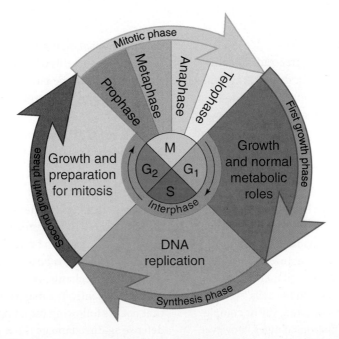

Figure 4-12 The cell cycle.

increased risk of cancer, the cell cycle will tempo-rarily halt to facilitate repair. This is known as *cell cycle arrest*. There are three main checkpoints for this arrest to take place (**Figure 4-13**): (1) at the boundary between G_1 and S, allowing the cell to "decide" whether cell division should continue, be delayed, or pass into quiescence; (2) during S, so that DNA replication is minimized until the DNA is fully repaired and the cell can "decide" if DNA duplication should continue; and (3) at the boundary between G_2 and mitosis, to ensure that after the radiation insult, the cell is now actually ready to undergo division and produce new cells.

These checkpoints are reliant on a number of protein complexes that are activated minutes after insult, such as *p53* (boundary between G_1 and S), ataxia telangiectasia mutated protein [ATM] (S phase) and DSB–cyclin B complexes (boundary between G_2 and mitosis). Some of these complexes serve as early sensors of damage or as mediators to facilitate subsequent repair. Certain individuals demonstrate a reduced ability to undergo these cell-cycle arrest mechanisms, particularly those with ataxia-telangiectasia, *BRCA1*, or *BRCA2* mutations.

Repair Mechanism 2: DNA Repair

As mentioned above, there are three distinct types of DNA lesions following radiation exposure: (1) base damage, (2) single-strand DNA breaks, and (3) double-strand DNA breaks. The first two of these are relatively easily repaired, since there is at least one strand that has remained intact and serves as a template for repair. The biologically important lesion is the double-strand DNA break; how this specific injury is repaired will be the focus here.

There appear to be two distinct pathways for repairing double-stranded DNA breaks: ***homologous recombination*** and ***non-homologous end joining***. Before we get into each type, a brief description of what is meant by DNA homology may be useful for the DNA-uninitiated. ***Homology*** simply means similarity in structure, and in the context of DNA means sequences of DNA that are very similar or identical to each other. In the case of

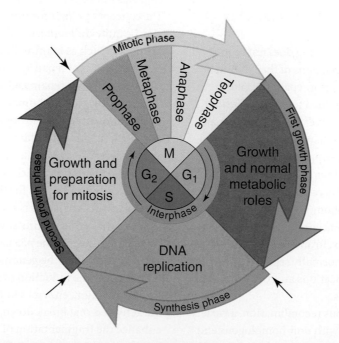

Figure 4-13 The cell cycle with arrows indicating the checkpoints.

double-strand breaks, homologous recombination relies on intact homologous DNA sequences being available; and non-homologous end joining, as you might expect, does not rely on such sequences.

Repair Mechanism 2: Homologous Recombination

Homologous recombination is a highly reliable and effective process for restoring the fidelity of the original DNA. It relies on there being available a healthy strand of DNA to serve as a template. Following a double-strand break, **cell cycle arrest** occurs to stop the damaged cell from reproducing itself. Then, **resection** (cutting away) of the broken ends of the DNA takes place. A homologous template is used, often from the overhang of the broken DNA strand, and this together with a healthy, similar strand of DNA (**strand invasion**) allows DNA synthesis to occur, and the formation and joining together (**ligation**) of a DNA molecule that is identical to the original before the radiation exposure. A variety of gene types are involved with this type of effective repair, including several RAD-51 type genes.

Repair Mechanism 2: Non-Homologous End Joining

Non-homologous end joining does not require homologous, healthy portions of the DNA to be available. With this type of repair, the ends of the strand breaks are joined together (**ligation**) using microhomologies (very short strand material) existing at the overhang towards the end of the strand break. If the opposing overhangs are perfectly compatible, then usually an efficient repair occurs, unless there are missing nucleotides. However, if the microhomologous material is not compatible, then an inaccurate repair is much more likely, leading to chromosomal translocations where genes that are normally separated are joined together. Such translocations are common features within cancerous cells.

As with homologous recombination, a variety of genes are involved with non-homologous end joining, including those responsible for producing

the KU, DNA-PK, XRCC4, and DNA ligase IV proteins. Importantly, any existing defects in these genes can lead to substantial increases in the radio sensitivity of the exposed individual as a result of being unable to repair the double-strand breaks.

Repair Mechanism 2: A Third DNA-Repair Option?

There is a third type of repair mechanism that has been shown in non-mammalian cells, but that may be relevant to humans. **Single-strand annealing** is a process that relies on elements of both non-homologous end joining and homologous recombination. It looks for identical DNA sequences on both strands close to the break and uses these sequences to generate identical sequences that are then used to produce the double-strand repair. It is a form of homologous recombination, except a healthy template is not involved. In addition, it does not preserve the efficiencies of homologous recombination, resulting in loss of sequences around the break and subsequent inaccurate DNA repair.

Repair Mechanism 3: Apoptosis

The concept of repair for primitive organisms may be quite different from that of higher-level organisms such as mammalians. For primitive beings, the aim of repair is at the cellular level, where attempts to repair each cell occur following damage. However, for humans, the focus is on the preservation of the whole organism, and if a cell or its genetic content is damaged—with its damaged progeny potentially leading to a tumor at a later stage that might kill the organism—then it is better to sacrifice the cell for the overall welfare of the organism. **Apoptosis** is such a sacrificial event, whereby the cell "commits suicide" to avoid serious consequences later. The *p53* gene, otherwise known as the "guardian of the genome," is fundamentally important to the induction of apoptosis. Further to *p53* induction, enzymes known as caspases are activated that break down cell structures and enhance the fragmentation of DNA. An example of an apoptotic cell is given in **Figure 4-14**).

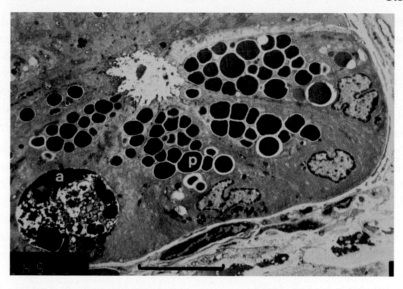

Figure 4-14 An apoptotic body (a) following radiation insult is shown within a cell at the base of the crypt of Lieberkuhn within the small intestine.

Repair Mechanism 4: Adaptation

The adaptive response that utilizes the above three repair mechanisms means that the effect of several subsequent (sometimes contiguous) doses of radiation is not simply additive; rather, adaptive changes can occur within 3–6 hours post-irradiation, which may reduce the level of insult finally inflicted. This was shown by Brennan et al. (1998), where a protracted dose of radiation (5 Gy) spread over 25 days produced adaptive responses within the intestinal tract, such as longer enterocyte microvilli, increased number of secretory cells, and greater levels of cell division. These changes then offset some of the damage, such as severely depleted numbers of enterocytes, that occurred when the same dose of radiation was presented over a period of minutes. It has been proposed that heightened communication between irradiated and non-irradiated cells that heighten this adaptive response may be at least in part responsible, along with the *p53* gene. However, other workers have shown that these adaptive or even protective mechanisms are not consistent across all cell types, and in addition, these mechanisms may not be present to any great level with radiations of high LET. Whether these adaptive responses should impact on our current understanding on low-dose risks is not clear.

Repair Mechanisms: Summary

Clearly, evolution has provided man with three effective processes of repairing damaged DNA following radiation insult. These processes are not independent of each other; for example, cell cycle arrest may occur, allowing DNA reparative activities such as homologous recombination to take place. However, the fidelity of repair, particularly with non-homologous end joining, is currently unknown, and there is evidence that damaged cells can go on to produce daughter cells. Without 100% repair, and the fact that the lowest doses encountered in diagnostic radiology will induce DNA change, dismissal of the LNT Model may be unwise. The next section of this chapter now considers the impact of damaged DNA that escapes the protective mechanisms described above.

How Long Does it Take for Damaged DNA to Manifest Itself in Man?

To sum it up in one sentence, the sequence of events following radiation insult is that (mainly) unrepaired double-strand breaks can lead to chromosomal aberrations, which can lead to genetic mutations, which may eventually lead to cancer or hereditary change. Let us look at this in a little more detail.

Chromosomal Aberrations

Double-stranded DNA breaks are the most likely causal agents of chromosomal aberrations, and subsequently gene mutations, that may lead to the induction of cancer. While the relationship between DNA damage and chromosomal aberrations is well established for higher radiation doses, and we assume that the prevalence of double-strand breaks increase linearly with dose, whether there is a direct relationship between low-dose–induced double-strand breaks and chromosomal aberrations is currently unknown. At this time, there is no strong evidence to support a dose threshold below which there would be no chromosomal aberrations or mutagenic change.

There are a variety of chromosomal aberrations, and these include translocations, inversions, dicentrics, centric rings, and substantial deletions (**Figure 4-15, A–E**). These names are given on the basis of the resultant chromosomal morphology. While it is possible (although not guaranteed) that the first two of these can be passed from one cell to its daughters and indeed are present in a range of tumor types, the remaining three types of aberrations will most likely result in the cell death.

Chromosomal aberrations vary in complexity, where increasing complexity involves increasing interchanges between a number of chromosomes. For low-LET radiation such as x-rays, such complex aberrations are dose-dependent and rely on several incidents of DNA damage. The impact of these complex aberrations is currently unclear and most likely result in cell death; however, at this time, the passing down of these complex changes from one generation to the next cannot be ruled out.

Genetic Mutations

The outcome from chromosomal aberrations in cells that survive are genetic mutations, including point mutations, where a single nucleotide base is replaced, to large deletions involving single or multiple genes. If not essential for cell survival, such mutations may be passed from generation to generation, with gene deletions being the primary change most likely to result in a cancer. While studying the impact of radiation dose on mutations is even more complex than the impact on chromosomal aberrations, the evidence to date supports a direct linear relationship down to a dose level of 200 mGy.

Induction of Cancer

The changes that occur in an irradiated cell to transform it into a cancerous cell relies on three main stages: (1) *initiation*, where a normal cell is changed into one that has the potential of becoming a cancer; (2) *progression*, where initiated cells undergo development of their neoplastic abilities via a variety of cellular events; and (3) *conversion*, where the cell is converted into a malignancy. Each of these stages will be considered below.

Initiation

Initiation events have been described above in terms of DNA changes, chromosomal aberrations,

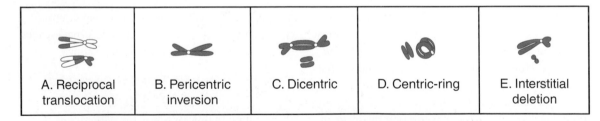

Figure 4-15 Chromosomal aberrations.

| A. Reciprocal translocation | B. Pericentric inversion | C. Dicentric | D. Centric-ring | E. Interstitial deletion |

and gene mutations. It has been considered for some time that this stage is the main carcinogenic effect of the radiation, and this has been confirmed by studies involving children's susceptibility to radiation, animal work that demonstrates that radiation has only a minor impact on the progression of cancer, and low-LET radiation studies exploring acute versus protracted doses and the decrease in risk associated with the latter. Recent studies involving rats and mice looking at a range of cancer types have further confirmed that the principal radiation effect is that involving initial DNA breaks and associated genomic mutations.

Progression

The progression stage is considered to be closely related to genomic instability that serves to compliment the changes presenting in the initiation stage; it results in cells from later generations demonstrating additional mutations compared with the initial radiation-induced mutations. Such instability can occur in up to 50% of irradiated cells, and it is this complimentary effect of genetic instability with initial post-irradiation mutations that drives the progression toward cancer formation. At doses encountered within diagnostic imaging departments, the level of induced instability is directly related to the dose delivered.

This genomic stability is supposed to be associated with telomeres, which are genes located at the end of the DNA that hold the DNA together, a little like the tight end of a shoelace. They have the critical function of protecting the chromosomes from erosion and interchromosomal fusion. Telomeric instability following irradiation has been reported in cancer cells; nonetheless, the specific mechanisms responsible for the complimentary effect of genomic instability and its specific role in contributing to tumorogenesis are still under investigation.

Conversion

The final stage conversion occurs when the irradiated cells eventually change into a tumor, an occurrence that may take many years to manifest.

Indeed, it is only a very small fraction of cells that were initiated that will reach this malignant state. The progression of cells to a malignancy, unfortunately, will be an ongoing event, since it appears that the genomic mutations and instabilities presented by the radiation insult cannot ever be eliminated with certainty.

In numerical terms, therefore, what are the stochastic risks of cancer following radiation exposure?

As mentioned earlier, the prudent approach to determining cancer risks associated with low-dose exposure relies on the LNT model. However, there is another factor known as the dose and dose rate effectiveness factor (DDREF), which the ICRP recommends should be used when calculating risks at low doses by extrapolating from high exposure levels. What the DDREF means is that at low doses or low-dose rates, the risks from low-dose exposures as calculated using the LNT model should be downgraded by a specified factor. Supported by epidemiologic, radiologic and experimental data, since 1990 the ICRP continues to recommend this factor, it having a value of 2; however, it is acknowledged that there are ongoing uncertainties around this figure.

The risk of cancer from exposure is calculated using data from the Life Span Study (LSS) from Japan, but also medical, environmental, and occupational data. It is presented using a parameter called the **detriment-adjusted nominal risk coefficient**. The **nominal risk coefficient** section of this parameter is calculated by averaging gender and age risk estimates across populations and focuses on cancer incidence for specific organs rather than lethality since misclassification is less likely with the former (ICRP 2007). The detriment portion takes into account the organs irradiated and the relative (weighted) detriment across different organs, taking into account lethality and years of life lost. This weighted detriment is them summed across all organs and should equal the total detriment to that exposure. All this is very well described in Annex 1 of ICRP (2007) and briefly summarized in **Table 4-1**.

Table 4-1 The required steps for arriving at detriment-adjusted nominal risk coefficient

Step	Description
1.	Calculate post-radiation cancer incidence risks for a variety of organs and other solid tumor types
2.	Apply DDREF
3.	Generalize risk across different populations
4.	Arrive at nominal risk coefficients
5.	Adjust for lethality
6.	Adjust for quality of life with non-fatal cancers
7.	Adjust for cancer-free life years lost
8.	Arrive at detriment-adjusted nominal risk coefficient

On the basis of the LNT model and the DDREF, the ICRP 103 publication (ICRP 2007) has issued an array of organ-specific and whole-organism risks. With regard to the latter, it has been calculated for the whole population that the detriment-adjusted nominal risk coefficient for cancer is 5.5% per sievert, with this value reducing to 4.1% per sievert for adults (adults being less radio sensitive than children; see below). The ICRP continue to emphasize that risk assessments based on these numbers should be applied to whole populations and not individuals.

Of course, the risk for individual organs in terms of cancer induction and subsequent lethality is highly variable when, for example, considering breast tissues versus liver tissue; therefore, the ICRP has provided data describing the relative risk across different organs. This is summarized in **Table 4-2**, which has been adapted from Annex 4 of ICRP 103 (ICRP 2007) and is presented in two parts: the first part for the whole population, the second for adults aged 18–64.

In the table are a number of columns. The first, the nominal detriment coefficient, simply describes the risk from 1 Sv of inducing a

cancer across 13 organ types plus data for other solid cancers. The second column summarizes the lethality (detriment) for each site, which is then multiplied by column one's nominal risk coefficient (with further consideration given to detriment from non-fatal cancers) to give a weighted nominal risk coefficient (Column 3). The figures in column 3 are then further adjusted by a weighting based on cancer-free life years lost (Column 4) to give the final detriment-adjusted nominal risk coefficient (Column 5). The final column (Column 6) demonstrates the relative detriment for each organ and other solid tumors, which totals a value of one for the whole body.

Hereditary Effects

Hereditary effects are stochastic effects, and the principles behind the induction of a cancer, such as induction of DNA damage, chromosomal aberrations, and gene mutations, are relevant here as well. The difference between these effects and the induction of cancer is that the effect is not seen in the individual exposed, but instead in the offspring of that individual. Just to be clear, this is not about irradiation of a fetus or embryo (that will be discussed at the end of the chapter); this is about the effects of exposure to an individual before the offspring has even been conceived.

The bottom line is that at present, there is no direct evidence for radiation-induced heritable effects in humans; however, there is good support that this effect occurs in animals. It is on the basis of this animal evidence that the current ICRP document continues to include risk estimates for hereditary effects, although these have been significantly downgraded for adults by a factor of 8 in ICRP 103 (2007) compared to the 1990 recommendations (ICRP 1991). This downgrading of heritable risks is further supported by the work of the UK Committee on Medical Aspects of Radiation in the Environment (COMARE), which in their seventh (COMARE 2002) and eighth report (COMARE 2004) indicated that it was highly unlikely that leukemia, solid tumors, miscarriage, or neonatal death were linked to preconception exposures. However, COMARE did highlight that one could not rule out

Table 4-2 A summary of the risk coefficients associated with 13 organs and other solid tumors;

Tissue	Nominal risk coefficient (cases /10,000/Sv)	Lethality fraction	Nominal risk adjusted for lethality and quality of life	Relative cancer free life lost	Detriment (relating to column 1)	Relative detriment
Whole population						
Bladder	43 (0.43%)	0.29	23.5 (0.24%)	0.71	16.7	0.029
Bone	7 (0.07%)	0.45	5.1 (0.05%)	1.00	5.10	0.009
Bone marrow	42 (0.42%)	0.67	37.7 (0.38%)	1.63	61.5	0.107
Breast	112 (1.12%)	0.29	61.9 (0.62%)	1.29	79.8	0.139
Colon	65 (0.65%)	0.48	49.4 (0.49%)	0.97	47.9	0.083
Gonads (Heritable)	20 (0.2%)	0.80	19.3 (0.19%)	1.32	25.4	0.044
Liver	30 (0.3%)	0.95	30.2 (0.3%)	0.88	26.6	0.046
Lung	114 (1.14%)	0.89	112.9 (1.13%)	0.80	90.30	0.157
Oesophagus	15 (0.15%)	0.93	15.1 (0.15%)	0.87	13.1	0.023
Other solid	144 (1.44%)	0.49	110.2 (1.10%)	1.03	113.5	0.198
Ovary	11(0.11%)	0.57	8.8 (0.09%)	1.12	9.9	0.017
Skin	1000 (10%)	0.002	4 (0.04%)	1.00	4.00	0.007
Stomach	79 (0.79%)	0.83	77 (0.77%)	0.88	67.7	0.118
Thyroid	33 (0.33%)	0.07	9.8 (0.1%)	1.29	12.7	0.022
Total	**1715 (17.2%)**		**565 (5.65%)**			**1.000**
Working age population (18–64 ages)						
Bladder	42 (0.42%)	0.29	23 (023%)	0.85	19.3	0.046
Bone	5 (0.05%)	0.45	3 (0.03%)	1.00	3.40	0.008
Bone marrow	23 (0.23%)	0.67	20 (0.2%)	1.17	23.9	0.057
Breast	49 (0.49%)	0.29	27 (0.27%)	1.20	32.6	0.077
Colon	50 (0.5%)	0.48	38 (0.38%)	1.13	43.00	0.102
Gonads (Heritable)	12 (0.12%)	0.80	12 (0.12%)	1.32	15.3	0.036
Liver	21 (0.21%)	0.95	21 (0.21%)	0.93	19.7	0.047
Lung	127 (12.7%)	0.89	126 (1.26%)	0.96	120.7	0.286

(Continues)

Table 4-2 A summary of the risk coefficients associated with 13 organs and other solid tumors; (*Continued*)

Tissue	Nominal risk coefficient (cases /10,000/Sv)	Lethality fraction	Nominal risk adjusted for lethality and quality of life	Relative cancer free life lost	Detriment (relating to column 1)	Relative detriment
Oesophagus	16 (0.16%)	0.93	16 (0.16%)	0.91	14.2	0.034
Other solid	88 (0.88%)	0.49	67 (0.67%)	0.97	65.4	0.155
Ovary	7 (0.07%)	0.57	6 (0.06%)	1.16	6.6	0.016
Skin	670 (6.7%)	0.002	3 (0.03%)	1.00	2.7	0.006
Stomach	60 (0.6%)	0.83	58 (0.58%)	0.89	51.80	0.123
Thyroid	9 (0.09%)	0.07	3 (0.03%)	1.19	3.4	0.008
Total	**1179 (11.8%)**		**423 (4.23%)**		**423**	**1.000**

Data from: ICRP, 2007.

Values are expressed in percentages. Column 1: **The nominal risk coefficient** describes the risk of cancer across the organ and tumor categories. Column 2: Summary of the lethality (**detriment**) for each organ and other solid tumors. The detriment is multiplied by the nominal risk coefficient (with further consideration given to detriment from non-fatal cancers) to give a **weighted nominal risk coefficient** (Column 3). This latter value is then further adjusted for each organ and other solid tumors based on cancer-free life years lost (Column 4) to give the final detriment-adjusted nominal risk coefficient (Column 5). The final column (Column 6) gives the relevant detriment for each organ and other solid tumors, which add up to a total of one for the whole body.

the influence of low statistical power (due to low exposed populations and low doses involved) on these results.

Radiation can manifest itself into three broad groups of hereditary effect:

- Mendelian disorders that result from mutations in single genes and can be:
  (1) autosomal dominant, which means that if the mutation is present in one parent, it can be transmitted to the offspring;
  (2) autosomal recessive, which means the disease or abnormality can be passed on only if it is present in both parents at the same gene location; or
  (3) X-linked recessive disease that only manifests in males but may be carried by females.
- Chronic disease such as diabetes or hypertension
- Congenital problems such as cleft palate or neural tube defects

UNSCEAR and ICRP have been constantly updating and revising the genetic risks, but on the latest available evidence, the current risk coefficients for the total population calculated by the ICRP (2007) is 0.16% per Gy for the *first* generation, increasing to 0.22 Gy for the first two generations. It is interesting to note that these risk coefficients are not that different from those presented in ICRP 60 in 1990. However, there is one big difference between the two ICRP publications, and that is around the *detriment-adjusted nominal risk coefficient*, which takes into account the chances of these risks manifesting in actual disease or abnormality in the offspring. Since 1990, much research has been done looking at the type of mutations that causes heritable diseases in humans and the type of mutations radiation causes in mice, and it is now believed that of the post-radiation multilocus mutations that occur, only a proportion of these will reach a living offspring. Corrections using parameters such as the potential recoverability correction factor are required to estimate hereditary disease in an offspring from radiation-mutations in a mouse, and hence we have the *detriment-adjusted nominal risk coefficient*. The detriment-adjusted nominal risk coefficient differences therefore between the 1990 and 2007 ICRP publications are substantial, due to the increase in knowledge around radiation-induced mutations and their impact on hereditary disease. These differences are shown in **Table 4-3**.

Total of All Stochastic Detriment-Adjusted Nominal Risk Coefficient: Cancer and Hereditable Effects

For completion the latest detriment-adjusted nominal risk coefficients (ICRP 2007) are shown for cancer, hereditary effects and the total values in **Table 4-4**). The 1990 (ICRP 1990) are also shown for comparison purposes.

Deterministic Effects

Deterministic effects[2] are symptomatic changes that occur with the cells that are directly affected

Table 4-3 Detriment-adjusted nominal risk coefficient for heritable effects

Exposed population	Hertiable effects	
	Present	ICRP 60 (1990)
Whole	0.2	1.3
Adult	0.1	0.8
(*Source:* ICRP, 2007)		

---

[2]Please note that deterministic effects are otherwise known as non-stochastic effects and these terms can be used interchangeably.

Table 4-4 Detriment-adjusted nominal risk coefficient for all stochastic effects

Exposed population	Cancer		Hertiable effects		Total	
	Present	ICRP 60 (1990)	Present	ICRP 60 (1990)	Present	ICRP 60 (1990)
Whole	5.5	6.0	0.2	1.3	5.7	7.3
Adult	4.1	4.8	0.1	0.8	4.2	5.6

Data from: ICRP, 2007

Values for adult and whole populations are shown, as well as the ICRP 1990 and 2007 values.

by the radiation. They are distinct from stochastic risks in that deterministic effects are measurable and can be predicted after specific levels of radiation. At radiation doses encountered in diagnostic departments, these effects were rarely encountered and almost considered irrelevant until the last two decades; however, with the advent of higher-dose procedures such as cardiac interventions and transjugular intrahepatic portosystemic stent shunting (TIPSS), where skin doses can be as high, deterministic changes, particularly within the skin, are being increasingly reported. An example of a progressive deterministic effect is shown in **Figure 4-16**.

As with stochastic changes, there are three main principles that should be applied to deterministic effects:

1. There is a threshold below which a clinically demonstrable effect will not occur. In other words, for a deterministic change to occur (e.g., skin reddening), a specific level of radiation must have been delivered (e.g., 2 Gy).

2. The level of the effect (e.g., the degree of skin reddening) is proportional to the radiation dose delivered.

3. Deterministic events occur following the irradiation of many cells.

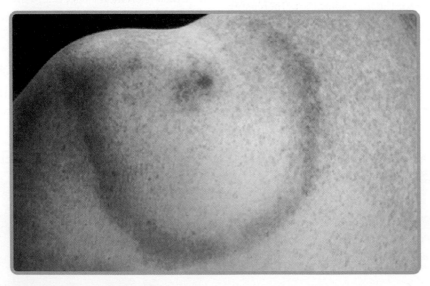

Figure 4-16 Example of a deterministic effect.
© zeckenrollen/Shutterstock.

Deterministic effects can be broken down into early or late effects. The *early effects* generally result from a number of cells being killed or removed following irradiation or as an inflammatory response. These early effects such as skin reddening (erythema) can occur within hours and are linked to capillary permeability and the release of histamine, with the effect being proportional to the dose received. Hair loss, hyperpigmentation, desquamation, and intestinal epithelial cell loss are other typical examples with some of these effects following from doses as low as 2 Gy.

Reactions that occur over a period of months and years after irradiation are known as *late effects* and include vascular insufficiency, skin necrosis, telangiectasia, ulceration, and cataract formation. These can be the direct result from cell loss, damage, or limited renewal or may be secondary to adjacent post-irradiation changes such as reduction in blood flow to the skin, leading to ulceration.

Examples of deterministic effects are given in **Table 4-5**, along with relevant threshold doses.

Factors Influencing Stochastic Risk or Deterministic Effects at Low-Dose Exposures

The mechanisms described above regarding DNA damage and chromosomal aberrations following direct exposure to a cell are the first part of the post-radiation story. However, it is very difficult to predict the eventual effect to the organism, even when the radiation type and dose are known, without considering a range of other factors that influence the degree of radiation damage and the risk of inducing a cancer. This section will consider these factors in order to understand for example why some cells are much more sensitive than others.

Radiosensitivity of the Cell

It is well known that certain cells react in a greater way to radiation than others; in other words, some cells are more radio sensitive than others. Even the most junior clinician or

Table 4-5 Deterministic effects with threshold doses

Effect	Dose (Gy)	Onset
Dermal atrophy (1st phase)	10	>12 weeks
Dermal atrophy (2nd phase)	10	>1 year
Dry desquamation	14	~ 4 weeks
Early transient erythema	2	Hours
Induration (invasive fibrosis)	10	-
Ischemic demal necrosis	18	>10 weeks
Late dermal necrosis	>12	>1 year
Late erythema	15	~ 8 -10 weeks
Main erythema	6	~ 10 days
Moist desquamation	18	~ 4 weeks
Permanent epilation	7	~ 1 week
Secondary ulceration	24	~ 6 weeks
Skin cancer	-	>5 years
Telangiectasia	10	>1 year
Temporary epilation	3	~ 3 weeks

Note: Dash (-) indicates not known

Data from: Koenig et al. 2001

technologist will be aware that breast, intestinal, and gonadal regions of the body are more sensitive to radiation than other regions. While it is commonly accepted that this is largely due to the proliferative nature of cells (how rapidly they divide), a concept that is generally (but not completely) true, this is not the whole story. Indeed, each proliferative cell is quite resistant to low levels of radiation for the majority of time; why this is, we will discuss this a little later.

For the time being, let us go back to the well-accepted principle that proliferative cells are more sensitive than cells that are not dividing. This idea was first proposed in 1906 by two radiobiologists, Bergonie and Tribondeau, who stated that *the radio sensitivity of cells is directly proportional to their level of reproductive activity (proliferation) and inversely proportional to their level of differentiation.*

There are some exceptions to this rule, namely oocytes and lymphocytes, which remain highly sensitive without dividing for reasons yet unknown, but generally, the proposal by Bergonie and Tribondeau holds true.

It is worth giving a practical example of this: In the small intestine, we have an array of different cell types. Some of these are rapidly dividing, and others are fully differentiated or mature, which means they have moved out of the proliferative stage. **Figure 4-17** shows a light microscopic cross-section of the small intestine; here, we can see the crypts of Lieberkuhn, which mainly contain a number of dividing cells that are not yet differentiated, i.e., they have not matured into a specific functional cell. As we move from the crypt to the villus—and most cells take this journey—these dividing cells become differentiated mature cells, one example being the enterocyte, which is responsible for nutrient absorption.

As we know, if a patient undergoes radiotherapy of the abdominal or pelvic regions, one of the

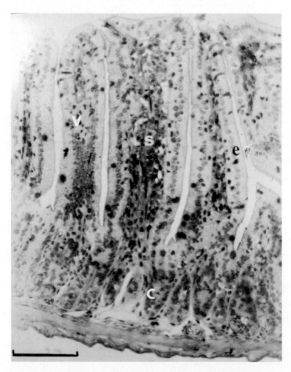

Figure 4-17 Light microscopic image of the small intestine. In the crypts (C), there are a number of dividing cells that are highly radiosensitive, but as they mature and move up the villus (V) and become highly differentiated, they become less responsive to radiation. Enterocytes (E) and stroma (S).

most important patient symptoms, such as diarrhea and vomiting, are related to the gastrointestinal tract. This is because the dividing cells within the crypt are highly sensitive to radiation and react strongly. However, the differentiated functional enterocytes within the villus are relatively resistant to radiation and shortly after irradiation look largely normal (**Figure 4-18**). However, at later time points when the damaged cryptal cells move into the villus compartment, the structure of the villus will change and the patient will exhibit symptoms (**Figure 4-19**). These temporal effects are discussed in some more detail under the kinetics section below.

Therefore, it should be clear that reproductive or proliferative cells are more sensitive to radiation than the functional differentiated cells with a couple of exceptions, named above. However, as stated above, this is not the whole story, since

a cell passing through the S part of the cell cycle (Figure 4-12) is relatively resistant to radiation compared with those passing through mitosis—and indeed, if one were to list the relative sensitivities in decreasing order, the sequence would be: mitosis, G_2, G_1 and S. The reasons for this are threefold:

1. During the mitotic portion of the cell cycle, there are fewer reparative agents.

2. The DNA material in mitosis is so close together that it is more difficult for reparative agents to get close to the damaged DNA to mediate repair processes following radiation insult.

3. There are more sulfhydryl-containing compounds outside mitosis. Sulfhydryl-containing compounds are free radical scavengers that help reduce the effects of reactive oxygen species on the cell.

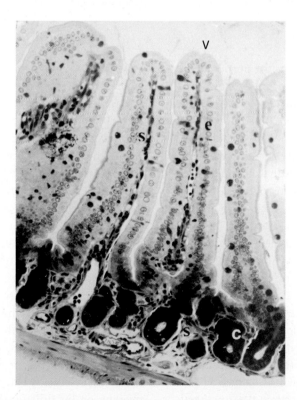

Figure 4-18 Light microscopic image of the small intestine shortly 6 hours following a radiation insult. Note how the crypts have been affected by the radiation; however, the villi look largely unscathed. Enterocytes (e) and lamina propria (l) are shown.

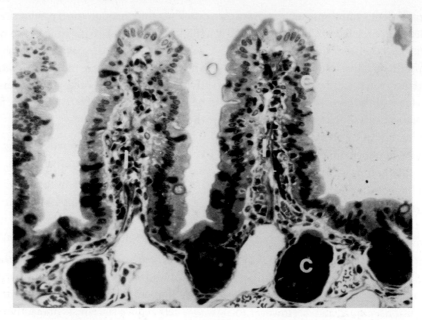

Figure 4-19 Light microscopic image of the small intestine shortly following a radiation insult (3 days post-irradiation). Compared with Figure 4-21, note how the crypts and villi have been effected by the radiation.

If mitosis is the radio-sensitive portion of the cell cycle, it is worth exploring the proportion of time within the cell cycle that is occupied by the mitosis. Fortunately (in terms of radio sensitivity), it is small. For example, if one considers the cell cycle of one the most rapidly dividing cells—the enterocytes within the intestinal epithelium—mitosis takes about 20 minutes of the 15 hours required for a completed cell cycle—about 0.02% of the entire process. This means that cells, even if they are reproductive, are at their most radio sensitive only for a brief period of time.

Kinetics

From the discussion above focusing on the small intestine, we can see that following a single irradiation event, a portion of the cells within the proliferative zone such as those located within the crypts of Lieberkuhn will be damaged (if the dose is high enough) and cells in the functional compartment will not. Therefore, immediately after exposure the irradiated individual may not experience obvious symptoms, since the non-affected cells within the villus, for example, are continuing to absorb nutrients and provide secretions. It is only when the affected cells within the crypt move into the functional component (e.g., within the villus) that the symptoms of diarrhea and vomiting become obvious.

To understand the timing of this transition within a specific tissue, one must understand the **_kinetics_** of that tissue. Continuing with the intestinal context, there are pluripotent stem cells located near the base of the crypt, which have the potential to produce cells that will continue to divide and produce one of the several types of intestinal cells such as the enterocyte—the cell responsible for intestinal absorption. This division of enterocyte precursor cells will continue, but in addition, these precursors will move towards the villus, eventually entering the villus compartment becoming fully functional, differentiated, non-dividing cells. These cells will continue to move up the villus, a little like people riding on an escalator, until they are ejected at the villous tip. The time taken from the bottom of the crypt to the base of the villus is around 3 to 4 days, with a similar (additional) time from the base to the top of the villus. These time points are important in context of the radiation response, since it is only when damaged cells reach the villus, or if there are so many killed cells within the crypt that the enterocyte population within the villus is not sufficiently replenished, that the irradiated individual will start to express the symptoms. As the villus has fewer fully functional cells, it starts to shrink in size. This can be seen in Figures 4-17, 4-18, and 4-19, where we can see the non-irradiated intestine (Figure 4-17) and the intestine at 6 (Figure 4-18) hours and 3 days after 5 Gy gamma irradiation (Figure 4-19). The effect on the villus at 3 days is very apparent, while little change (within the villus) is evident at the earlier time point.

Finally, with regard to the intestinal example and Figures 4-17 through 4-19, these changes are following much higher doses of radiation than we will encounter in diagnostic imaging departments, and it is unlikely that light microscopic changes would be evident in the intestine below 50 mGy. However, the example provided serves to demonstrate the importance of kinetics to the timing when post-radiation symptoms are expressed.

Presence of Oxygen

Increased presence of oxygen within irradiated cells will increase the effect of radiation. The reason behind this has been alluded to previously in the section describing reactive species, where we described the peroxyl free radical, which is created when the hydrogen free radical combines with oxygen. This free radical can live longer than the other free radicals and therefore cause damage farther from its site of origin. The formation of the peroxyl free radical is much more likely to occur when increased oxygen is available. The degree of increased radio sensitivity associated with oxygen is known as the *oxygen enhancement ratio* (OER), which has a value of ~2:1 (**Figure 4-20**).

The OER is of much interest in radiation therapy since a solid tumor with little access to oxygen can require radiation doses 2 to 3 times higher for a similar effect when a tissue is well oxygenated. This has paved the way for a whole field of research around angiogenesis, which is the formation of new blood vessels so that increased oxygen can be brought to hypoxic tumors. The OER, however, decreases with decreasing dose, and due to the lack of research looking at very low doses, the relevance of this phenomenon to diagnostic exposures is unknown.

Dose Rate

When the time over which a dose of radiation is delivered is increased, generally a reduction of radiation effect is reported due to opportunities for repair and adaptive mechanisms as described earlier. This is well known and is called the ***dose rate effect factor*** (DREF); supporters of the LNT Model highlight the importance of applying the DREF when estimating the effects of radiation at low doses by extrapolating from high-dose exposures. While the dose rate is a critically important determinant of radiation effect in high doses of radiation, such as those delivered in radiotherapy, there is little evidence describing its relevance in diagnostic levels of exposure.

Radioprotectants and Radiosensitizers

Radioprotectants and radiosensitizers are exogenous or endogenous agents that reduce or enhance the effects of radiation. Radioprotectants can work at a number of levels, in that they can reduce oxygen consumption, scavenge free radicals, boost repair mechanisms, and modulate inflammatory and death pathways (Koukourakis 2012). Producing effective radioprotectants has gained much interest from a variety of stakeholders, in particular, the air travel industry, the US military, and radiation therapy professionals, where the aim for the latter is to protect normal healthy tissue from the deleterious effects of radiation, while maintaining tumoricidal effects. Amifostine, the

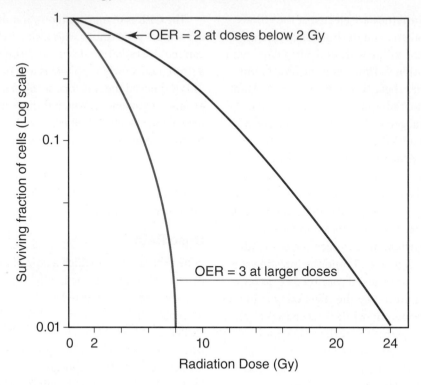

Figure 4-20 The oxygen enhancement ratio (OER). The blue curve indicates the lesser radiation doses required to kill cells compared with the red curve.

only clinically accepted radioprotectant, works by scavenging free radicals and alleviating some of the reactive oxygen species effects detailed earlier in this chapter. Another investigational agent, W-2721, one of the most effective radioprotectants, works on the same level and reduces the toxic effects of radiation by a factor of 2; however, the side effects of nausea, vomiting, and hypotension are severe.

Radiosensitizers, on the other hand, enhance the effects of radiation, and as discussed, one of the most effective radiosensitizers is the increased presence of oxygen, leading to a greater production of peroxyl free radicals. In radiation therapy, the ideal agent would be able to substantially increase the effects of radiation within the tumor with no side effects on normal tissue; however, this ideal agent does not as yet exist. Current radiosensitizers utilize a variety of mechanisms, including

increasing the production of free radicals, decreasing DNA repair, promoting cell cycle arrest, and targeting enzymes required for DNA metabolism. An agent that is clinically one of the most effective, 5-fluorouracil, has proven to potentially increase radiation effects by a factor of 3 or more (Byfield 1989). This agent works as an analogue of uracil (one of the bases within RNA), thus interfering with RNA synthesis.

Changes in Non-Irradiated Cells

The focus in the section above looking at the mechanisms of changes within the irradiated cells fails to consider that changes may occur within non-irradiated cells as a result of the radiation exposure. These changes fall into two categories: genomic instability and bystander effects.

Genomic Instability

Genomic instability occurs in the offspring of irradiated cells. This is distinct from mutations that are immediately apparent within the first generation of offspring, and also distinct from the type of instability described above in the progression stage of the development of cancer following irradiation. Rather, this is an instability that will be apparent within the genes of the offspring of irradiated cells, but will not manifest itself as a biologically important change until many generations later. The types of changes that can eventually occur include chromosomal aberrations and genetic mutations potentially manifesting themselves as a malignant transformation, although this type of transformation appears to be very rare. The instability can occur with either low- or high-LET radiation, and at low and high radiation doses, although the effect becomes saturated with the higher doses. However, the evidence to date regarding genomic instability is largely *in vitro* (in cell cultures) and while some data are available for genomic instability in mouse models following irradiation, its presence within humans has yet to be proven.

Bystander Effect

The bystander effect occurs when non-irradiated cells close to the radiation field undergo change even though they were not directly exposed. This was first shown in 1992 (Nagasawa & Little, 1992), where chromosomal aberrations were shown in 20–40% of cells exposed to alpha particles, even though only 0.1–1% of cells were actually directly exposed. This finding has since been shown by a number of different research teams, and it is proposed that the changes occur following the release of chemical agents, such as cytokines, by the irradiated population with increased frequency of changes occurring at very low levels of radiation. The involvement of the *p53* gene within the irradiated cells and the generation of reactive oxidative species are all likely mediating agents.

The type of change within bystander cells is different from those cells directly exposed to radiation, with about 90% of the change being point mutations, unlike the predominant partial or total gene deletions mainly encountered within directly irradiated cells.

Epigenetics

It is possible that changes can occur within DNA that do not result in altering the sequence of DNA bases. Such changes are described within the field of *epigenetics* and can manifest for example as changes to the methylation pattern within adenine or cytosine bases. While DNA sequences may remain unaffected, such epigenetic changes can have an impact upon gene expression. It is accepted that environmental influences can affect the *epigenome*, particularly during developmental periods of humans such as gestation, early years of one's life, and puberty; however, the effect of radiation on the epigenome has not been fully explored (Dauer et al. 2010). Nonetheless, some early work has demonstrated that high doses of radiation can lead to epigenetic changes, resulting in increased cancer risks. Research into lower-dose effects on the epigenome is required.

Effects of Radiation on Children, Embryos, and Fetuses

Before completing this chapter, some consideration must be given to the fact that children and fetuses are more susceptible to radiation effects compared with adults. This is due to a number of reasons, but not least is that their cells are more proliferative (so a greater proportion are passing through mitosis at any given time point); also, they will generally live for more years post-exposure than adults, which offers a greater opportunity to express any long-term effects such as cancer, and repair mechanisms are not so well developed as in adults. The NRPB (2011) provides data suggesting that the increased sensitivity of a young child can be up to 10 times that of elderly individual.

With specific reference to the unborn child, it is important to clarify some facts around this, as this is often a contentious issue for parents and clinicians. The first point worth noting is that a fetus in utero probably has the same level of risk of radiation-induced cancer as a young child, which is 3 times that of the whole population. It is important to note that there are certain gestation periods that are more sensitive than others. In particular, from 8 to 15 weeks is the most sensitive time frame, as this is where the period of maximum organogenesis and central nervous system development occurs. While in animals there appears to be a threshold of around 100 mGy for a deleterious effect, from data provided by the Japanese bomb victims, in humans this threshold appears to be closer to 300 mGy. It has been suggested that there can be a drop of 25 IQ points for every 1 Gy received during this gestational period; however, the impact of any reduction in IQ with doses below 100 mGy would be clinically irrelevant. Finally, there are recent data that have demonstrated the lethal effects of radiation prior to the conceptus being implanted, but it is calculated that the number of such events at doses below 100 mGy would be very low. Once again, this topic has been very well reviewed by the ICRP and the reader is directed to ICRP 90 (ICRP 2003) for a fuller treatment.

Summary of Key Concepts

1. **Stochastic and deterministic effects.** The first thing to note when one considers the impact of radiation on biological tissue is that the effects can be divided into two main categories: **stochastic effects**, which are focused on the risks associated with inducing certain effects such as cancer within the exposed individual and hereditary changes apparent in the future offspring of individuals exposed to radiation, and **deterministic effects**, which are direct effects on the cells that are irradiated, resulting in symptoms such as skin reddening or ulceration.

2. **Factors and complexities behind describing stochastic changes.** Stochastic effects are concerned with the risks associated with radiation exposure, such as cancer within the exposed individual or hereditary changes passed on to an individual's offspring. There is no guarantee whatsoever that these changes will occur following irradiation.

3. **Changes that occur leading to deterministic effect.** Deterministic effects are symptomatic changes that occur with the cells that are directly affected by the radiation. They are distinct from stochastic risks in that deterministic effects are measurable and can be predicted after specific levels of radiation.

4. **Factors that affect radio sensitivity.** The mechanisms regarding DNA damage and chromosomal aberrations following direct exposure to a cell are the first part of the post-radiation story. However, it is very difficult to predict the eventual effect to the organism, even when the radiation type and dose are known, without considering a range of other factors that influence the degree of radiation damage and the risk of inducing a cancer. We must consider these factors in order to understand for example why some cells are much more sensitive than others.

5. **Radio sensitivities of children and fetuses in utero.** The fact is that children and individuals in utero are more susceptible to radiation effects compared with adults. This is due to a number of reasons, but not least is that their cells are more proliferative (so a greater proportion are passing through mitosis at any given time point). Also, they will generally live for more years post-exposure than adults, so have a greater opportunity to express any long-term effects such as cancer, and their repair mechanisms are not so well developed as in adults.

Discussion Questions

1. Contrast stochastic with deterministic effects.
2. Discuss the factors that contribute and impact stochastic effects.
3. Discuss the factors that affect radio sensitivity of cells and tissues.

References

BEIR. Health risks from exposure to low levels of radiation: BEIR VII, Phase 2. Committee to Assess Health Risks from Exposures to Low levels of Ionizing Radiation, Board of Radiation Effects, Research Division on Earth and Life Studies, National Research Council of the National Academies. Washington, DC: National Academies Press; 2006.

Brennan PC, Carr KE, Seed T, McCullough JS. Acute and protracted radiation effects on small intestinal morphological parameters. *Int J Radiat Biol*. 1998;73:691–698.

Brenner DJ, Hall EJ. Cancer risks from CT scans: Now we have data, what next? *Radiology*. 2012;265:330–331.

Byfield JE. 5-Fluorouracil radiation sensitization — A brief review. *Investigational New Drugs*. 1989;7:111–116.

Committee on Medical Aspects of Radiation in Environment (COMARE). Parents occupationally exposed to radiation prior to conception of their children. A review of the evidence concerning the incidence of cancer in their children. Seventh Report. Chilton, UK: National Radiological Protection Board; 2002.

Committee on Medical Aspects of Radiation in Environment (COMARE). Review of pregnancy outcomes following preconceptual exposure to radiation. Eighth Report Chilton, UK: National Radiological Protection Board; 2004.

Dauer L, Brooks AL, Hoel DG, Morgan WF, Stram D, Tran PH. Review and evaluation of updated research on the health effects associated with low-dose ionizing radiation. *Radiat Prot Dosimetry*. 2010;140:103–136.

International Commission of Radiological Protection (ICRP). Biological effects after prenatal irradiation (embryo and fetus). ICRP publications 90. *Ann ICRP*. 2003;33(1/2).

International Commission of Radiological Protection (ICRP). The 2007 Recommendations of the International Commission on Radiological Protection. ICRP Publication 103. *Ann ICRP*. 2007;37(2-4).

Koenig TR, Wolff D, Mettler FA, Wagner LK. Skin injuries from fluoroscopically guided procedures. Part 1, characteristics of radiation injury. *AJR Am J Roentgenol*. 2001;177:13–20.

Koukourakis MI. Radiation damage and radioprotectants: New concepts in the era of molecular medicine. *Br J Radiol*. 2012;85:313–330.

Munro TR. The relative radio sensitivity of the nucleus and cytoplasm of Chinese hamster fibroblasts. *Radiat Res*. 1970;42:451–470.

Nagasawa H, Little JB. Induction of sister chromatid exchanges by extremely low doses of alpha-particles. *Cancer Res*. 1992;52:6394–6396.

Pearce MS, Salotti JA, Little MP, McHugh K, Lee C, Kim KP, et al. Radiation exposure from CT scans in childhood and subsequent risk of leukaemia and brain tumours: A retrospective cohort study. *Lancet*. 2012;380:499–505.

Pierce DA, Shimizu Y, Preston DL, Vaeth M, Mabuchi K. Studies of the mortality of atomic bomb survivors. Report 12, Part 1. Cancer: 1950–1990. *Radiat Res*. 1996;146:1–27.

Preston DL, Ron E, Tokuoka S, Funamoto S, Nishi N, Soda M, Mabuchi K, Kodama K. Solid cancer incidence in atomic bomb survivors: 1958–1990. *Radiat Res*. 2007;168:1–64.

Wall BF, Haylock, R, Jansen JTM, Hillier MC, Hart D, Shrimpton PC. Radiation risks from medical X-ray examinations as a function of the age and sex of the patient. Chilton, UK: Health Protection Agency Centre for Radiation, Chemical and Environmental Hazards HPA-CRCE-028; 2011. (Available at https://www.gov.uk/government/uploads/system/uploads/attachment_data/file/340147/HPA-CRCE-028_for_website.pdf; Retrieved August 17, 2015.)

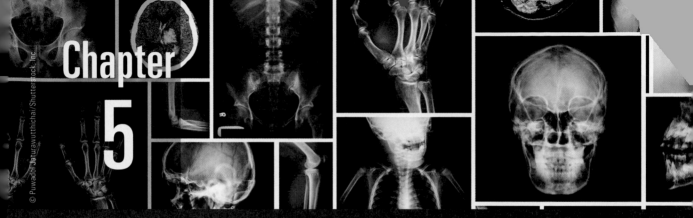

Chapter 5

Radiation Protection Practice

Outline

- Introduction
- Dose Risks in Diagnostic Imaging
- Justification
  - What is justification?
  - How is justification implemented?
- Optimization
  - What is optimization?
  - Why might non-optimization be evident?
  - Non-implementation of findings in the literature
  - Optimization initiatives
- Optimization and cost
- Optimization: Image quality versus diagnostic efficacy
- Radiation Dose Limits
- Radiation Detection and Measurement
  - Thermoluminescent dosimetry (TLDs)
  - Dose-area product meters (DAPs)
  - Solid-state meters
  - Radiochromic film
- References

Objectives

On completion of this chapter, you should be able to:

1. Identify the cancer risks for common, non-fluoroscopic and non-CT examinations.

2. State and discuss two well-known principles have been adopted within legislative, regulatory, and advisory documents to promote keeping the risk to patients as low as reasonably achievable.

3. Discuss the essential considerations of the principles of justification and optimization.

4. Explain briefly what is meant by the term "non-optimization."

5. Identify new technologies that play a role in dose optimization.

6. Discuss a number of optimization initiatives.

7. Differentiate between *image quality* and *diagnostic efficacy* in the optimization process.

8. Explain what is meant by dose limits.

9. State the dose limits for occupational individuals and members of the public.

10. Identify and discuss four methods of radiation detection and measurement.

Introduction

Every radiation exposure in medical imaging departments will introduce a risk of inducing a cancer, but it should present a benefit to the patient as long as the exposure is justified. The responsibility of the radiographer or radiologic clinician is to ensure that the radiation dose is minimized and the benefit maximized for each examination that takes place. The "as low as reasonably achievable" (ALARA) principle should be applied each time we expose the patient, meaning that the radiation risk is kept to a low level, but not to the extent where the diagnostic efficacy of the examination is compromised—and techniques and technologies have been developed around this objective.

But there is more: Systems and policies must also in place to ensure that the radiation dose to individuals who are *not* patients, but who nonetheless may be exposed as a result of diagnostic examinations in their workplace, is also kept as low as possible. Such individuals include healthcare workers, people transporting patients (e.g., first responders, family members, etc.), and other people in the vicinity at the time of the exposure. In this context, radiation protection standards have evolved.

Three main systems are in place to maintain good protective standards: (1) *justification* to make sure that there is a good reason for performing each x-ray examination; (2) *optimization,* which will promote the best possible methods and technologies for imaging the patient at the lowest dose; and (3) *dose limits* for those other individuals who may inadvertently (and without any direct benefit) undergo radiation exposures during patient examinations. With regard to dose limits, it is very important to highlight that these limits or dose constraints *do not apply to the patient*; if the examination dose is justified, then that dose is delivered. Admittedly, we do have diagnostic reference levels for patients to offer guidance levels for doses that should be administered, but these are not dose limits (**Figure 5-1**).

The three principles of justification, optimization, and dose limits are the focus of a number of recent legislative, regulatory, and advisory documents addressing radiation protection. For example, in the European Council Directive 97/43/EURATOM *On Health Protection of Individuals Against the Dangers of Ionizing Radiation in Relation to Medical Exposure and Repealing Directive 84/466/Euratom* (ECD 1997; Teunan 1998), which has been adopted into national legislation in a number of European states, articles 3 and 4 are dedicated (respectively) to justification and optimization. In the European Council Directive 96/29/Euratom *Laying Down Basic Safety Standards for the Protection of the Health of Workers and the General Public Against the Dangers Arising from Ionising Radiation* (1996), again incorporated within national legislation across Europe, Chapter I of Title IV deals with justification and optimization, whereas Chapter II of the same Title focuses on describing specific dose limits. These and other legislative or advisory documents will be discussed throughout this chapter (ARPANSA 2008; ICRP 2007).

Finally, a fundamental component of good radiation protection standards is **effective dosimetry**; i.e., methods of measuring radiation doses to patients, workers and other exposed individuals. These methods range from personal dosimetry devices, which are worn at all times by individuals working with radiation, to the more sophisticated electronic dosimeters—a fundamental tool for quality assurance procedures ensuring radiation protection standards. Dosimetric methods will be considered toward the end of this chapter.

Dose Risks in Diagnostic Imaging

Before appropriate radiation protection methods can be described, we need to put into context the risks that are associated with medical imaging. As has been discussed elsewhere, the risk of inducing a cancer using doses typically encountered in diagnostic imaging departments is low. The majority of non-fluoroscopic and non-CT examinations involve effective doses somewhere between 0.0001 mSv for a dorsiplantar projection of the foot, up to 0.5 mSv for an anteroposterior (AP) projection of the abdomen. These doses for a 20-year-old

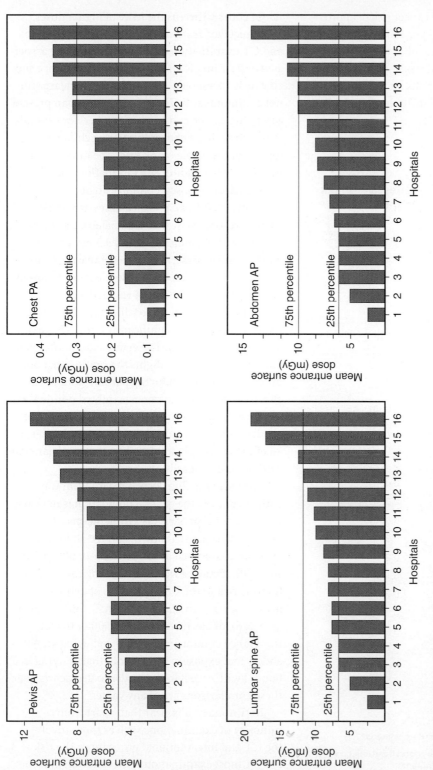

Figure 5-1 The 75th percentile demonstrates DRL values for a number of examinations.

Data from: Johnston DA, Brennan PC. Br J Radiol. 2000 Apr;73(868):396–402.

individual equate to a fatal cancer risk of approximately 1 per billion and 3.5 per 100,000, respectively (yet we must still remember to take great care in assessing individual risks). A summary of effective doses and cancer risks for these types of examinations are provided in **Tables 5-1** and **5-2**), respectively (Wall et al. 2011).

Table 5-1 A summary of effective doses for common non-fluoroscopic and non-CT examinations

Radiograph	103 (mSv)
Abdomen AP	0.43
Both hips AP	0.19
Cervical spine AP	0.018
Cervical spine Lat	0.012
Chest Lat	0.038
Chest PA	0.014
Femur AP	0.011
Femur Lat	0.001
Foot (dorsi-plantar)	0.0001
Foot (olique)	0.0001
Head AP	0.033
Head Lat	0.016
Head PA	0.02
Knee AP	0.0001
Knee Lat	0.0001
Lumbar spine AP	0.39
Lumbar spine Lat	0.21
Lumbo-sacral joint Lat	0.17
Pelvis AP	0.28
Shoulder (Axial)	0.004
Shoulder AP	0.007
Single hip AP	0.087
Thoracic spine AP	0.24
Thoracic spine Lat	0.14

AP = Antero - posterior

PA = Postero - anterior

Lat = Lateral (average of left and right lateral)

HPA 2011, page 6 © Crown copyright. Reproduced with permission of Public Health England.

Of course, there is the issue of higher doses being received from interventional investigations and CT examinations, notwithstanding the associated deterministic effects that may occur once specific dose thresholds are exceeded (which are still not commonplace). These higher doses can present a risk that can be considerably higher; for example, risk of inducing a cancer to a young child undergoing CT of the whole trunk might be in excess of 1 in 1000. Other high-dose examinations can deliver typical effective doses; coronary angiography and whole-trunk CT can produce doses of 3.9 mSv and 10 mSv, respectively, with associated cancer risks in a 50-year-old male of 1.9 and 3.5 per 10,000. A more complete description of effective doses and cancer risks for these higher dose examinations are given in **Tables 5-3** and **5-4** respectively.

You will see from these tables that the lifetime risk of cancer varies significantly between ages and gender. The level of variation depends on the examination type. This highlights the caution that one must apply when employing parameters such as effective dose and detriment-weighted nominal risk coefficients, which, averages the parameters over genders, ages, and indeed different populations in an effort to provide single values that clinicians can work with more easily.

Presenting such risks in a meaningful way to patients or even the general population is not easy, since the concept of risk is a difficult one. If we take the cancer risk following an AP abdominal exposure, estimated at roughly 1 in 30,000 (3.5 in 100,000), it may be worth comparing this with the lifetime risk to the US population of dying from heart disease (1 in 5), cancer (1 in 7), falling down (1 in 246), or electrocution (1 in 5000). In fact, the chance of inducing a cancer following an AP abdominal exposure is similar to that of dying in a flood. I will leave it to the reader to decide whether these comparisons are of any value.

In summary, it is clear that, apart from a minority of examinations such as those involving CT and interventional procedures, the risk is low for most examinations. The question must be

Table 5-2 A summary of cancer risks for common non-fluoroscopic and non-CT examinations

Examination	Sex	Age at exposure (y)									
		0–9	10–19	20–29	30–39	40–49	50–59	60–69	70–79	80–89	90–99
Head	M	12	8.5	5.9	4.4	3.2	2.2	1.3	0.6	0.3	0
(AP+PA+Lat)	F	11	7.7	5.3	3.7	2.9	1.8	1	0.5	0.2	0
Cervical spine	M	2.7	1.9	1.2	0.9	0.6	0.4	0.2	0.1	0.1	0
(AP+Lat)	F	6.2	3.7	2.2	1.3	0.8	0.5	0.3	0.2	0.1	0
Chest	M	1.3	1.1	0.9	0.8	0.7	0.6	0.5	0.3	0.1	0
(PA)	F	1.9	1.6	1.4	1.3	1.2	1.1	0.8	0.5	0.2	0
Thoracic spine	M	30	24	20	17	16	13	9.7	6.1	2.6	0.1
(AP+Lat)	F	65	50	40	34	30	25	18	11	4.2	0.1
Abdomen	M	55	44	35	27	21	15	9.3	4.8	1.7	0.1
(AP)	F	49	39	31	25	20	14	9.4	5.2	1.8	0
Pelvis	M	31	25	20	16	13	9.4	5.9	3	1	0
(AP)	F	24	19	16	13	10	7.8	5.2	2.9	1	0
Lumbar spine	M	72	56	43	34	26	19	12	6.1	2.3	0.1
(AP+Lat)	F	65	51	41	32	26	19	12	6.8	2.4	0.1
Knee	M	0.011	0.008	0.005	0.004	0.003	0.002	0.001	0	0	0
(AP+Lat)	F	0.008	0.006	0.004	0.003	0.002	0.001	0.001	0	0	0
Foot	M	0.0049	0.0035	0.0024	0.0017	0.0012	0.0007	0.0004	0.0002	0	0
(AP+Lat)	F	0.0036	0.0026	0.0019	0.0013	0.0009	0.0006	0.0003	0.0002	0	0

Table 5-3 A summary of effective doses for fluoroscopic and CT examinations

Examination	103 (mSv)
Coronary angiography	3.9
Femoral angiography	2.3
CT Abdomen	5.6
CT Abdomen + Pelvis	6.7
CT Chest	6.6
CT Chest + Abdomen + Pelvis	10

HPA 2011 © Crown copyright. Reproduced with permission of Public Health England.

asked, however: If the risk is already low, is it still important or worth the effort to further protect the patient (or staff) by having radiation protection standards? While we will look at this question in more depth as this chapter progresses, the simple response is to ask ourselves that if we *can* produce images of equal diagnostic efficacy at lower risks to the patient (even if that risk is already very low), as radiographers and clinicians, do we not have that responsibility to the patient? Particularly if we can reduce (or even remove) exposures at minimum (or no) extra cost or effort?

Two well-known principles have been adopted within legislative, regulatory, and advisory documents to promote keeping the risk to patients as low as reasonably achievable: *Justification* and *Optimization*. Each of these principles will now be considered.

Justification

What is Justification?

Each x-ray exposure must have a good medical reason for performing it. Irradiating individuals introduces a risk, yet this risk is acceptable if it is outweighed by the benefit that is provided diagnostically by the resultant image or images. In other words, there must be good *justification* regarding the exposure; in the words of the International Commission on Radiological Protection (ICRP 2007), it should "*do more good than harm for the*

patient." The whole issue of justification has been well argued by Matthews et al. (2008), which will be referenced in this section.

First, let us look at how legislation or guidance documents define justification. In the European Council Directive 97/43/EURATOM, Article 3 (ECD 1997; Teunan 1998) defines justification thus:

> *Medical exposure … shall show a sufficient net benefit, weighing the total potential diagnostic or therapeutic benefits it produces, including the direct health benefits to an individual and the benefits to society, against the individual detriment that the exposure might cause, taking into account the efficacy, benefits and risks of available alternative techniques having the same objective but involving no or less exposure to ionizing radiation.*

The same document makes it quite clear that if the exposure cannot be justified, then it should be prohibited.

In its *Initiative to Reduce Unnecessary Radiation Exposure from Medical Imaging* (FDA 2012), the Food and Drug Administration within the United States presents a similar definition of justification:

> *The imaging procedure should be judged to do more good than harm (e.g., detriment associated with radiation induced cancer or tissue effects) to the individual patient. Therefore, all examinations using ionizing radiation should be performed only when necessary to answer a medical question, treat a disease, or guide a procedure. The clinical indication and patient medical history should be carefully considered before referring a patient for any x-ray examination.*

Other documents from a variety of other countries, including Australia in its *Radiation Protection in the Medical Applications of Ionizing Radiation* (ARPNSA 2008), similarly highlight the importance of justification (and optimization).

Table 5-4 A summary of cancer risks for fluoroscopic and CT examinations

Examination	Sex	Age at exposure (y)									
		0–9	10–19	20–29	30–39	40–49	50–59	60–69	70–79	80–89	90–99
Coronary angiography	M	330	290	250	230	210	190	150	94	41	2.1
	F	430	390	370	360	370	330	270	170	66	1.7
Femoral angiography	M	280	220	170	140	110	85	56	32	14	1.6
	F	210	170	140	110	110	73	45	24	8.8	0.5
CT head	M	250	190	130	100	80	57	36	20	9	1.2
	F	190	140	100	77	71	46	27		4.8	0.3
CT chest	M	530	440	350	300	260	220	160	99	42	2.2
	F	1100	860	680	560	490	390	290	180	68	1.7
CT abdomen	M	670	530	400	310	240	170	110	56	21	1.5
	F	610	480	380	300	240	170	110	59	20	0.6
CT abdomen + pelvis	M	850	670	520	410	320	230	150	78	29	1.9
	F	740	590	470	370	310	230	150	80	28	0.8
CT chest + abdomen + pelvis	M	960	780	630	520	440	340	240	140	58	3.3
	F	1500	1100	910	740	640	500	260	210	80	2.1

HPA 2011 © Crown copyright. Reproduced with permission of Public Health England.

It should be stressed that a number of the well-known perspectives on justification rely on the details contained within the ICRP 103 (ICRP 2007) recommendations.

How is Justification Implemented?

Justification is implemented at two main levels: First, at a broad level, the use of a specific examination or a specific imaging tool must be considered justifiable by an industry and/or governmental accreditation board before it can be adopted by health services, screening programs, imaging departments, insurance providers, and so on. The second point of justification is specific to each patient: Before any individual exposure takes place, the radiographer or clinician must be satisfied that there is a good medical benefit for providing such an exposure. Both broad and specific implementation will be considered here. Of course, it can be argued (as in ICRP [2007] and Matthews et al. [2008]) that there is a more fundamental level of justification, which is that the introduction of x-rays at all must demonstrate a net benefit compared with any detriment.

Broad Implementation of Justification

In the European legislation (1997), justification at the broader level should be evident (1) whenever *a new or alternative method* of method imaging that uses ionizing radiation is being proposed, and (2) for *all existing methods when new data regarding efficacy has been made available.*

When a new or alternative method of imaging is being proposed, it must be carefully evaluated to make sure that an overall benefit will accrue to the population on whom this technology or technique will be used. A modern example may help explain this: In most countries (**Figure 5-2**), breast cancer screening uses mammography as the first-line tool via 2-dimensional cranio-caudal (CC) and medio-lateral oblique (MLO) images taken of each breast (**Figures 5-3**).

Over the last few years, there has been increasing evidence that a new modality—digital breast tomosynthesis (DBT), which presents the images

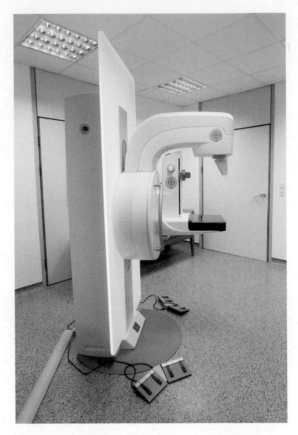

Figure 5-2 Typical mammographic equipment used in breast screen imaging.
© zlikovec/Shutterstock

in discrete slices or as 3-dimensional images (Alakhras et al. 2013; **Figure 5-4**) may offer important benefits in terms of increased cancer detection rates and lower numbers of false positives (e.g., cases where an anomaly is identified by the radiologist as a cancer that later proved to be normal or benign tissue). A study by Skaane et al. (2013) involving over 12,000 women whose breast images were interpreted using mammography alone or mammography combined with DBT concluded that there were significant benefits when the new approach was used with this population of women.

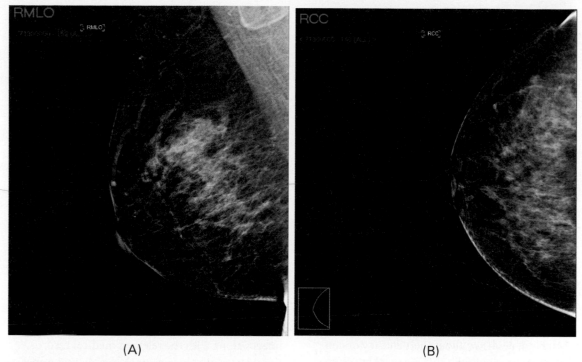

(A)   (B)

Figure 5-3 CC (A) and MLO (B) images typically produced for each woman presenting at a breast screening clinic.

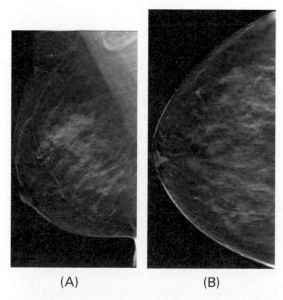

(A)   (B)

Figure 5-4 (A) MLO projection of the breast (digital). (B) CC projection of the breast.

While these results and others looking at DBT clearly offer a good basis for a justifying this new technology, more data are required before a full justification to replace mammography is presented. These data would include:

- Full radiation dose assessment so any increased risk to women being examined is understood
- Impact on radiographic and radiologic work practices, since longer examination times may result in fewer women being x-rayed
- Full health economic assessment, to make sure that a specific population's financial situation can support implementation of this new tool
- Whether the new tool will actually replace the old or serve as an adjunct technology

It is also important to make sure that evidence is relevant to the population to which a new technology or technique is being introduced. Again using the mammography example, while there is encouraging data on DBT coming out of the United States, Europe, and Australia, will this be useful to women in the Middle East and Southeast Asia, for example, where the types of cancer and the age profile of women with breast cancer can be very different from those in the Western world? It is often critically important that individual states or countries introduce their own evidence to support a change in practice or equipment when their circumstances are different, rather than simply (and conveniently) relying on data that has been produced from elsewhere.

While rigorous studies are usually performed to explore whether a novel practice or technology should be implemented, often there is less emphasis on justifying current activities. Let us remind ourselves again that, according to at least one set of legislation, "existing types of practices involving medical exposure may be reviewed whenever new, important evidence about their efficacy or consequences is acquired." This means that if a new, scientifically robust study demonstrates that the *current* method of x-raying an abdomen in the AP position is not optimal and might be improved if a mobile patient was placed in the posteroanterior (PA) position, then the current practice of using AP positioning should be reviewed. Unfortunately, in the experience of this author, review of common radiographic procedures rarely takes place, even though evidence does emerge from time to time of potentially better ways of x-raying our patients. This discussion does cross over to optimization of techniques, and the argument of needing to have systems in place to revisit long-established procedures will continue. A good example of an effective review system that covers UK health delivery much more broadly is the one implemented by the National Institute for Health and Care Excellence (NICE), where specific topics are referred to NICE for consideration; these are effectively reviewed, and recommendations for best practice are provided based on the latest evidence. It is difficult to see how current radiographic practices can be thoroughly justifiable without a similar, albeit more focused, system of review. With the risks associated with radiographic exposures setting up an effective review system should be, in the opinion of the author, an issue of priority for international, national, and local professional and regulatory bodies.

Individual Implementation of Justification

According to the European legislation (ECD 1997; Teunan 1998), "all individual medical exposures shall be justified in advance, taking into account the specific objectives of the exposure and the characteristics of the individual involved." This level of justification occurs, therefore, each time we examine a patient radiologically, and it means that before any exposure is performed, a good clinical reason for that exposure must be provided. To facilitate justification, the European legislation is clear that all relevant prior details, such as previous images along with the relevant medical records, should be available and considered so that unnecessary exposures are avoided.

So who is responsible for making sure that each individual exposure is justified? While this responsibility may vary from jurisdiction to jurisdiction, at least in a number of European states, this role appears to fall into two categories: The person requesting the exposure and the person with the responsibility to perform the examination. The person requesting the exposure must provide sufficient clinical reason for the procedure. In the UK and Ireland in the early 2000s, to make sure that referrers such as general practitioners (GPs) and hospital-based medical doctors were equipped with the necessary information to allow an appropriate referral, each received a set of referral guidelines (Royal College of Radiologists 2003). These guidelines have been subsequently updated (Royal College of Radiologists 2007).

While in the United States, according to the FDA, the referrer has the primary responsibility for justifying the examination, in Europe the second category of persons—those with responsibility for delivering the examination—is also critically important to the individual justification process. This importance was highlighted when it was shown in three European member states that significant numbers of medical exposures for common radiographic examinations did not have sufficient referral justification (Bell and McLaughlin 2001; Triantopoulou et al. 2005; Morris-Stiff et al. 2006). The European legislation therefore specifically refers to an individual described as a *practitioner* who will be involved in the justification process, that practitioner being defined as a "medical doctor, dentist, or other health professional who is entitled to take clinical responsibility for an individual medical exposure." It has been debated as to whether the radiographer or radiologic technologist is in the position to be either the practitioner or someone who acts as an interface between the prescriber and the practitioner, particularly when the clinical information provided by the prescriber is insufficient. Whatever the official role might be—and this will vary from one locality to another—it is clear that the person who is responsible for delivering the radiation, most likely the radiographer or technologist, will contribute importantly to the justification process since, ultimately, according to 97/43/EURATOM (ECD 1997; Teunan 1998), "if an exposure cannot be justified it should be prohibited."

The emphasis above has focused on demonstrating the need for clinical justification before any exposure is performed. However, there are two important exceptions to this clinical justification. The first involves the provision of x-ray images, particularly of the chest, for immigration, employment, or medico-legal purposes. In such instances, we do not have a good *clinical* justification for each individual exposure, but nonetheless these are performed on a reasonably regular basis. The European legislation simply says that justification for these procedures is the need for "special attention" (1997). The second exception is when x-ray exposures are performed for research purposes; however, these exposures should be (and usually are) approved by rigorous ethical application

process and restricted to the specific protocols approved by the ethics committee in line with local and national policy.

Optimization

What is Optimization?

Optimization of x-ray procedures means employing technologies or techniques that can reduce the radiation dose to patients (and staff) while not sacrificing in any way the clinical information (relevant to the patient's condition) provided by performing the examination. European Council Directive 97/43/EURATOM (ECD 1997; Teunan 1998) describes optimization thus:

> All doses due to medical exposure for radiological purposes...Shall be kept as low as reasonably achievable consistent with obtaining the required diagnostic information taking into account economic and social factors.

The question was posed earlier: If the risk to patients from an array of medical x-ray procedures is low, is it worth us putting time and effort into making sure that we present an even lower risk by optimizing exposures? A second question was posed as well: If producing images of equal diagnostic efficacy at lower risks to the patient is possible, do radiographers and clinicians have a duty or responsibility to the patient to keep those risks to a minimum, particularly if lower dose measures are not costly or inconvenient? To the author, this latter proposition is a good enough reason to lower the doses wherever possible, but other arguments are presented now, starting with a real and modern-day context.

One of the most frequently discussed examinations when it comes to benefit versus risk is the breast cancer screening mammogram. The value of this examination is hotly debated, with the majority of the evidence coming down on the side of supporting breast cancer screening strategies. However, there is a persistent anti-screening argument: In addition to the issue of overdiagnosis, the other often-quoted concern associated with x-raying well women is the radiation dose delivered during the screening with its associated risk of inducing a cancer. Radiation protection practices are particularly tightly controlled in breast screening, and subsequently the typical mean glandular dose (MGD) for a mammogram is around 3–5 mSv. According to the nominal risk coefficient stated within ICRP 103 (ICRP 2007), this would mean that in a cohort of 1 million women, each receiving the above dose, the risk would be about 30 to 50 induced breast cancers *per million examinations*—a number increasing by a factor of between 7 and 10 over a set period in which women receive repeated screenings (say, 20 years). This should be balanced against the estimated 5000 breast cancer deaths prevented per 1 million women by the breast screening program (Marmot et al. 2012). Would it make much difference if the radiation protection standards were not as tight, and the resultant doses increased by, say, a factor of 3 or 4 (which is the typical variation seen across centers for other examination types)? While clearly the risk would increase by around a factor of 3–4, the overall revised risk of approximately 90–150 cases per million women examined (compared with 30–50) is still arguably very low; however, to the women in that group of 40 to 100 additional women whose cancer would be induced at the higher level exposure, this is an important change, particularly if it indicates sloppiness and center-dependent variations when it comes to radiation control measures. An indicator of success with breast screening programs is high attendance rates among at-risk women—greater than 70%, for example—and if women learned that the control on radiation doses was not as rigorous as it could be, it could impact attendance rates.

Other reasons for optimizing radiation delivery in diagnostic imaging departments include:

1. Radiation, while generally poorly understood, does introduce (perhaps a disproportionate level of) fear. Therefore, if the radiologic community can demonstrate rigid controls on radiation levels, it should ultimate reduce patient anxiety *and* parent/caregiver anxiety.

2. The background data justifying the need for diagnostic reference levels already show that variations between departments for the same examination and similar patient size are excessive, and radiation protection standards must be rigorously applied across all departments to make sure that reported dose variations are minimized.

3. Some radiation doses are not insignificant, as shown elsewhere. Therefore, the stochastic and deterministic risks for the relatively high-dose examinations should be kept to a minimum wherever possible.

4. If we do not implement radiation protection standards, the most vulnerable of our society is at greatest risk. Children have a greater radio sensitivity than adults, and since they would normally live for a greater number of years post-exposure, they have more opportunity to express any induced cancers.

5. In many regions, including the European states, United States, Canada, and Australia, it is a legislative requirement that radiation protection standards should be implemented.

The ICRP suggest that the implementation of *diagnostic reference levels* is a key way of optimizing exposures in medical imaging, something with which the authors totally agree. However, over-reliance on reference levels is not good, since showing that one hospital's radiation dose for CT head is below the acceptable 75th percentile value may fail to demonstrate this dose results from an optimized procedure, as it may be possible to further reduce dose while not affecting the diagnostic efficacy of the examination (or conversely, the dose could be too low to produce a suitable image for an adequate diagnosis). The authors of this text are not convinced that the imaging community has been as diligent as it could be to ensure that doses to patients are as low as reasonably achievable. Three contexts will be given to support this argument, each focusing on one of three common reasons for non-optimization: (1) Reliance on traditionally employed, well established procedures; (2) acceptance of new technologies; and (3) non-implementation of findings in the literature that might support lower doses.

Why Might Non-Optimization be Evident?

Reliance on Traditionally Employed, Well-Established Procedures

In radiography, we have been fortunate to have a number of important and highly influential pioneers who have led the way in the area of devising and publishing effective positioning and technical criteria for most examinations performed day-to-day. One such person was Kitty Clarke, (**Figure 5-5**) who not only founded one of the first schools in radiography in the 1930s, but published the seminal textbook *Positioning in Radiography* in 1939, which transformed the radiographic practice and is still being published in a revised form today.

While the importance of that textbook is not debated, fundamental components of techniques that were proposed in 1939 may not have the same

relevance or need as today. Let us look at one example—the distance of the x-ray source to the image receptor (or film as it was in 1939), which for many non-erect positions was recommended to be 100 cm. In 1939, this distance was possibly more necessary than today due to the lower power available to x-ray tubes, and therefore the need to keep the x-ray source within close vicinity of the receptor, but with today's technology, is this distance necessary? And more important, will maintaining it result in an optimized examination? Let us consider the science for a moment.

Geometric un-sharpness is one of the key sources of poor definition within radiographic images. It arises from the finite size of the focal spot that can be anywhere between 0.1 and 2 mm, which leads the edge of an object being displayed as a slightly blurred entity (**penumbra**) as opposed to a very sharp point. This is displayed in **Figures 5-6** and **5-7**. The size of this penumbra is dependent on three key factors: (1) The size of the focal spot; (2) the distance between the focal spot and the object being irradiated; and (3) distance between the object and the image receptor.

This can be summarized as:

$$U_g = \frac{S_{fs} \times D_{o \to i}}{D_{S \to o}}$$

where U_g is geometric unsharpness, S_{fs} is focal spot size, $D_{o \to i}$ is distance from the object to the image receptor, and $D_{S \to o}$ is distance from the focal spot to the object.

The important thing to note here is that as the focal spot to object distance ($D_{S \to o}$ above), *increases*, the geometric unsharpness *decreases*; in other words, as we increase the distance between the x-ray source and the patient (and other factors remain unchanged), the image should get sharper. (Whether this will improve diagnostic efficacy in all situations would require examination specific observer studies.) One way of increasing the source to patient distance ($D_{S \to o}$) is by increasing the distance from the x-ray source to image receptor, since the patient to image receptor distance should remain constant.

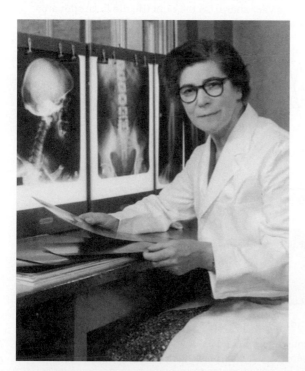

Figure 5-5 Kitty Clarke, a radiographic pioneer.

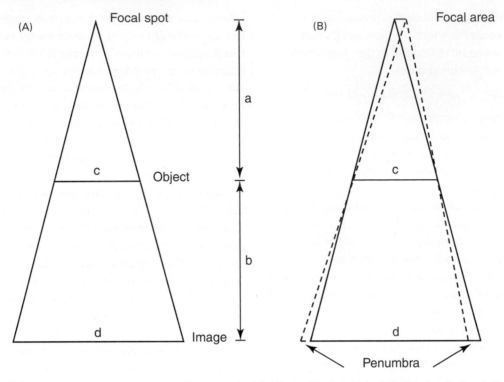

Figure 5-6 Geometric unsharpness. In the figure on the left (A), the focal spot size is infinitely small and therefore the reproduction of the edge of the object being irradiated is very sharp. On the right (B), the focal spot area demonstrates a definite width resulting in a penumbra or blurred reproduction of the edge.

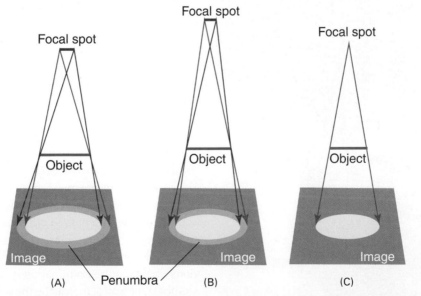

Figure 5-7 Illustration of the impact of increasing the source-to-image receptor distance on image quality. In A, the penumbra can easily be seen resulting from the geometric unsharpness generated by the focal spot size. In B, this unsharpness has been reduced as a result of the increased source-to-receptor distance; however, a penumbra is still evident when compared with an ideal infinitely small focal spot size (C).

While the positive implication for image quality is very evident when one uses a longer source-to-patient distance (by increasing the source-to-receptor distance), it can be asked what this has to do with optimization, since there has been no reduction in dose. There are two answers to this: first, if we go back to the European definition of optimization a few paragraphs above, we see that it does not automatically say that *reductions* in doses will be achieved; rather, that they will be kept *as low as reasonably achievable* while obtaining the required diagnostic information. The second half of this means that *providing the information for an accurate diagnosis is fundamental to optimization*, and techniques that involve increasing the source-to-patient distance, potentially improving image quality and better defining pathologic appearances, should be investigated rigorously. Second, as it happens, a dose reduction advantage with this technique *has* been argued for in the literature due the effect of the Inverse Square Law, where an effective dose reduction of 33% has been observed when the source-to-receptor distance is increased from 100 cm to 130 cm (while the patient-to-receptor distance remained constant) for pelvis examinations. While the extent of the dose reduction associated with increasing the source-to-patient distance is debated (Huda et al. 2005; Brennan and O'Leary 2006), and an awareness of the type of collimation that needs to be used to reap the full benefits of this technique is required (Poletti and McLean 2005; O'Leary and Brennan 2006), the potential overall benefit to the patient of increasing the distance (which incurs little or no additional cost) should have led to a rigorous reevaluation of the traditional distance of 100 cm. This has not happened.

It should be acknowledged that with an increased source-to-receptor distance, one needs to consider the constraints imposed by table unit position, grid focus specifications, and the height of the radiologic technologist!

Acceptance of New Technologies

When new technologies are being proposed, it is important that they are introduced in a careful way so they are used to their full potential at the lowest risk to the patient. There may be a flurry of research activity, often supported by manufacturers, to demonstrate the efficacy of new equipment, but this does not usually translate into regular departmental or even national reviews of the technology to ensure that optimal usage is in place, and that the technology is indeed useful to the specific environment in which the equipment is placed.

Two examples might help—the first around the issue of non-optimized use. The introduction of digital technology is probably the greatest change within medical imaging that we have seen since x-rays were discovered in 1895. A lot of important research was initially performed—for example, the DMIST trial in mammography (Pisano et al. 2008)—to make sure that the new technology offered benefits to the patient and clinicians. However, while the efficacy of digital acquisition was made clear, regular follow up studies are rarely evident to make sure that computed (CR) (**Figure 5-8**) or direct radiography

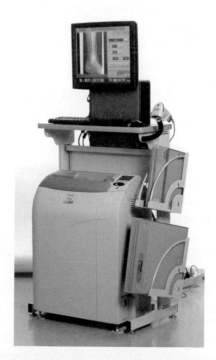

Figure 5-8 Computed radiography system.
Courtesy of Fuji

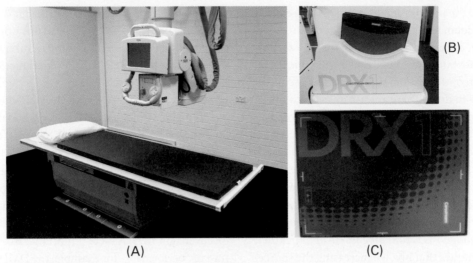

Figure 5-9 Direct radiography system. X-ray tube and table (A). DR battery and charger (B). DR cassette (C).

(DR) (**Figure 5-9**) systems with a variety of *potential* benefits are being used in a way that maximizes (or even realizes) those benefits.

Specifically around exposure factors, the reader may be aware that the materials used in digital receptors and their attenuation properties are quite different from those contained within rare-earth intensifying screens and films. The materials used in rare-earth screens had K-edge values of around 52 and 39 for gadolinium- and lanthanum-based phosphors, respectively, compared with values closer to 37, 35, and 13, respectively, for barium-, cesium-, and selenium-based materials used with digital acquisitions in CR (barium) and DR (cesium and selenium). If we wish to maximize the attenuation of x-rays by the image receptors, we should be using x-ray beams with energy profiles so that the mean, median or effective beam energy emerging from the patient is at or just above the K-edge of the receptor materials. In other words, due to the generally lower K-edge with digital technologies compared with intensifying screens, it is possible that the kVp selection should be lower than that used with screens. Of course, the potentially higher skin doses with lower energies would need to be

investigated, but there appears to be a paucity of clinical-based research investigating this, and therefore exposure factors traditionally used for many years with film are often being used in the context of digital imaging. If we are matching emergent energies with K-edge of the receptors in a more efficient way, this would mean greater attenuation of x-rays and potentially dose savings, since the x-rays would be captured more effectively. It is this level of complexity that often exists within imaging that demands ongoing, clinically relevant research. Until this work is done, we cannot be sure that the exposures being employed are optimized and that the potential dose savings or image quality enhancements often quoted with digital technology are being maximized.

The second example addresses the issue of making sure that the new technology is suitable to each environment in which it is placed. Initial efficacy research cannot examine all possible application situations for novel equipment. When digital breast tomosynthesis (DBT) was being introduced, there was a plethora of research published demonstrating DBT's benefits in terms of sensitivity and specificity, with some of the most impressive and important work being performed in collaboration with industry (Skaane et al. 2013). At the time of this writing (2013), due to these research outputs, in the opinion of the authors, it is likely that DBT (quite rightly) will play a critical role in breast imaging in the future and will have an important place within breast screening strategies. However, without debating the potential value of DBT, specific benefits to women in particular environments are as yet unclear. For example (again at the time of writing), it appears that DBT is being introduced in the Middle East, a region in which the age of the women being screened and the nature of their breast tissue, as well as the profile of the cancers encountered in this population, are quite different from these factors in women on whom most of the DBT studies have been performed. Research needs to be done on the specific populations who will be utilizing this new technology to see if the benefits described elsewhere are relevant to these different groups of women. In addition, the technology may be introduced into new environments within developing countries where radiologists and radiographers may not have the same level of expertise or training as those involved in the original research studies; ongoing reviews and work are necessary to ensure that women being examined or not being affected in a deleterious way following the technology change. Simple acceptance of new technology without the relevant, tailored, supporting evidence should not happen.

Finally, research-funding agencies must take some responsibility for these issues of optimal usage of equipment and suitability of new technologies for different populations. In most environments there is (quite rightly) much emphasis on providing monies to support studies focusing on innovative ideas; unfortunately, the same emphasis is not placed on making sure we are getting the most benefit out of the new technology at the lowest patient risk once this new technology has been installed. Until this imbalance is addressed, it is difficult to see how one can make sure of maximum diagnostic yield at lowest radiation risk to the patient.

Non-Implementation of Findings in the Literature
Again, a simple radiographic example may be useful here. A study performed some time ago demonstrated the potential benefit of performing a PA rather than an AP projection for the abdomen (Brennan and Madigan 2000). While this proposed change in technique could clearly only be performed on reasonably mobile patients, the benefits were significant, with reductions of around 40% in patient entrance surface dose and internal phantom dose, respectively, and no change in image quality. The reason proposed for this reduction in dose was the decreased patient diameter due to tissue displacement and the radioprotective nature of anatomy located at the posterior part of the patient. While this technique had no apparent cost or social implications, widespread adoption of this technique has not occurred.

Poor translation of research findings into practice within medicine is not uncommon. It appears that performing scientifically valid studies and publishing resultant findings in important peer-reviewed journals is not enough; systems or process must be in place to make sure that the latest important findings relevant to a particular discipline are regularly reviewed and implemented whenever appropriate. The value of bodies such as NICE has been considered earlier in this chapter, and this type of arrangement—albeit on a smaller scale—needs to be in place within radiology and radiography to maximize translation of best practice. This body would have the potential to take responsible for reviewing and implementing current and new technology and practice and should consist of experts from a variety of bodies including consumer groups facilitating a multidisciplinary. Sadly, at this time, such organizations are not common.

Optimization Initiatives

Some national initiatives that are focused on image optimization are in place in different countries and are responsible for highly effective initiatives such as the implementation of diagnostic reference levels in the UK by the Health Protection Agency, formally known as the National Radiological Protection Board. Other bodies include Image Gently in the United States, which focuses on optimizing procedures for children; NEXT in the United States, which looks at keeping radiation risks as low as possible for a variety of examinations; and ARPANSA, which looks at CT reference levels in Australia. These are the type of activities that will lead to important optimization benefits within radiology and radiography, but should be evident more widely if widespread optimization is to be in place.

Optimization and Cost

Before implementation of any new optimized procedure or equipment—even if significant dose reductions are shown and/or improved image quality—two issues that are referred to in the European legislation should be considered: *economic and social factors*. Economic clearly means how much it would cost; while the increased source-to-receptor distance example shows that in some cases, the cost is minimal (apart perhaps from some increased wear and tear on the x-ray tube due to having to increase the exposure at the greater distances), the cost for other techniques may be more significant. An interesting example of how a cost-benefit analysis can be performed across a country and what parameters should be included in such an analysis was provided by Ginsberg et al. (1998) when the use of rare-earth screens was being proposed for widespread use in Israel. While the context is outdated, the approach is still very relevant today. The social factors are harder to define, but the acceptability of introducing the technique from a clinician and patient perspective must form an important part. To return to our example of the increased source-to-receptor distance: in implementing this change, the new technique should present little or no difficulty for the patient; however, for staff, there is the challenge of smaller staff members being able to raise the x-ray tube to a level to accommodate

the increased source-to-receptor distance. While this specific challenge should be easily overcome with the availability of a step or similar tools, other optimizing techniques may present much more challenging circumstances. All costs and social considerations must be carefully examined before clinical implementation.

Optimization: Image Quality Versus Diagnostic Efficacy

Finally, for clarity, the author would like to differentiate between *image quality* and *diagnostic efficacy*, as both these terms have been used in this chapter. Increased image quality refers to a circumstance in which the appearance of the image shows an improvement, either subjectively to the observer or measurably, which could be related to increased contrast or sharpness, for example. However, increased diagnostic efficacy goes a step further: It describes a situation where there is now an *increase in the level of clinical information that is provided* to the radiologist or other expert observer so that diagnosis is improved. While increased image quality improves the likelihood that diagnostic efficacy will be improved, it is important to be clear that for a variety of reasons, this is not always the case.

Radiation Dose Limits

Obviously, imposing dose limits is another way to limit radiation risks; however, this is not an option for patients undergoing medical imaging. The bottom line is that if a diagnosis is needed for the future well being of the patient, the radiation that is required must be administered. In fact, a dose limit could potentially be an obstacle to diagnosis.

On the other hand, there are dose limits for workers and members of the public (perhaps family members accompanying patients) that should be adhered to. Those published by the ICRP and other national or international agencies are summarized in **Table 5-5**. If these values are exceeded, appropriate measures should be put into place to minimize

Table 5-5 Dose limits for workers and members of the public

Measure	Occupational exposure	Members of the public
ICRP (2007)		
Effective dose	20 mSv per year, averaged over 5 years	1mSv
Lens of the eye	150 mSv	15 mSv
Skin	500 mSv	50 mSv
Hands & feet	500 mSv	—
United States (REF AND DETAILS, NEED TO BE ADDED)		
Effective dose	50 mSv	1mSv
Lens of the eye	150 mSv	15 mSv
Skin	500 mSv	50 mSv
Hands & feet	500 mSv	50 mSv
Under 18 year olds		
Effective dose	1 mSv	—
Lens of the eye	15 mSv	—
Skin	50 mSv	—
Hand & feet	50 mSv	—
European Union (1996)		
*Workers, apprentices and students (aged 18 or over)		
Effective dose	100 mSv over a five year period, maximum of 50 mSv in any one year	1mSv
Lens of the eye	150 mSv	15 mSv
Skin	500 mSv	50 mSv
Hands, forearm, feet & ankle	500 mSv	—
Apprentices and students (aged 16 & 17)		
Effective dose	6 mSv	—
Lens of the eye	50 mSv	—
Skin	150 mSv	—
Hand & feet	150 mSv	—
Australia (2008)		
Effective dose	20 mSv per year, averaged over 5 years	1mSv
Lens of the eye	150 mSv	15 mSv
Skin	500 mSv	50 mSv
Hands & feet	500 mSv	—
Canada (2008)		
Whole body (Effective dose)	20 mSv per year, averaged over 5 years	1mSv
Lens of the eye	150 mSv	15 mSv
Skin	500 mSv	50 mSv
Hands	500 mSv	50 mSv
All other organs	500 mSv	50 mSv

Key: * = In the European Union, workers are classified into Category A or B. Category A workers are those who could receive an annual effective dose greater than 6 mSv or an equivalent dose to the lens, skin or extremities that is larger than 3/10s of the limits described within the table. Category B are all other workers

Unless otherwise stated these are annual values. Apart from the effective doses, other values are dose equivalents.

reoccurrence, and the exposed individual should be monitored for any adverse sequelae.

Obviously, special consideration must be given to pregnant patients requiring medical diagnostic exposures. It is important to note that there is no evidence that exposure to an unborn child from diagnostic radiologic examination presents any risk to the child of pre- or postnatal death, growth malformations, or mental impairment (ICRP 2007). In fact, the risk to an unborn child of a stochastic event is the same as any young child (ICRP 2007). Nonetheless, to minimize the risk, it is important that a patient informs the radiologist or radiographer prior to any exposure so that special consideration is given to optimize the procedure. A potential procedure would be as follows: If an x-ray procedure is likely to provide a radiation dose of more than, for example, 1 mSv to the unborn child, then specific justification for the need of that examination needs to be performed along with an assessment of (1) the risk to the unborn child if the examination is performed and (2) risk to the woman if the examination is not performed. If it is decided that the examination should go ahead and an optimized procedure is identified, the risks to the child are usually explained to the women and to the referrer of the examination *before* the examination has been performed. The estimated radiation dose delivered will be recorded.

Radiation Detection and Measurement

The principles of radiation protection—justification, optimization, and dose limits (particularly the last two)—rely on effective methods on measuring radiation dose. There are a number of ways of doing this, but the main methods used in diagnostic imaging departments are:

- thermoluminescent dosimetry;
- dose-area product technology
- solid-state meters
- radiochromic film

Each of these will be considered in turn. It is important to emphasize that the dose quantity measured with most current commercial units used in diagnostic imaging departments is the air kerma.

Thermoluminescent Dosimetry

Overview

Thermoluminescent dose (TLD) meters can be used for patient and staff radiation measurements. They are made of a variety of materials but commonly come as lithium fluoride or lithium bromide, and in recent years, some have been doped with copper or manganese to increase the sensitivity to radiation. They are usually small chips around a few millimeters in diameter, but are available in other sizes and in powder form (**Figure 5-10**).

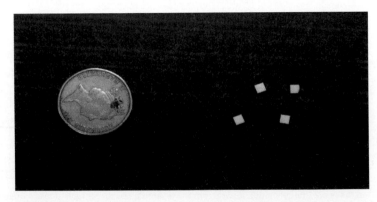

Figure 5-10 Thermoluminescent dosimeters beside an Australian dollar coin. The coin is about 2 cm in diameter.

This range of sizes offers much versatility and facilitates measurements on the entrance surface of patients, for example, without any adverse image quality effects, as well as at a range of body locations for staff such as the tips of fingers. They are also useful for measurements at a variety of locations inside an anthropomorphic phantom.

TLDs: How Do They Work?

TLDs work on the principle that when they are exposed to ionizing radiation such as x-rays or gamma rays, electrons within the dosimeter crystals are moved to a higher energy level and are trapped there as a result of deliberately added impurities such as manganese. The electrons remain in this higher-energy state until heat is applied, whereupon they move back to their normal position and release the excess energy in the form of light. The number of light photons that are released are counted, and following appropriate calibration procedures, the radiation dose can be calculated based on light photon number. TLDs offer the advantage of being able to measure backscattered radiation from the exposed individual, which may account for up to an additional 40% of dose (air kerma).

Modern TLDs such as lithium fluoride doped with manganese (LiF: Mg, Ti) have the capability to record doses as low as 10 µGy and as high as 1 Gy, whereas copper-doped versions (LiF; Mg, Cu, P) can extend this range from 1 µGy to 20 Gy. TLDs can record x-ray photons with energies above 5 keV.

Patient Measurements

For patient dose measurements, TLDs are usually placed on the patient surface at the central entrance point of the radiation (**Figure 5-11**).

In case of erroneous recordings of dose, sometimes two or three TLDs are positioned at the same time. They are placed in a black plastic sachet, which protects the TLD from dirt and grease, but more importantly represents the stratum corneum of the skin, which is made up of dead cells. This means that the radiation amount that reaches the

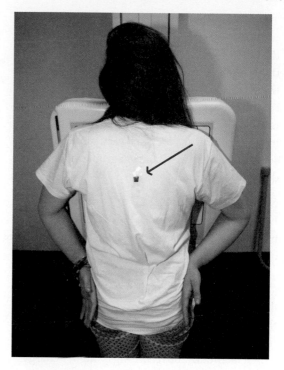

Figure 5-11 TLD placed on the entrance surface of the patient at the center of the x-ray beam.

TLD represents the radiation amount that would have reached the first living layer of patient tissue. From this position, the entrance surface dose to the patient can be calculated, from which effective doses can be determined.

Patient measurements with TLDs can only be used effectively for non-fluoroscopic examinations. During fluoroscopic procedures such as barium swallows or cardiac angiography, the patient moves considerably throughout the examination, and since the TLD is usually on a fixed patient position, this means that the TLD will change its distance from the x-ray source—it may sometimes be on the entrance surface and other times on the exit surface, and may even be outside the x-ray beam's field for some of the exposure. This allows for much misinterpretation when faced with resultant dose values; a better alternative is the dose-area product (DAP) meter discussed below.

One other examination type that TLDs are not suited for is mammography. In mammography, the beam energies are traditionally much lower than in other fields of radiography, meaning that there is the possibility that the TLD will be seen on resultant images. This would present with certain challenges, since breast pathologies such as microcalcifications are often very subtle, and the superimposition of a TLD image may have serious deleterious effects.

Staff Measurements

For measuring staff doses, the TLD is placed in a badge-like structure (**Figure 5-12**), which can come in a variety of forms.

One type contains two TLD discs, one thin (40 microns) and one thick (90 microns). The thin disc has no plastic badge covering and allows the measurement of low-energy doses, while the thicker disc is covered by a thick layer of plastic, which facilitates the recording of higher energy exposures. Under normal circumstances, the badge is worn close to the gonadal areas, and when lead rubber aprons are being worn, the dosimeters are worn under the protective apron to better represent the radiation dose actually being received by the organs. The doses received are usually very low, and in the large majority of cases, there is no reading on the TLD. During interventional procedures, where doses are generally higher and exposure times are longer compared with other fluoroscopic examinations, staff may wear a further TLD dosimeter close to the thyroid if a protective collar is not worn; indeed, the Health Protection Agency in the UK has a dosimeter that can be positioned at the thyroid that is calibrated to assess radiation dose levels to the lens of the eye. It has been proposed that TLDs positioned in regions of the body that are not usually covered by protective garments are possibly more valuable that those positioned underneath aprons, where the dose is nearly always at an immeasurably low level. A recent survey of radiology departments in 13 European countries demonstrated that the practice in five of these countries was to wear a single TLD outside the lead apron at the position of the collar.

Calibration

Each dosimeter must be calibrated to facilitate useful TLD dose measurements; otherwise, there is no way of knowing how many light photons equals how much radiation dose. To do this, before any patient or staff exposure takes place, the TLDs are irradiated using a known level of radiation dose, usually a batch at a time. The light photons released are then counted, and a ratio between light photons and the known radiation dose is calculated, which then facilitates all future calculations. After this procedure, the TLDs are cleared of any remnant excess energy before they are used to measure patient or staff doses. It is critically important to note that TLDs are calibrated at a specific x-ray beam, which means that they should only be used at or close to this specific energy.

TLD Reading

Following exposure, the TLDs are then heated (*thermo*luminescent) to release light (thermolu-*minescent*). This is done using a TLD reading oven (**Figure 5-13**) using hot nitrogen gas.

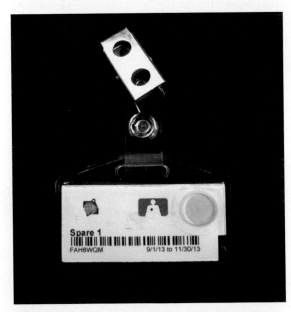

Figure 5-12 Thermoluminescent dosimeter badge.

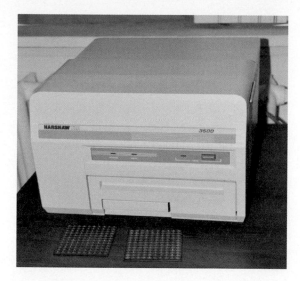

Figure 5-13 Thermoluminescent dosimeter reader.

Traditionally, TLD reading was a very tedious process, with only one TLD being read at any one time; however, modern units can now read up to 280 dosimeters within an hour. Within each heating oven, there is a particular cycle that consists of a pre-heating stage (up to 165°C), a reading stage (up to 300°C), and an annealing stage. The aim of the latter stage is to clear the TLD of any remnant recording of dose so that when used for a specific patient measurement, the vast majority of the reading on the TLD results from that patient exposure.

Uncertainty with TLD Measurements
While TLDs for patient measurements are cheap, around $5 each, anyone who has used them will be aware that there are a number of uncertainties around their measurements. These uncertainties arise from a variety of sources and include:

1. **TLD signal fade**. This is where dose information that is stored on the TLD in the form of electrons trapped at higher energy levels starts to decrease even before reading of the TLD. Depending on the type of TLD, the type of exposure and the type of annealing process, the level of fading can vary between 1% in a year to 7% in the first couple of weeks.

2. **Non-linear response of TLDs to radiation dose**. This is particularly a problem at the lower and higher dose readings, but manufacturers would argue that with modern-day TLDs and readers, the linearity is within 5% for doses between 10 µGy and 1 Gy.

3. **Dependency of TLDs on radiation beam energy**. TLDs are highly sensitive to the level of energy to which they are exposed. This means, for example, that if a batch of TLDs is calibrated at 80 kVp, then strictly speaking, one should only use the TLDs close to this beam energy. In practice, however, this adherence to a single energy value is difficult, since patients come in a variety of sizes and conditions and therefore require a variety of energy settings.

4. **The validity of the calibration**. As mentioned above, TLDs must be calibrated before use, so that the radiation dose that the patient (or staff member) has been exposed to can be calculated from the number of light photons being released. However, this is far from a perfect science; for example, when it was said above that for calibration TLDs are exposed to an *known level of radiation dose*, that known dose is only as reliable as the measuring provided by a unit such as a solid-state dosimeter. These dosimeters are prone to error and need to be regularly calibrated to some primary or secondary source to make sure that their dose readings are valid.

5. **Variations in TLD reader performance**. Unfortunately, if two TLDs are exposed to the same level of radiation, one will not necessarily get the same reading from each dosimeter if they are read by different machines. The performance of the reader can vary depending on age, the rigor and recency of calibration, the model type and level of precision offered, and the technical support.

These sources of error are not insignificant, but for radiation doses between 0.1 mGy and 11 mGy, overall uncertainty should not be larger than 25%

at the 95% confidence level between beam energies of 50 kVp with 2.5 mm Al equivalent and 120 kVp with 5 mm Al equivalent. On the one hand, it is reassuring that these conditions should cover *most* exposure conditions encountered within diagnostic imaging centers; on the other hand, an uncertainty of 25% means that real changes or differences in radiation doses between patients or experimental conditions would need to be sizable if they are not to be obscured by uncertainty. Also, the lower dose at which any reasonable level of certainty remains (0.1 mGy) is actually not that low, and certainly this dose and below would be relevant for some chest and pediatric imaging and would be close to values demonstrated for exit patient doses and internal phantoms measurements. An often-quoted solution to this low-dose inaccuracy (or even sometimes non-reading) is to expose the same TLD to several exposures across 5 or 10 patients and then take the mean value; however, this averaging approach comes with its own difficulties.

Some of these uncertainties may be alleviated by a new technology: optically stimulated luminescent dosimetry (OSL). These are made of aluminum oxide crystal detectors (Al_2O_3) that, following radiation exposure, can release details on the dose received by using *light* stimulation and not heat (**Figure 5-14**).

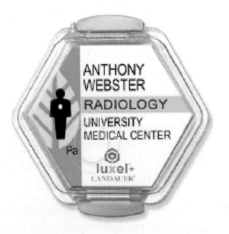

Figure 5-14 Optically stimulated luminescent dosimeter (OSL).

Following irradiation, the dosimeter is stimulated by a laser (green) light, and the emitted blue light is then amplified using a photomultiplier tube and send on for absorbed dose estimation. While a number of the inaccuracies and inconveniences associated with heating the TLDs are removed, the other key advantage of OSLs are that they can be placed on the site of investigation in mammography without any effect on image display. The use of OSLs can be seen in **Figure 5-15**. The apparatus in this case being designed to facilitate real-time dosimetry readings in mammography (Aznar et al. 2005): the OSL is attached to the readout and display electronics using fiber links and is stimulated using a green laser light.

Dose-Area Product Meters (DAPs)

Overview

Dose-area product dosimetry is possibly the most common method of patient dosimetry currently being carried out. The arrangement requires an ionization chamber to be attached to the output of the x-ray tube (**Figure 5-16, A** and **B**); however, the facilitation of readings that are generated automatically following exposure (**Figure 5-17**) makes this a highly attractive option, where placement of dosimeters on patients and elaborated reading processes are not required.

Indeed, in the European Union, it is a requirement that this type of dosimeter should be available with all new x-ray equipment:

> *If new radiodiagnostic equipment is used, it shall have, where practicable, a device informing the practitioner of the quantity of radiation produced by the equipment during the radiological procedure. Euratom 97 43 (1997).*

DAP Meters: How Do They Work?

DAP meters, as the name suggests, simply relies on measuring the amount of radiation interacting with the ionization chamber (located at the x-ray tube) (**Figure 5-16**) and multiplying this value by the area of exposure. Resultant doses are expressed

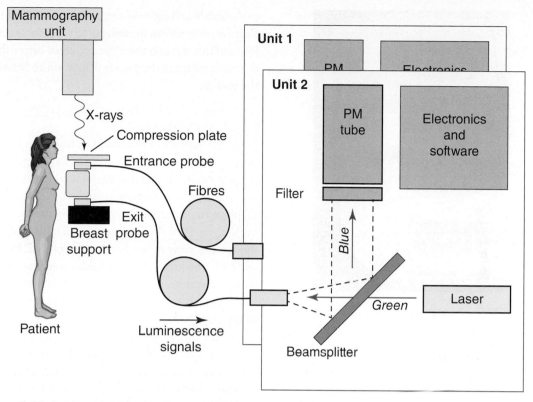

Figure 5-15 An example of the placement of OSLs in mammography for real-time dosimetry. An OSL is placed at the entrance and exit surface of the breast, and these are attached to the read and display electronic using fibers.

Reproduced from: http://bjr.birjournals.org/content/78/928/328.figures-only; Aznar MC, Hemdal B, Medin J, Marckmann CJ, Andersen CE, Bøtter-Jensen L, Andersson I, Mattsson S. In vivo absorbed dose measurements in mammography using a new real-time luminescence technique. Br J Radiol. 2005 78(928):328–34.

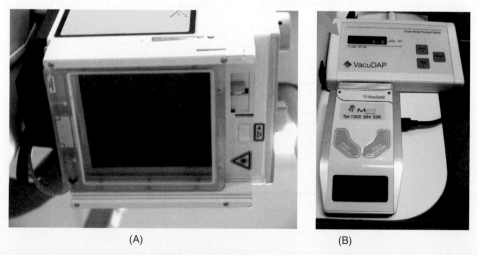

(A)   (B)

Figure 5-16 Photograph of a DAP ionization chamber (A) and readout unit (B, see arrow).

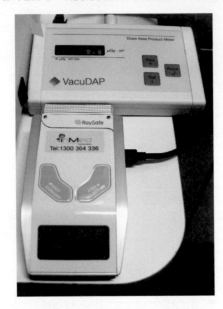

Figure 5-17 DAP readout unit (see arrow).

using the unit of Gycm²; however, modern units in addition simultaneously record DAP rate and irradiation time. The ionization chamber is simply a radiation detector, which contains air, the particles of which require energies of around 34 eV to ionize, thus creating an ion pair (**Figure 5-18**).

So, for example, if the chamber is exposed to a photon with an energy of about 34 keV, approximately 1000 ion pairs will be created—1000 electrons and 1000 positive ions—and these will be attracted

to the anode and cathode, respectively. In reality, the electron output from the ionization chamber is very low, and this signal is therefore amplified before the dose data is sent to the display device, which informs the operator.

Location of the Ionization Chamber and Associated Advantages

Since the ionization chamber is attached to the output of the x-ray tube, it must be as transparent as possible so that it does not attenuate too many x-rays, nor interfere with the light beam diaphragm device. However, it is this attachment to the x-ray tube that makes it so versatile and follows the x-ray tube wherever it is placed. In addition, the location of the ionization chamber at the x-ray tube, but at the patient side of the collimators facilitates two important requirements: firstly that the ionization chamber is positioned perpendicular to the x-ray beam; secondly that the ionization chamber captures the whole area of the x-ray beam, in other words however large the collimated field, the area of the ionization chamber is always larger than this. As mentioned above, the resultant dose value given is therefore the product of the absorbed dose at the chamber and the area of exposure, so for example if a dose of 5 mGy is delivered over an area of 2 cm × 2 cm, the dose-area product (DAP) reading will be 20 mGycm². If, however, the area is increased to 4 cm × 4 cm

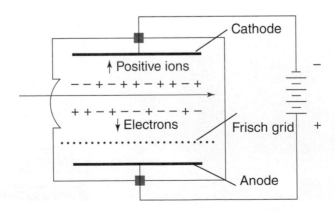

Figure 5-18 A diagram of a part of an ionization chamber. Some ion pairs are shown and these will be attracted to one of the two electrodes.

and the dose remains the same, the DAP reading is now 80 mGycm². One key consequence of measuring the DAP in this way and at the x-ray source is that, regardless of the distance that the patient is from the x-ray tube, the radiation dose will remain constant if the beam is appropriately collimated.

Here is an example:

Imagine a patient at 100 cm from the DAP's ionization chamber and the area of exposure *at the DAP meter* required to expose the abdomen is 4 cm × 4 cm. The absorbed dose at the DAP is 2mGy, resulting in a DAP reading of 32 mGycm². If the distance between the patient and the chamber is increased to 200 cm, because of the nature of the divergent beam, the collimation field will have to be made smaller to ensure a constant x-ray field on the patient's surface, otherwise the whole patient could be irradiated. In fact, the field would have to be reduced to 2 cm × 2 cm. However, since the patient's distance from the x-ray tube has doubled, the dose at the patient has been reduced by a factor of 4 in accordance with the Inverse Square Law; therefore, to maintain an adequate dose at the patient, the exposure and hence the dose at the chamber will have to be increased by a factor of 4, to 8 mGy. At this new patient position, simple calculations will demonstrate that the DAP reading will be 32 mGycm², which is identical to the original exposure at 100 cm and reflects the fact that because of the interdependence of radiation dose and area of exposure as distance changes, the dose at the entrance of the patient has remained the same, regardless of the distance. A simple dose reading at the chamber without considering the area of exposure would not have been adjusted in the same way. A photograph of a patient being examined at two distances is shown in **Figure 5-19**.

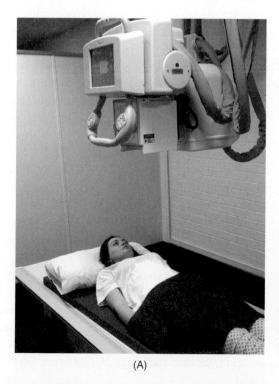
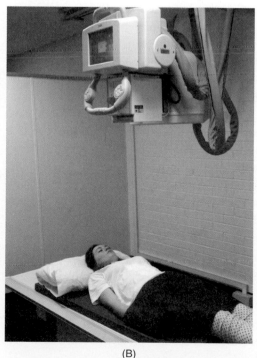

(A)   (B)

Figure 5-19 Increasing distance for an AP lumbar spine examination. (A) normal distance (100 cm); (B) increased distance (130 cm).

Traditionally, the connection between the DAP's ionization chamber and the display device that demonstrates the subsequent readings had to be long enough to facilitate positioning of the x-ray tube in all possible locations within the x-ray room; however, modern versions using wireless Bluetooth technology have provided a technological solution to this challenge.

DAP Limitations

Because readings happen with minimum input from the radiographer or radiologist (making them very convenient) and the inclusion of the area of exposure as well as the dose, it is likely that this form of dosimetry will be the main method used for widespread patient dosimetry of the future. However, DAPs do not come without their limitations. First, DAP meters need to be regularly calibrated. A study performed in UK hospitals (Crawley et al. 2001) demonstrated that the DAP reading given on 31% of the 41 units measured was more than 10% away from the true DAP value, with miscalibration being more apparent for under-couch (50%) rather than over-couch (23%) tube locations. There were no differences between the level of miscalibration between the DAP units that came with the x-ray equipment and those fitted retrospectively. While it was acknowledged in the paper that air pressure and temperature could have, in theory, an impact of up to 5% on the readings, the units measured were highly unlikely to have been subjected to such extreme climatic variations. It was recommended that DAP calibrations should be performed at intervals of no less than 6 months.

The second limitation is around the actual measurement that is performed with DAP meters. Because of the location of the ionization chamber, the dose measured is that at the output of the x-ray tube and not that at the patient, and one must question how accurately the dose displayed therefore represents the actual patient dose. An example of where this can become a problem is when an object is placed between the DAP chamber and the patient, resulting in a DAP reading that implies a higher dose to the patient than what the patient actually received. This becomes an issue when under-couch tubes are employed and the x-ray table is positioned between the patient and the x-ray source, and attempts to measure patient skin or effective dose therefore require complex calculations.

A third limitation is that while DAP meters are useful for the calculation of the stochastic risks of the radiation exposures,, in recent years with increasing interventional doses, more emphasis is on skin dose. DAP readings have certain limitations here, since they do not distinguish between a large-field, low-dose exposure and a small-field, high-dose exposure. In other words, without further measuring devices such as TLDs or radiochromic film (discussed below), the exposure to specific skin sites is not properly assessed.

A final issue with the position of the DAP chamber is that subsequent readings cannot include the backscatter proportion (up to an extra 40%) that can be accounted for with TLDs placed on the patient's surface.

Nonetheless, while these limitations around DAP values representing patient exposures are acknowledged, work looking at the level of agreement between DAP readings and patient entrance dose when calculating effective dose have shown good agreement (Theocharopoulos et al. 2002). It is interesting to note also the conclusions of another study that compared the effective dose resulting from DAP and TLD measurements (Yakoumakis et al. 2001). Both methods were argued to be useful ways of calculating effective dose, although the DAP readings resulted in values that were up to 38% higher than those generated from TLD readings. The authors concluded that since the increased levels with the DAP readings were most likely related to the large exposure areas sometimes used by radiographers, resulting in fields that were in fact larger than the image detector area, DAP readings may be a more accurate way of calculating effective dose.

Uncertainty with DAP Measurements

DAP measurements, like TLDs, are subject to certain uncertainties; however, it has been stated that these uncertainties should not be greater than ± 25% at the 95% confidence level for doses between 10 Gycm^2 to 10^3 Gy/cm^2 for x-ray energies between 50 kVp (2.5 mm Al) and 120 kVp (5 mm Al).

Solid-State Meters

Solid-state meters have the convenience of being placed wherever in the x-ray room one requires measurements along with the immediate display of dose data. They come as an electronic base unit, sometimes with additional probes; however, their size imposes certain limitations (the Unfors XI model pictured later in this chapter is approximately 14 cm × 7.5 cm × 3 cm).

Solid-state dosimeters have been around for a century. The modern types rely on semiconductor technology, the physics of which are beyond the scope of this text, but will be summarized here.

First, one must understand the terms *valency* and *conduction bands* within an atom. The outer orbital electrons in an atom are arranged in the form of an electron cloud. Some of these are tightly bound to the atom, and these are said to be located in the valency band, while others are free to move over reasonably large distances and are known to be located within the conduction band. The number of electrons contained within the conduction band will determine the object's conductivity; typically, metals such as copper have high numbers of electrons within this band. Insulators or semiconductors have no or very few electrons in the conduction band and therefore have low conductivity. The energy difference between electrons within these two bands is low, ranging from several eV to close to 1 eV in semiconductors.

Due to the low energy differences between bands, semiconductors may find some electrons within the conduction band, but the number of these electrons is amplified by the deliberate introduction of impurities within the structure, which serve as electron donors or electron receivers just below the conduction band. If a donor is provided, it means that electrons can move into the conduction zone at very low energies, and since the presence of electrons in the conduction zone facilitate conduction, this is known as a n-type (n = negative) semiconductor. Alternatively, the presence of a receiver encourages the movement of electrons from the valence band to this acceptor, leaving electron vacancies in the valence band which are known as holes; this is known as a p-type (p = positive) semiconductor. With both n- and p-type semiconductors the energy to create this electron movement is very small, ~1–3 eV, so irradiation of these devices can easily be detected at energy levels much less than those relevant to ionization chambers (34 keV). In practice, these n- and p-type semiconductors in circuits are joined together as shown in **Figure 5-20,** and any ionizations resulting from radiation interactions will result in an electrical current being created, which will indicate the level of the original irradiation.

Without getting into the intricacies of the potential semiconductor arrangements, one can see that semiconductors can serve as sensitive (and robust) detectors of radiation and have been proven to be highly efficient, with a response that is linear to the level of exposure. These types of dosimeters can be small in size, serving as a tool for personal dosimetry (**Figure 5-21**), or larger, making them relevant to much wider applications. (**Figure 5-22**).

Modern-type solid-state dosimeters are capable of recording many different types of data, including dose, dose rate, kVp levels, half-value layer, and more. The output reading is immediately available on the detector unit and can be distributed to a database via wire or Bluetooth technology. It has the ability to record doses over

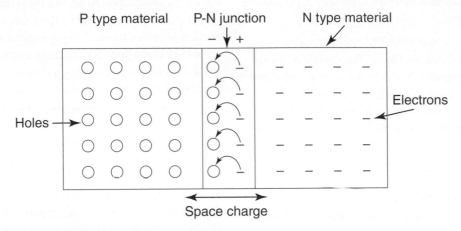

Figure 5-20 N- and p-type semiconductors in a circuit.

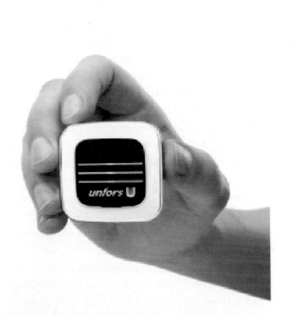

Figure 5-21 A solid-state dosimeter using semiconductor technology.

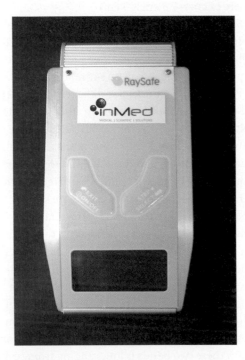

Figure 5-22 A RaySafe dosimetry tool.

a huge range—from 10 nGy to 1000 Gy—and is sensitive from 35–160 kVp, with units specific for mammography covering a 22–40 kVp range. Quoted uncertainties for dose readings for these meters are 5% for the standard units and 2% for mammography.

While these units are highly effective, there are three main limitations: (1) cost as these units can cost up to $10,000 or more; (2) they cannot be used in real-time imaging, as they attenuate x-rays and the unit would be visible on the image; and (3) they do not measure backscatter radiation.

Radiochromic Film

When one talks of radiation hazards within diagnostic x-ray departments, traditionally the focus has been on stochastic effects, with deterministic effects such as skin lesions being the domain of radiation therapy centers. In recent years, however, certain procedures within diagnostic radiology—particularly those including interventional components—have been changing this focus, since the prolonged exposures and high doses associated with those techniques are leading to skin burns and similar deterministic changes being reported. This means that for these examinations, skin dose monitoring requires serious consideration—in addition, of course, to the usual dose measuring that goes on. Unfortunately, the previously mentioned dosimeters have certain limitations when it comes to measuring skin doses: DAP and solid-state meters cannot be placed at the skin surface during a procedure, and while one or a number of TLDs can be positioned on the skin, movement of the patient into multiple different positions would require a high number of TLD placements for a comprehensive series of measurements. One potential solution to providing skin doses is to use clever methods of calculation to estimate skin dose from other dose

recording metrics (Jones and Pasciak 2012), and previous workers have shown good to fair levels of correlation between maximum skin dose and DAP and fluoroscopic time measurements (Chida et al. 2006). While such calculations appear to be reasonable approaches for estimating a single parameter such as peak skin dose and can be done retrospectively once a procedure has been shown to be prolonged, comprehensive description of the spatial distribution of the dose across the skin surface requires an alternative strategy. This is the role of the radiochromic film.

Radiochromic film is a medium that is sensitive to radiation and will change its color depending on the level of exposure it has received, without any complex chemical processing (**Figure 5-23**). Typically, it consists of an active radio-sensitive layer around 0.03 mm thick sandwiched between two polyester layers. While its greatest use is in radiation therapy, types now available are suitable for diagnostic purposes, with the range of products

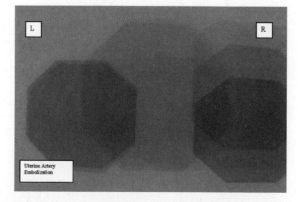

Figure 5-23 Radiochromic color change following an uterine artery embolization interventional procedure. The different colors represent different doses, which then can be profiled graphically.

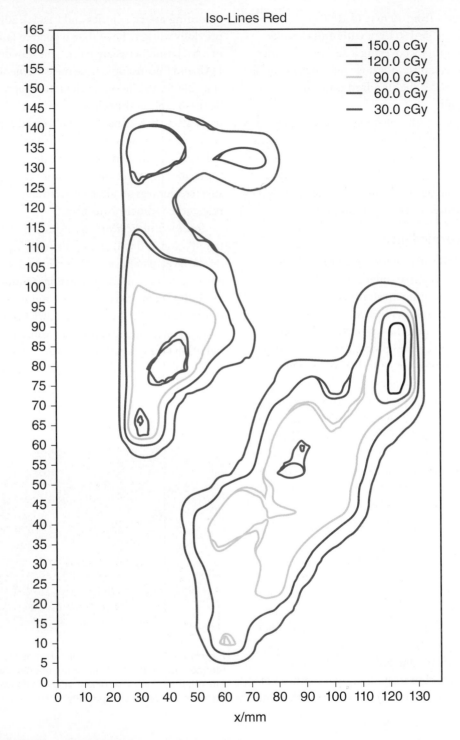

Figure 5-24 Profiling of radiation dose in two dimensions.

Courtesy of David Lewis, Ashland Specialty Ingredients (2011).

available facilitating the recording of doses from as low as 1 mGy up to 15 Gy. The spatial resolution—that is, the ability to demonstrate in fine details which part of the skin was exposed to which dose—is continually improving.

Clearly the color on the film that represents the dose must be accurately read if precise conclusions about spatial exposure distributions are to be made. Subjective opinions about the color will only go so far, and equipment such as calibrated densitometers or flatbed scanners are required for more accurate descriptions. Once scanned or measured appropriately, contour images can be produced demonstrating the specific dose distributions (**Figure 5-24**).

It is important to note that radiochromic film does have certain limitations that require careful consideration by the user. Its sensitivity to light and high temperature (>60°C), and the fading of colors post-irradiation mean that strict protocols must be adhered to if accurate measurements are to be made. Also, detailed information of the position of the film on the patient is required if information on doses deducted from the film's coloring will be precisely allocated to specific skin regions. Finally, since the film size can vary from 12.5 cm^2 × 12.5 cm^2 to 20 cm^2 × 20 cm^2, several films would need to be placed for a comprehensive measurement (which may not be the easiest thing in a complicated interventional procedure).

Summary of Key Concepts

1. **Risks associated with diagnostic imaging**. Every radiation exposure in medical imaging departments will introduce a risk of inducing a cancer, but should present a benefit to the patient as long as the exposure is justified. The responsibility of the radiographer or radiologic clinician is to ensure that the radiation dose is minimized and the benefit maximized for each examination that takes place.

2. **Justification and optimization principles**. Each x-ray exposure must be justified: it should have a good medical reason for performing it. As referred to many times within this text, irradiating individuals introduces a risk; however, this risk is acceptable if it is outweighed by the benefit that is provided diagnostically by the resultant image or images. Optimization of x-ray procedures means employing technologies or techniques that can reduce the radiation dose to patients (and staff) without sacrificing in any way the clinical information (relevant to the patient's condition) provided by performing the examination.

3. **Current radiation dose limits**. There are dose limits for workers and members of the public (e.g., family members accompanying patients) that should be adhered to. Examples of these are published by the ICRP and other national or international agencies. If these values are exceeded, appropriate measures should be put into place to minimize reoccurrence, and the exposed individual should be monitored for any adverse sequelae.

4. **Merits and applications of different dose measurement alternatives**. The principles of radiation protection—justification, optimization and dose limits (particularly the last two)—rely on effective methods on measuring radiation dose. There are a number of ways of doing this, but the main methods used in diagnostic imaging departments are thermoluminescent dosimetry; dose-area product technology; solid-state meters; and radiochromic film.

Discussion Questions

1. Discuss rationally the risks associated with radiation doses delivered during diagnostic x-ray procedures.

2. Debate the justification and optimization principles.

3. Discuss the variations in current radiation dose limits.

References

Alakhras M, Bourne R, Rickard M, Ng KH, Pietrzyk M, Brennan PC. Digital tomosynthesis: a new future for breast imaging? *Clin Radiol.* 2013;68:225–236.

Australian Radiation Protection and Nuclear Safety Agency. *Radiation Protection in the Medical Applications of Ionizing Radiation.* Victoria NSW: ARPANSA; 2008. (Available at http://www.arpansa.gov.au/publications/codes/rps14.cfm; Retrieved August 18, 2015.)

Aznar MC, Hemdal B, Medin J, Marckmann CJ, Andersen CE, Bøtter-Jensen L, Andersson I, Mattsson S. In vivo absorbed dose measurements in mammography using a new real-time luminescence technique. *Br J Radiol.* 2005;78:328–334.

Bell RE, McLaughlin RE. Ionising radiation (medical exposure) regulations (Northern Ireland) 2000 and their implications for accident and emergency (A&E) doctors in training. *Ulster Med J* 2001;70(No. 1):19e21.

Brennan PC, Madigan E. Lumbar spine radiology: analysis of the posteroanterior projection. *Eur Radiol.* 2000;10(7):1197–1201.

Brennan PC, McDonnell S, O'Leary D. Increasing film-focus distance (FFD) reduces radiation dose for x-ray examinations. *Radiat Prot Dosimetry.* 2004;108(3):263–238.

Chida K, Saito H, Otani H, Kohzuki M, Takahashi S, Yamada S, Shirato K, Zuguchi M. Relationship between fluoroscopic time, dose-area product, body weight, and maximum radiation skin dose in cardiac interventional procedures. *AJR Am J Roentgenol.* 2006;186:774–778.

Crawley MT, Mutch S, MSc, Nyekiova M, Reddy C, Weatherburn H. Calibration frequency of dose–area product meters. *Br J Radiol.* 2001;74:259–261.

Dowsett DJ, Kenny PA, Johnston RE. *The Physics of Diagnostic Imaging*, 2nd edition. London: Hodder Arnold; 2006.

European Commission. On health protection of individuals against the dangers of ionizing radiation in relation to medical exposure and repealing directive 84/466/EURATOM. European Council Directive 97/43/EURATOM; 1997.

European Commission. Laying down basic safety standards for the protection of the health of workers and the general public against the dangers arising from ionising radiation. European Council Directive 96/29/EURATOM; 1996.

Ginsberg GM, Schlesinger T, Ben-Shlomo A, Kushilevsky A, Margaliot M, Oren M, Finkleman M, et al. An economic evaluation of the use of rare earth screens to reduce the radiation dose from diagnostic X-ray procedures in Israel. *Br J Radiol.* 1998;71(844):406–412.

Health Canada. *Radiation Protection in Radiology – Large Facilities. Safety Procedures for the Installation, Use and Control of X-ray Equipment in Large Medical Radiological Facilities.* Safety Code 35; H128-1/08-545E. Ottawa: Health Canada; 2008. (Available at http://www.hc-sc.gc.ca/ewh-semt/pubs/radiation/safety-code_35-securite/index-eng.php; Retrieved August 18, 2015.)

Huda W, Ogden KM, Brennan PC, O'Leary D. Comments on 'Increasing film-focus distance (FFD) reduces radiation dose for X-ray examinations' by P.C. Brennan, S. McDonnell and D. O'Leary. *Radiat Prot Dosimetry.* 2005;113(4):453–435.

International Commission on Radiological Protection. The 2007 Recommendations of the International Commission on Radiological Protection. ICRP Publication 103. *Ann. ICRP* 2007;37(2-4).

Jarvinen H, Buls N, Clerinx P, Jansen J, Miljanic S, Nikodemova D, Ranogajec-KomorMand d'Errico F. Invited Editorial. Overview of double dosimetry procedures for the determination of the effective dose to the interventional radiology staff. *Radiat Prot Dosimetry.* 2008;129:333–339.

Jones AK, Pasciak AS. Calculating the peak skin dose resulting from fluoroscopically guided interventions. Part I: Methods. *J Appl Clin Med Phys.* 2011;12:3670.

Marmot MG, Altman DG, Cameron DA, Dewar JA, Thompson SG, Wilcox M, and The Independent UK Panel on Breast Cancer Screening. The benefits and harms of breast cancer screening: An independent review. *Br J Cancer.* 2013;108(11):2205–2240.

Matthews K, Brennan PC. Justification of x-ray examinations: General principles and an Irish perspective. *Radiography.* 2008;14:249–235.

Morris-Stiff G, Stiff RE, Morris-Stiff H. Abdominal radiograph requesting in the setting of acute abdominal pain: temporal trends and appropriateness of requesting 1. *Ann R Coll Surg Engl.* 2006;88(3):270e4.

O'Leary D, McDonnell S, Brennan PC. Increasing film focus distance (FFD) reduces radiation dose for X-ray examinations. *Radiat Prot Dosimetry.* 2004;108:263.

Pisano ED, Hendrick RE, Yaffe MJ, Baum JK, Acharyya S, Cormack JB, et al.; DMIST Investigators Group. Diagnostic accuracy of digital versus film mammography: exploratory analysis of selected population subgroups in DMIST. *Radiology.* 2008;246(2):376–383.

Poletti JL, McLean D. The effect of source to image-receptor distance on effective dose for some common X-ray projections. *Br J Radiol.* 2005;78:810–815.

Royal College of Radiologists. Making the best use of a department of clinical radiology: guidelines for doctors. 5th ed. London: Royal College of Radiologists; 2003.

Royal College of Radiologists. iRefer Making the best use of clinical radiology. London: Royal College of Radiologists; 2007.

Skaane P, Bandos AI, Gullien R, Eben EB, Ekseth U, Haakenaasen U, et al. Comparison of digital mammography alone and digital mammography plus tomosynthesis in a population-based screening program. *Radiology.* 2013;267:47–56.

Teunen D. The European Directive on health protection of individuals against the dangers of ionising radiation in relation to medical exposures (97/43/EURATOM). *J Radiol Prot.* 1998;18(2):133–137.

Theocharopoulos N, Perisinakis K, Damilakis J, Varveris H, Gourtsoyiannis N. Comparison of four methods for assessing patient effective dose from radiological examinations. *Med Phys.* 2002;29:2070–2079.

Triantopoulou Ch, Tsalafoutas I, Maniatis P, Papavdis D, Raios G, Siafas I, et al. Analysis of radiological examination request forms in conjunction with justification of X-ray exposures. *Eur J Radiol.* 2005;53:306e11.

Wall BF, Haylock R, Jansen JTM, Hillier MC, Hart D, Shrimpton PC. HPA-CRCE-028: Radiation Risks from Medical X-ray Examinations as a Function of the Age and Sex of the Patient (2011).

Yakoumakis E, Tsalafoutas IA, Nikolaou D, Nazos I, Koulentianos E, Proukakis C. Differences in effective dose estimation from dose-area product and entrance surface dose measurements in intravenous urography. *Br J Radiol.* 2001;74:727–734.

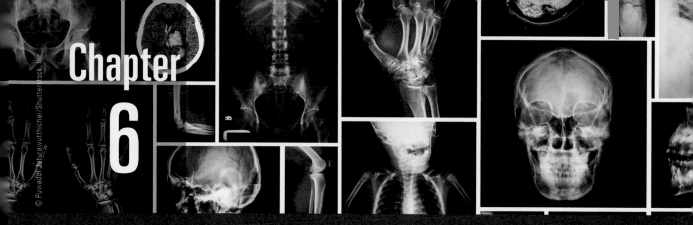

Chapter 6

Radiation Protection Organizations

Outline

- Introduction
- International Organizations
  - International Commission on Radiological Protection (ICRP)
  - International Commission on Radiation Unit and Measurement (ICRU)
  - United Nations Scientific Committee on the Effects of Atomic Radiation (UNSCEAR)
  - Radiation Effects Research Foundation (RERF)
  - Biological Effects of Ionizing Radiation Committee (BEIR)
- National Organizations
  - National Council on Radiation Protection and Measurement (NCRP)
- Center for Devices and Radiological Health (CDRH)
- Radiation Protection Bureau-Health Canada (RPB-HC)
- National Radiological Protection Board-United Kingdom (NRPB-UK)
- Definition of Terms Used in Reports
  - ICRP's Definitions
  - NCRP's Definitions
  - RPB-HC's Definitions
- Radiation Protection Recommendations—Common Elements
- References

Objectives

On completion of this chapter, you should be able to:

1. Identify five major international radiation protection organizations and explain the role of each one.

2. Identify four national radiation protections and explain the role of each one.

3. State the definitions of "shall," "should," and "must" as used in radiation protection reports of the International Commission on Radiological Protection (ICRP, the National Council on Radiation Protection and Measurements (NCRP), and the Radiation Protection Bureau-Health Canada (RPB-HC).

4. Describe the common elements of radiation protection recommendations for diagnostic x-ray imaging.

Introduction

The safety standards, guidelines, and recommendations cited in this book for the prudent use of radiation in medicine are based on the work of dedicated, knowledgeable individuals who are members of various radiation protection and related organizations throughout the world. Because of the citations from several of these organizations, it is important to become familiar with the activities and contributions of these various groups.

The purpose of this chapter is to explore the nature of these organizations in terms of their contributions to radiation protection. Specifically, the overall goals will be stated and the major activities of groups relevant to diagnostic radiology will be described briefly. Furthermore, specific reports dealing with radiation protection considerations for diagnostic radiology will be identified. Finally, the meanings of the words "should," "shall," and "must" as used in these reports will be defined.

In general, radiation protection organizations are divided into those that operate at an international level and those that serve a national function. In addition, some of these bodies deal primarily with the biological effects of radiation, while others focus on radiation protection principles, concepts, and practices.

International Organizations

There are several international organizations of relevance to radiation protection; however, only five of them will be highlighted in this section. They are:

- International Commission on Radiological Protection (ICRP)
- International Commission on Radiation Units and Measurements (ICRU)
- United Nations Scientific Committee on the Effects of Atomic Radiations (UNSCEAR)
- Radiation Effects Research Foundation (RERF)
- Biological Effects of Ionizing Radiation Committee (BEIR)

International Commission on Radiological Protection (ICRP)

The ICRP represents a very important body for diagnostic radiology because it makes major recommendations on radiation protection based on information provided by organizations concerned primarily with the biological effects of radiation, such as the BEIR, UNSCEAR, and RERF.

The ICRP was formed in 1928 by the Second International Congress of Radiology and was then referred to as the International X-Ray and Radium Protection Committee. Its primary activity at that time was to ensure radiation safety standards in radiology. The ICRP assumed its present name in 1950 to reflect more accurately its expanded role in radiation protection. The ICRP bases its recommended radiation protection measures on fundamental principles, and it leaves to the various national radiation protection bodies, the task of devising safety standards, regulatory procedures and practice guidelines that best address that country's needs (Berry 1987).

The ICRP is made up of individuals who are experts in radiology, physics, radiobiology, health physics, radiation protection, genetics, biochemistry, and biophysics. The commission is also actively involved with several other organizations including the ICRU, the World Health Organization (WHO), the International Atomic Energy Agency (IAEA) and the International Radiation Protection Association (IRPA).

The first recommendations of the ICRP were published in the *British Journal of Radiology* in 1928. These recommendations addressed x-ray and radium protection. This was followed by subsequent recommendations until 1959, when the first report—that is, Publication I, entitled "Recommendations of the International Commission in Radiological Protection"—was published by Pergamon Press in Oxford, England. Later, the general recommendations were published in 1964 (Publication 6), 1996 (Publication 9), 1977 (Publication 26), and in 1990 (Publication 60); each publication reflected the ongoing changes and evolution of radiation protection philosophy.

In 1977, Publication 26 — Recommendations of the ICRP, *Annals of the ICRP* introduced the International System of Radiological Protection based on "the current understanding of the science of radiation exposures and effects; and value judgements. These value judgements take into account societal expectations, ethics, and experience gained in application of the system" (ICRP 2013). In particular, this publication was significant because it introduced what was referred to as the current system of radiation protection, based on three principles as follows:

1. Principle of justification.
2. Principle of optimization.
3. Application of dose limits.

Furthermore, this publication introduced the terms **stochastic** and **non-stochastic** to describe genetic and somatic effects of radiation. In accordance with this new system of radiation protection, the goals of the ICRP are intended to minimize stochastic effects to an acceptably low level of risk, and to prevent non-stochastic (now referred to as **deterministic**) effects.

In 1991, the ICRP revised its recommendations once again and Publication 26 was superseded by Publication 60, "1990 Recommendations of the International Commission on Radiological Protection," released in the *Annals of the ICRP*. In this publication, some major changes were made based on the results of BEIR Committee Report V, *Health Effects of Exposure to Low Levels of Ionizing Radiation*. The 1990 ICRP recommendations identified that the risks of radiation to be about three to four times greater than had been previously estimated. This major finding prompted the ICRP to make several recommendations of importance to radiation protection. One such recommendation relates to reducing the dose limit to occupationally exposed individuals from 50 mSv (5 rems) to 20 mSv (2 rems) per year, averaged over defined periods of 5 years.

In 2007, the ICRP once again revised its recommendations, which were adopted in March 2007, in Germany, following a period of eight years of discussion with scientists, regulators, and users all over the world. These recommendations have been published in *ICRP Publication 103: The 2007 Recommendations of the International Commission on Radiological Protection* (Valentin 2007). The major features of the 2007 recommendations as summarized by Valentin (2007) are:

- Update radiation and tissue weighting factors
- Maintain the principle of justification, optimization, and application of dose limits
- Maintain individual dose limits
- Reinforce the principle of optimization
- "Include an approach for developing a framework to demonstrate radiological protection of the environment" (p. 11)
- "Evolving from the previous process-based approach using practices and interventions, by moving to a situation-based approach applying the fundamental principles of justification, and optimization of protection to all controllable exposure situations, which the present recommendations characterize as planned, emergency, and existing exposure conditions." (p. 11)

The ICRP, as of August 2015, has about 147 publications available to interested users. For example, ICRP Publication 123 is entitled "Assessment of Radiation Exposure of Astronauts in Space," a report that is obviously of interest to astronauts and to the National Aeronautics and Space Administration (NASA). Similarly, the following recent reports are important not only to radiologists but also to radiologic technologists as well:

1. ICRP Publication 93: Managing Patient Dose in Digital Radiology. *Ann ICRP*. 31(1), 2004.
2. ICRP Publication 102: Managing Patient Dose in Multi-Detector Computed Tomography (MDCT). *Ann ICRP*. 2007;37(1).
3. ICRP Publication 103: 2007 Recommendations of the International Commission on Radiological Protection (users Edition). *Ann ICRP*. 2007;37(2-4).

4. ICRP Publication 113: Education and Training in Radiological Protection for Diagnostic and Interventional Procedures. *Ann ICRP*. 2009;39(5).

5. ICRP Publication 117: Radiological Protection in Fluoroscopically Guided Procedures outside the Imaging Department. *Ann ICRP*. 2010;40(6).

6. ICRP Publication 121: Radiological Protection in Paediatric Diagnostic and International Radiology. *Ann ICRP*. 2013;42(2).

7. ICRP Publication 127: Radiological Protection in Ion Beam Radiotherapy. *Ann ICRP*. 2014;43(4).

8. ICRP Publication 128: Radiation Dose to Patients from Radiopharmaceuticals: A Compendium of Current Information Related to Frequently Used Substances. *Ann ICRP*. 2015;44(2S).

9. ICRP Publication 129: Radiological Protection in Cone Beam Computed Tomography (CBCT). *Ann ICRP*. 2015;44(1).

Finally, the ICRP works in conjunction with its "sister body," the ICRU, and has "official relationships" with organizations such as UNSCEAR, WHO, and IRPA, among others.

International Commission on Radiation Unit and Measurement (ICRU)

The ICRU was established in 1928 with the goal of developing recommendations that would be accepted by the international community. The ICRU deals primarily with establishing radiation quantities and units, measurement procedures, and the use of data to ensure uniform reporting. The ICRU is also active in occupational radiation protection, e.g, radiation therapy and medical imaging, including radiology, CT, and nuclear medicine.

The ICRU encourages national organizations to develop their own procedures for standards, and also recommends that countries pay careful attention to the universal concepts relating to radiation quantities and units for radiation protection.

The most recent report the ICRU has contributed to radiology is Report 74: Patient Dosimetry for X-Rays used in Medical Imaging (ICRU 2005).

United Nations Scientific Committee on the Effects of Atomic Radiation (UNSCEAR)

UNSCEAR was established in 1955 by the General Assembly of the United Nations and is made up of expert radiologists from around the world. There are 27 countries that provide scientists to serve on this committee. The committee has the task of examining current available data on the risks of natural and artificial radiation from sources as diverse as RERF, major epidemiological studies, and animal studies. UNSCEAR also makes it a priority to stay abreast of recent developments in radiobiology as a means of keeping track of biological effects at both the systemic and cellular levels. Furthermore, this committee also makes predictions about the incidence of biological effects among the general population.

UNSCEAR has published major reports from 1977 to 2012. Generally, the purpose of these reports is to assess the risks of radiation exposure using the available biological evidence. Examples of these reports include:

1. UNSCEAR 2012 Report: *Biological mechanism of radiation actions at low doses.*

2. UNSCEAR 2010 Report: *Summary of low-dose radiation effects on health.*

3. UNSCEAR 2008 Report: *Source and effects of ionizing radiation*, in two volumes. While Volume 1 deals with medical radiation exposures, exposures of the public and workers from various sources, Volume 2 addresses exposures in accidents, health effects due to radiation from the Chernobyl accident, and effects of ionizing radiation on non-human biota.

4. UNSCEAR 2006 Report: *Effects of ionizing radiation*, in two volumes. Volume 1 looks at epidemiological studies of radiation and cancer, etc. Volume 2 deals with delayed effects

of exposure to ionizing system, and sources-to-effects assessment for radon exposures in homes.

5. UNSCEAR 2001 Report: *Hereditary effects of ionizing radiation*.

Radiation Effects Research Foundation (RERF)

The RERF is a scientific research institution championed by the government of Japan, and obtains support from the United States of America. The overall objective of RERF is "to conduct research and studies for peaceful purposes on medical effects of radiation and associated diseases in humans, with a view to contributing to maintenance of the health and welfare of the atomic bomb (A-bomb) survivors and to the enhancement of the health of all humankind" (RERF 2013). The survivors refer to those humans of the atomic bombings of the cities of Hiroshima and Nagasaki during World War II.

It is important to note that the RERF data are purely statistical in nature (Brown 1989). Once these data are made available in scientific publications, other organizations pore over it in an effort to evaluate new risk models and predictions with the ultimate goal of devising new recommendations for radiation protection procedures.

Biological Effects of Ionizing Radiation Committee (BEIR)

The BEIR committee was formed by the National Research Council (NRC) organized by the US National Academy of Sciences (NAS), and in this regard, the BEIR committee is not "strictly" an international committee (Brown 1989).

The BEIR committee has evolved from BEIR I to the most recent BEIR VII, with each committee charged with the specific responsibility of advising the United States (US) government on the health effects of radiation exposures. In 1986, the BEIR V committee was formed "to conduct a comprehensive review of the biological effects of ionizing radiations focusing on information that had been reported since the conclusion of the BEIR III study

and, to the extent that available information permitted, provide new estimates of the risks of genetic and somatic effects in humans due to low-level exposures of ionizing radiation" (NRC, 1990, p. vi).

Using information provided by RERF, the BEIR V Report concluded that the risks of radiation exposure are about three to four times greater than had been previously estimated in the BEIR III Report (NRC, 1990). The results of this BEIR study, as presented in the BEIR V Report entitled *Health Effects of Exposure to Low Levels of Ionizing Radiation*, have significant implications for radiation protection. It is with these results that the ICRP made recent recommendations on standards and guidelines for radiation protection.

The last report published is BEIR Report VII, Phase 2-2006: *Health Risks from Exposure to Low Levels of Ionizing Radiation, Phase 2*. A brief summary of this report provided by the NRC (2005) is as follows:

> *In general, BEIR VII supports previously reported risk estimates for cancer and leukemia, but the availability of new and more extensive data have strengthened confidence in these estimates. A comprehensive review of available biological and biophysical data supports a "linear-no-threshold" (LNT) risk model — that the risk of cancer proceeds in a linear fashion at lower doses without a threshold and that the smallest dose has the potential to cause a small increase in risk to humans... (p. 1)*

National Organizations

National organizations are those that provide recommendations on medical radiation protection for their respective countries. The major organizations to be described briefly in this section are those of the US, Canada, and the United Kingdom (UK).

The US organizations include the National Council on Radiation Protection and Measurements (NCRP), the Center for Devices and Radiological Health (CDRH), and the Food and Drug

Administration (FDA). While the Canadian organization of importance is the Radiation Protection Bureau-Health Canada (RPB-HC), the UK organization is the National Radiological Protection Board (NRPB). An important point to note here is that there are additional organizations such as the US Nuclear Regulatory Commission (USNRC), and the Canadian Nuclear Safety Commission (CNSC). Since these two organizations deal with all aspects of nuclear safety, they will not be considered further in this text.

National Council on Radiation Protection and Measurement (NCRP)

The NCRP is a non-profit organization chartered by the US Congress in 1964 to replace the Advisory Committee on X-Ray and Radiation Protection, the original agency founded in 1929.

The NCRP is organized into a main committee and other scientific subcommittees and is made up of expert scientists in radiation protection. These subcommittees study and prepare reports on specific radiation protection issues and then submit them to the main committee for approval and publication. The NCRP has produced more than 150 scientific reports, a few of which will be listed later in this section.

The Charter of the Council (Public Law 88-376) has issued four major objectives as follows:

1. *"Collect, analyze, develop and disseminate in the public interest information and recommendations about (a) protection against radiation, and (b) radiation measurements, quantities, and units, particularly those concerned with radiation protection;*

2. *Provide a means by which organizations concerned with the scientific and related aspects of radiation protection, and of radiation quantities, units and measurements may cooperate for effective utilization of their combined resources and to stimulate the work of such organizations;*

3. *Develop basic concepts about radiation quantities, units, and measurements, about*

the application of these concepts, and about radiation protection;

4. *Cooperate with the International Commission on Radiological Protection, the Federal Radiation Council, the International Commission on Radiation Units and Measurements and other national and international organizations, governmental and private, concerned with radiation quantities, units, and measurements and with radiation protection." (NCRP, 2010, p. 1-2)*

The NCRP is not a government organization; however, its recommendations on radiation protection are often considered by local, state, and federal governments.

The NCRP has published quite a large number of proceedings, Lauriston S. Taylor lectures, commentaries and substantive reports. Recent important reports of relevance to radiologic technologists are as follows:

1. Report No. 133: *Radiation Protection for Procedures Performed Outside the Radiology Departure* (2000).

2. Report No. 147: *Structural Shielding Design for Medical X-Ray Imaging Facilities* (2004).

3. Report No. 149: *A Guide to Mammography and Other Breast Imaging Procedures* (2004).

4. Report No. 157: *Radiation Protection in Educational Institutions* (2007).

5. Report No. 160: *Ionizing Radiation Exposure of the Population of the United States* (2009).

6. Report No. 168: *Radiation Dose Management for Fluoroscopically-Guided Interventional Medical Procedures* (2010).

7. Report No. 174: *Preconception and Prenatal Radiation Exposure-Health Effects and Protective Guidance* (2013).

Center for Devices and Radiological Health (CDRH)

The CDRH was created by merging the Bureau of Radiological Health (BRH) and the Bureau of

Medical Devices (BMD) to assume responsibility for all medical devices including radiation-emitting equipment, such as diagnostic x-ray tubes. The CDRH is of interest to radiologic technologists because it is a federal organization (US Public Health Service) that also plays a major role in evaluating population exposure to x-rays, as well as other diagnostic imaging modalities, and radiation therapy.

The CDRH aims to minimize unnecessary radiation exposure by assuming regulatory control of the performance of x-ray equipment. This goal is accomplished by providing technical and biological background information and advice to the medical profession and to the general public.

Radiation Protection Bureau-Health Canada (RPB-HC)

Radiation protection in diagnostic x-ray imaging is addressed by RPB-HC, a federal government organization. The RPB has an x-ray section and a non-ionizing radiation section. While the x-ray section addresses safety procedures and presents equipment and installation guidelines, the non-ionizing radiation section deals with safety issues relating to microwaves, radio waves, and lasers.

A major and significant publication of the RPB is Safety Code 35: Radiation Protection in Radiology–Large Facilities: *Safety Procedures for the Installation, Use, and Control of X-Ray Equipment in Large Medical Radiological Facilities* (2008).

This Safety Code 35 (SC-35) "brings Canada's standards in line with the standards that have been in place for many years in European countries, the United States, and internationally." (Bjarnason et al. 2013, p. 6)

The major goals of SC-35 are to:

1. Minimize patient exposure to ionizing radiation, while ensuring the necessary diagnostic information is obtained and treatment provided.

2. Ensure adequate protection of personnel operating x-ray equipment.

3. Ensure adequate protection of other personnel and the general public in the vicinity of areas where x-ray equipment is used (Health Canada, 2008, p. 6).

The SC-35 Report is divided into three major sections as follows:

- Section A: Responsibilities and Protection
- Section B: Facility and Equipment Requirements
- Section C: Quality Assurance Program

National Radiological Protection Board- United Kingdom (NRPB-UK)

The NRPB was a radiation protection agency in the UK charged with the goal of conducting radiation protection research and providing technical advice on the safe use of ionizing and non-ionizing radiations. Its functions were assumed by Public Health England's Radiation Protection Service in 2005. During its operation, NRPB's research activities covered a wide scope of topics (such as internal dosimetry, radon hazards, epidemiology and molecular biology and medical x-rays), technical advice range from optimization of radiation protection, transport of radioactive materials, personnel dosimetry, and education courses, to conducting radiation surveys (O'Riordan 2010).

The NRPB published several reports which can be viewed on the UK National Archives website (accessed in August 2015) at http://webarchive.nationalarchives.gov .uk/20140721185223/http://www.hpa.org.uk /Publications/Radiation/NPRBArchive/.

Definition of Terms Used in Reports

There are three terms used in specific Reports of the ICRP, NCRP, and RPB-HC and they include "*shall*," "*should*," and "*must*." These terms are used in selected recommendations of these three organizations. In **Table 6-1**, the terms used by each of these organizations are given, and each of

Table 6-1 Terms used by three radiation protection organizations to indicate the nature of their recommendations

ICRP	NCRP (US)	RPB (Canada)
Shall	Shall	Must
Should	Should	Should

the terms, as defined by each organization, has a special meaning.

ICRP's Definitions

The meanings of terms *shall* and *should* as defined by the ICRP (2007) in their Radiation Protection Reports are as follows:

> "*Shall: Necessary or essential for radiation protection*
> *Should: To apply, whenever reasonable, in the interest of improving radiation protection.*" (p. 5)

Likewise, the negatives of these terms carry distinct meanings.

NCRP's Definitions

The NCRP (2000) defines these terms in their reports as follows:

> "*Shall: indicates a recommendation that is necessary or essential to meet the currently accepted standards of radiation protection. Should: indicates an advisory recommendation that is to be applied when practicable and is equivalent to 'is recommended' or 'is advisable.'*" (p. 4)

RPB-HC's Definitions

In Canada, RPB-HC (2008) defines the terms *must* and *should* in SC-35, as follows:

> "… must *indicates a requirement that is essential to meet the currently accepted standards of protection, while* should *indicates an advisory recommendations that is*

highly desirable and is to be implemented where practicable." (p. 3)

Radiation Protection Recommendations– Common Elements

With respect to radiation protection recommendations as stated in specific reports of the ICPR, NCRP, and RPB-HC SC-35, there are common elements that outline the same guiding principles. For example, with respect to the recommendation of holding patients, the guiding principles are as follows:

1. Restraining device *should* be used to immobilize patients during examinations.

2. Individuals holding patients *shall* and *must* be protected by wearing lead aprons and lead gloves.

3. No part of the shielded body of those who hold patients is in the direct path of the primary beam.

In this particular example, holding patients, it appears that both national organizations (NCRP, and RPB-HC) have adopted the recommendations of the ICRP. In situations where the national recommendations differ from what is proposed by the international organization (ICRP), the national recommendations should be more stringent, and definitely not below the standards and guidelines of the ICRP. For example, the ICRP recommends a total x-ray beam filtration of 2.5 mm aluminum equivalent for equipment operating above 70 kVp. National organizations must either adopt this recommendation or provide a more stringent one, in which case, the total filtration at the same kVp will be greater than 2.5 mm but not less.

While the primary goal is to know the major recommendations, guidelines, and standards of the safe used of radiation in imaging patients, the secondary goal is to become familiar with the common elements inherent in these radiation protection guidelines, standards, and recommendations.

Summary Of Key Concepts

1. This chapter explored the nature of both selected international and national radiation protection organizations with specific reference to their contributions to radiation protection and the major activities of groups relevant to diagnostic radiology. In addition, specific reports dealing with radiation protection considerations for diagnostic radiology were identified.

2. International organizations include the Commission on Radiological Protection (ICRP), International Commission on Radiation Units and Measurements (ICRU), United Nations Scientific Committee on the Effects of Atomic Radiations (UNSCEAR), Radiation Effects Research Foundation (RERF), and the Biological Effects of Ionizing Radiation Committee (BEIR).

3. Of these, The ICRP represents a very important body for diagnostic radiology because it makes major recommendations on radiation protection based on information provided by organizations concerned primarily with the biological effects of radiation, such as the BEIR, UNSCEAR, and RERF.

4. The ICRP has produced numerous reports, including:
   - ICRP Publication 93: Managing Patient Dose in Digital Radiology. *Ann ICRP.* 2004; 31(1).
   - ICRP Publication 102: Managing Patient Dose in Multi-Detector Computed Tomography (MDCT). *Ann ICRP.* 2007;37(1).
   - ICRP Publication 103: 2007 Recommendations of the International Commission on Radiological Protection (users Edition). *Ann ICRP.* 2007;37(2-4).
   - ICRP Publication 113: Education and Training in Radiological Protection for Diagnostic and Interventional Procedures. *Ann ICRP.* 2009;39(5).
   - ICRP Publication 117: Radiological Protection in Fluoroscopically Guided Procedures outside the Imaging Department. *Ann ICRP.* 2010;40(6).
   - ICRP Publication 121: Radiological Protection in Paediatric Diagnostic and International Radiology. *Ann ICRP.* 2013;42(2).
   - ICRP Publication 127: Radiological Protection in Ion Beam Radiotherapy. *Ann ICRP.* 2014;43(4).
   - ICRP Publication 128: Radiation Dose to Patients from Radiopharmaceuticals: A Compendium of Current Information Related to Frequently Used Substances. *Ann ICRP.* 2015;44(2S).
   - ICRP Publication 129: Radiological Protection in Cone Beam Computed Tomography (CBCT). *Ann ICRP.* 2015;44(1).

5. The current system of radiation protection based on three principles as follows:
   - Principle of justification
   - Principle of optimization
   - Application of dose limits

6. The ICRU deals primarily with establishing radiation quantities and units, measurement procedures, and the use of data to ensure uniform reporting. The ICRU is also active in occupational radiation protection, e.g., radiation therapy and medical imaging including radiology, CT, and nuclear medicine.

7. UNSCEAR makes predictions about the incidence of biological effects among the general population, and in general, the purpose of their reports is to assess the risks of radiation exposure using the available biological evidence.

(Continues)

8. The RERF is a scientific research institution championed by the government of Japan, and obtains support from the United States of America. The overall goal of RERF is to conduct research about the effects on the survivors of the 1945 atomic bombings of the cities of Hiroshima and Nagasaki in Japan.

9. Using information provided by RERF, the BEIR committee examines the risks of radiation exposure, which have significant implications for radiation protection. It is with these results that the ICRP made recent recommendations on standards and guidelines for radiation protection.

10. The US national organizations include the National Council on Radiation Protection and Measurements (NCRP), the Center for Devices and Radiological Health (CDRH), and the Food and Drug Administration (FDA). While the Canadian organization of importance is the Radiation Protection Bureau-Health Canada (RPB-HC), the UK organization was the National Radiological Protection Board (NRPB) until 2005, but its functions have since been assumed by Public Health England (PHE).

11. The NCRP has published a number of important reports of relevance to radiologic technologists such as:
    - Report No. 133: *Radiation Protection for Procedures Performed Outside the Radiology Departure* (2000).
    - Report No. 147: *Structural Shielding Design for Medical X-Ray Imaging Facilities* (2004).
    - Report No. 149: *A Guide to Mammography and Other Breast Imaging Procedures* (2004).
    - Report No. 157: *Radiation Protection in Educational Institutions* (2007).
    - Report No. 160: *Ionizing Radiation Exposure of the Population of the United States* (2009).
    - Report No. 168: *Radiation Dose Management for Fluoroscopically-Guided Interventional Medical Procedures* (2010), and
    - Report No. 174: *Preconception and Prenatal Radiation Exposure-Health Effects and Protective Guidance* (2013).

12. The goal of the CDRH is to minimize unnecessary radiation exposure by assuming regulatory control of the performance of x-ray equipment. This goal is accomplished by providing technical and biological background information and advice to the medical profession and to the general public

13. There are three terms used in specific Reports of the ICRP and the NCRP: "*shall*," "*should*," and "*must*." These terms are used in selected recommendations of these three organizations. The ICRP's definitions are as follows:
    - "*Shall*: Necessary or essential for radiation protection
    - *Should*: To apply, whenever reasonable, in the interest of improving radiation protection." (p. 5)

    The NCRP defines these terms in their reports as follows:
    - "*Shall*: indicates a recommendation that is necessary or essential to meet the currently accepted standards of radiation protection.
    - *Should*: indicates an advisory recommendation that is to be applied when practicable and is equivalent to "is recommended" or "is advisable."

14. While the primary goal is to know the major recommendations, guidelines, and standards of the safe used of radiation in imaging patients, the secondary goal is to become familiar with the common elements inherent in these radiation protection guidelines, standards, and recommendations.

Discussion Questions

1. Discuss the role of the ICRP and identify several major reports of relevance to the technologist. State the three major principles of radiation protection established by the ICRP.

2. Identify several national radiation protection organizations and discuss the role of the NCRP and the CDRH in the US.

3. Outline the definitions of "shall," "should," and "must" as used in the reports of the ICRP and the NCRP.

4. Describe briefly what is meant by the common elements of the various radiation protection reports of the ICRP and the NCRP.

References

Berry RJ. The international commission on radiological protection. An historical perspective. In Russell J, Southwood R (Eds). *Radiation and Health.* New York, John Wiley and Sons; 1987.

Brown D. International bodies of importance for radiation protection practices in Canada. *Bull Can Radiat Prot Assoc.* 1989;10:9–15.

Bjarnason TA, Thakur Y, & Aldrich JE. Health Canada safety code 35: Awareness of the impacts for diagnostic radiology. *Can J Radiologists.* 1987;64:6–9.

Health Canada. *Radiation protection in radiology – Large facilities: Safety code 35.* Ottawa: Government of Canada; 2008. (Available at: http://www.hc-sc.gc.ca/ewh-semt/pubs /radiation/safety-code_35-securite/index-eng .php; Retrieved August 20, 2015.)

International Commission on Radiation Units and Measurements, Inc (ICRU). Patient Dosimetry for X Rays used in Medical Imaging (Report 74). J ICRU 2005;5(2). (Available at http://www.icru .org/home/reports/patient-dosimetry-for-x-rays -used-in-medical-imaging-report-74; Retrieved August 20, 2015.)

International Commission on Radiological Protection (ICRP). 1990 Recommendations of the ICRP (Publication No. 60). Elmsford, New York, Pergamon Press; 1991.

International Commission on Radiological Protection (ICRP). About the ICRP. (Available at www.icrp .org; Retrieved August 20, 2015.)

NRC BEIR Committee. *The effects on populations of exposure to low levels of ionizing radiations.* Washington, DC: National Academy of Sciences /National Research Council; 1990.

NRC. BEIR VII: *Health risks from exposure to low levels of ionizing radiation.* Washington, DC: National Academies Press; 2005.

NCRP (2010). Our Mission. (Available at www .ncrponline.org/AboutNCRP/Our_Mission .html; Retrieved August 20, 2015.)

NCRP. NCRP Report No. 133: *Radiation protection for procedures performed outside the radiology department.* Bethesda, MD; 2000.

O'Riordan, MC. The NRPB Era. *J Radiol Prot.* 2010;30(1):85–92.

RERF. Radiation Effects Research Foundation. (Available at www.rerf.jp/intro/establish /index_e.html; Retrieved August 20, 2015.)

Valentin J. (Ed.) International Commission of Radiological Protection (2007). The 2007 Recommendations of the International Commission Radiological Protection. St. Louis, MO: Elsevier-Mosby; 2007.

Wambersie A, Zoetelief J, Menzel HG, Paretzke H. The ICRU (International Commission on Radiation Units and Measurements). Its contribution to dosimetry in diagnostic and interventional radiology. *Radiat Prot Dosimetry.* 2005:117(1-3):7–12.

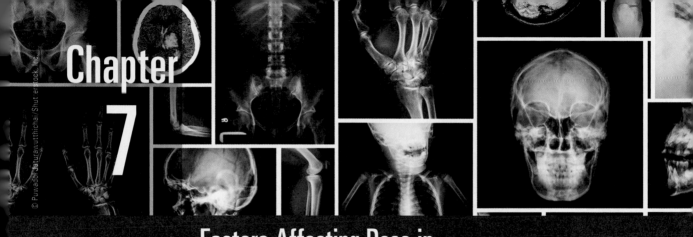

Chapter 7

Factors Affecting Dose in Radiographic Imaging

Outline

- Introduction
- System Components Affecting Dose: An Overview
  - Radiographic systems: Exposure components
- Clinical Factors
  - Responsibility of referring physicians
  - Role of the technologist
  - Role of the radiologist
  - Responsibility of the patient
  - Responsibilities and radiation protection
- Technical Factors in Radiography
  - Exposure technique factors
  - Automatic exposure control
  - X-ray generator waveform
- Filtration
- Collimation and field size
- Beam alignment
- Source-to-image receptor distance/source-to-skin distance
- Patient thickness and density
- Anti-scatter grids
- Sensitivity of the image receptor
- Film processing
- Repeat radiographic examinations
- Repeat rates in digital radiography
- Shielding radio-sensitive organs
- References

Objectives

On completion of this chapter, you should be able to:

1. Describe the major components affecting the dose for radiography imaging systems.
2. Discuss the overall responsibilities of the physician, technologist, radiologist, and the patient in radiation protection.
3. List 15 technical factors affecting the dose to the patient in radiographic imaging.
4. Explain how each of the 15 factors identified in objective 3 above affects the dose in radiographic imaging.

Introduction

Radiation protection in diagnostic radiology is mainly concerned with optimization of the radiation dose to the patient and minimizing radiation dose to personnel and members of the public. Furthermore, radiation protection of the patient depends on *good clinical judgment*, *proper design of the equipment*, *good operational practice*, and *competent interpretation of patient images* (ICRP 1982). These four requirements still hold true today. While good clinical judgment refers primarily to the patient's physician, it is linked to the first principle of radiation protection advocated by the ICRP, justification (discussed at length elsewhere). The proper design of equipment is undertaken so that manufacturers and end users alike can comply with regulatory international and national radiation protection requirements. Good operational practice and competent interpretation of the patient's images are directed to users of the equipment, such as technologists and radiologists. These latter three requirements are consequently linked to the ICRP's optimization principle.

In addition, radiation protection of the patient requires knowledge of (1) biological effects, (2) physical factors, (3) technical factors, and (4) procedural factors. Physical and biological factors are beyond the scope of this chapter and are described elsewhere; this chapter will address the technical and procedural factors. Specifically, this chapter will review imaging system exposure components affecting dose for radiographic and fluoroscopic systems, clinical factors, and several technical factors—some that are under the direct control of the operator (factors related to exposure technique, for example), and others that are not (e.g., x-ray generator waveform). Factors affecting the dose in digital radiography (DR) and computed tomography (CT) will not be addressed here, as they are described in detail elsewhere.

System Components Affecting Dose: an Overview

Radiographic Systems: Exposure Components

The general components of radiographic imaging systems affecting the dose to the patient are illustrated in **Figure 7-1**.

It is clear that the components include the x-ray generator, the x-ray tube, x-ray beam filter, the x-ray beam collimator, the x-ray beam area—or *field-of-view* (*FOV*) as it is sometimes called—patient thickness and density, table top, scattered radiation grid, the image receptor (detector) image processing, source-to-skin in distance (SSD), source-to-image receptor distance (SID) and finally, the users (technologists and radiologists) who have direct control of the x-ray beam quantity (mAs) and quality (kVp) needed for the examination.

The important considerations with respect to the radiation dose are as follows:

1. The technologist selects the exposure technique factors (kVp, mAs) for the appropriate patient examination.

2. These exposure technique factors are subsequently applied to the x-ray generator to produce the appropriate beam quantity (mAs) and beam quality or penetrability (kVp). The efficiency of x-ray generation depends on the type of generator used; x-ray generators have evolved from single-phase to three-phase, to high-frequency generators. The voltage waveforms of these generators and how they relate to patient exposures will be highlighted later in the chapter.

3. The mAs and kVp are applied to the x-ray tube, which produces a beam of x-rays that is used to image the patient. This is a broad beam (*open-beam geometry*) that must first be filtered and subsequently be collimated to the area of interest on the patient.

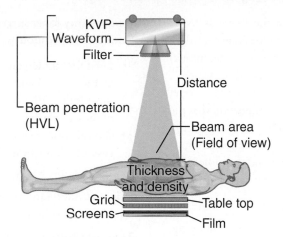

Figure 7-1 The general components of an x-ray imaging system affecting dose to the patient, including factors under the direct control of the operator.

Courtesy of Dr. Perry Sprawls, PhD, FACR, FAAPM, Distinguished Emeritus Professor, Emory University; Director, Sprawls Educational Foundation. Reproduced by permission.

4. During the exposure, the beam is fixed in one position (area of interest defined by the collimation) on the patient.

5. The beam passes through the patient, table top, and grid, and subsequently falls upon the image receptor. The radiation dose depends on the tissue thickness and density, the attenuating properties of the table, the characteristics of the scattered radiation grid used and the sensitivity of the image receptor.

6. The latent image obtained on the image receptor must be rendered visible, which is a function of the image processor. This can be either a chemical processor for film-screen radiography or a computer for digital radiography.

7. Additional factors that influence the dose delivered to the patient are the SSD, SID, the x-ray beam, and the light beam of the collimation system, which must be in perfect alignment. These will be described in detail later in this chapter.

Clinical Factors

Clinical factors refer to the overall responsibilities of the individuals involved in exposing patients to radiation. These responsibilities relate not only to the prescription of the x-ray examination but also to the non technical, procedural aspects such as patient care, communications, and comfort. The individuals who shoulder the responsibility for determining the nature and extent of a patient's radiologic examination are the *referring physician*, the *radiologist*, and the *technologist*.

The patient first sees the referring physician (usually a family physician or the emergency physician) who prescribes the x-ray examination based on a physical/clinical examination of the patient. Next, the patient arrives in the radiology department and, depending on the type of procedure, may come in contact with the technologist and/or radiologist, or both. While the technologist is responsible for conducting the radiographic examination, the radiologist assumes full responsibility for performing fluoroscopic examinations, with the assistance of the technologist.

Responsibility of Referring Physicians

Having examined the patient clinically, the referring physician prescribes the x-ray examination. Generally, the physician indicates on a requisition form the clinical justification for the x-ray examination. For example, a chest x-ray is justified if the patient suffers from (or is suspected to have) an inflammatory disease (e.g., pneumonia), a traumatic problem (e.g., pneumothorax) or a neoplastic disease (e.g., bronchogenic carcinoma) of the respiratory system. It is important that the physician provides enough clinical data regarding the patient's condition, since this information enables both the technologist and the radiologist to carry out the most appropriate x-ray examination.

Role of the Technologist

The role of technologists in diagnostic imaging is clear. They must first be educated and trained in the art and science of diagnostic imaging and must maintain an understanding of new instrumentation and procedures. Technologists apply the knowledge of anatomy and physiology, physics, instrumentation, radiobiology and radiation protection, pathology, and radiographic technique and positioning to the successful completion of an x-ray examination. Communication and interpersonal skills and the application of ethical principles are also vital skills of the technologist. The technologist must use the clinical information provided by the patient's physician in conjunction with the protocols for x-ray examinations established by the imaging department.

Role of the Radiologist

One of the primary roles of radiologists is the performance of fluoroscopic examinations with the assistance of a technologist. Radiologists often communicate with the referring physician in order to tailor the examination to the needs of the patient (Sierzenski et al. 2014). They also communicate to the patient all details related to the procedure. The radiologist and the technologist work together to expedite the examination and to ensure patient safety and comfort before, during, and after the examination.

Responsibility of the Patient

In addition to the responsibilities highlighted above, the patient must also assume some degree of

responsibility for ensuring that the examination is conducted expeditiously. This means that patients:

- must first understand the instructions provided by the technologist and/or radiologist;
- must follow all instructions during the conduct of the examination;
- should cooperate with personnel to ensure successful completion of the examination.

The technologist should always ensure the patients understand the significance of these requirements before and during the examination.

Responsibilities and Radiation Protection

It is absolutely clear that the responsibilities outlined briefly above play a significant role in radiation protection of the patient in diagnostic imaging. So important are these responsibilities that they are often identified and stated in Radiation Safety Codes of most countries. For example, the Radiation Protection Bureau-Health Canada (RPB-HC) Safety Code 35 (2008) features an entire section addressing "Responsibilities of Personnel"; the parties identified and described include the owner of the facility (usually a radiologist or medical center), a responsible user (a trained individual who can operate x-ray equipment), the x-ray equipment operator, medical physicist, referring physician, and an information systems specialist. Furthermore, with respect to the referring physician, the Safety Code 35 states that "the main responsibility of the referring physician/practitioner is to ensure that the use of x-rays is justified …. [the referring physician] should be confident that the procedure will improve patient diagnosis and/or treatment sufficiently in comparison with alternate, non-x-ray utilizing methods of diagnosis and/or treatment; be aware of the risks associated with x-ray procedure" (p. 9).

Another example of responsibilities of personnel in radiation protection is noted in the Federal Guidance Report No. 14 (EPA 2012) on *Radiation Protection Guidance for Diagnostic and Interventional*

X-ray Procedures. In the section on "Communication among Practitioners," the recommendation is as follows:

> *[W]henever possible, the Radiological Medical Practitioner should review all examination requests requiring fluoroscopy, CT, and other complex or high dose studies before the examination is given and preferably before it is scheduled. For this reason, it is important that a thorough and accurate patient history be included with each examination request. Based upon the clinical question, history and relevant available previous studies, the Radiological Medical Practitioner should direct the examination using standard protocols, with any appropriate addition, substitution or deletion of views or sequences. It is preferable that changes in the examination be done in consultation with the Referring Medical Practitioner."* (EPA 2012, p. 21)

Technical Factors in Radiography

There are several technical factors affecting patient dose in diagnostic radiography, some of which are under the direct control of the technologist and others that are not. These factors are illustrated in Figure 7-1. The type of x-ray generator and x-ray tube characteristics cannot be controlled by the technologist; however, those under the direct control of the technologist include the exposure technique factors, collimation and field size, beam alignment, SID, SSD, and image receptor. Each of these factors will now be described briefly.

Exposure Technique Factors

Recall that during x-ray production, electrons are "boiled off" the filament of the cathode of the x-ray tube and are accelerated across the tube to strike the target of the x-ray tube anode. Upon striking the target, a beam of x-rays is produced. This beam, the useful beam, is a heterogeneous beam of radiation that is transmitted through the patient and the table top to produce an image on the image receptor.

The photons of a heterogeneous beam have different energies ranging from low to high. Whereas the high-energy photons pass through the patient to strike the image receptor and produce the image, the low-energy photons do not have enough energy to penetrate the patient. They are absorbed by the patient and subsequently contribute to unnecessary patient dose.

Exposure technique factors are characterized by the tube potential energy, measured in kilovolts (kVp); the tube current, measured in milliamperes (mA); and the exposure time in seconds (s). The kV not only represents the speed of the electrons striking the target but also the energy of the photons (that is, the *quality* of the x-ray beam) emanating from the x-ray tube. The mA, on the other hand, reflects the flow of electrons across the tube and is the primary determinant of the *quantity* of photons falling upon the patient. The exposure time refers to the duration (in seconds) of the exposure of the patient to the radiation beam.

These three factors (tube potential energy, tube current, and time) not only determine the quality (kV) and quantity (mA × s = mAs) of the radiation beam needed to image the patient, but they also affect the dose to the patient. Additionally, these factors are under the direct control of the technologist, who must be able to optimize the dose and work within the philosophy that doses should be "as low as reasonably attainable" (ALARA). This can be accomplished through the selection of the best possible combination of kVp and mAs needed to conduct the examination without compromising the image quality needed to make a diagnosis.

Tube Potential Energy (kVp)

The tube potential energy, or kVp, affects the penetrating power of the x-ray beam. A beam produced using a high kVp is much more penetrating than a beam produced by a low kVp. Wolbarst et al. (2013) offer explanations for the differential in deposited dose as a function of the penetrating power of the beam:

1. With low-kVp techniques, a higher dose is deposited in a larger area of the patient because the photons do not have enough energy to penetrate the entire thickness of the patient.

2. With high-kVp techniques, a lower dose is deposited in the tissues because the photons have adequate energy to penetrate the tissues and get to the image receptor.

Additionally, Wolbarst (2005) also explained that when considering the two interactions of radiation with matter that are of importance in radiology—the photoelectric effect and the Compton effect (described in detail elsewhere)—the photoelectric effect predominates at lower kVp techniques, particularly in tissues with high atomic numbers, such as bone. As a result, there is more absorption of the radiation beam (dose) in tissues with high atomic numbers.

Tube Current (mA)

The tube current, or mA, primarily affects the quantity of radiation coming from the x-ray tube. Because the quantity of radiation is directly proportional to the mA, doubling the mA doubles the radiation quantity (hence the dose) to the patient. Unlike kVp, which has an exponential relationship with dose, there is a linear relationship between mA and dose. For example, if the mA is held constant, the dose increases by about 50% if the kVp is increased from 120 kVp to 140 kVp. On the other hand, the dose decreases by about 65% if the kVp is reduced from 120 kVp to 80 kVp (Kaza et al. 2014).

Exposure Time

The dose delivered to the patient during a radiographic examination is directly proportional to the exposure time. Recall the following relationship

from any radiologic physics text (Bushong 2013, for example).

$$\text{Exposure} = \text{Exposure Rate} \times \text{Time}$$

Thus, if the exposure time is doubled, the exposure (dose) to the patient will also be doubled.

Radiation Quantity (mAs)

The quantity of radiation administered to the patient, mAs, is the product of mA and time, measured in seconds (s). The quantity of radiation is influenced by the mAs of the exposure technique. Such quantity is directly proportional to the mAs; hence, if the mAs is double, the quantity of radiation (dose) doubles. Techniques based on high kVp require a subsequent reduction in mAs; hence, high-kVp techniques result in reduced dose to the patient.

Automatic Exposure Control

Automatic exposure control (AEC) timing systems were developed to solve exposure technique problems experienced with manual exposure timing systems. Such problems arise as a result of variations in patient sizes, patient pathologies, and aging of the x-ray tube, for example. AEC systems ensure that a preselected amount of radiation reaches the image receptor, and in this manner provide correct exposures regardless of the problems mentioned above. The result of this is that repeat exposures are subsequently reduced. AEC systems are not completely "fail-safe," and therefore the operator must be trained in the correct use during radiographic imaging employing AEC.

X-Ray Generator Waveform

Once exposure technique factors are set on the control panel of the x-ray unit by the technologist, they are applied to the x-ray generator during the exposure time. As such, the x-ray generator plays an important role in delivering a dose of radiation (as defined by the exposure technique factors) suitable for the examination.

X-ray generators have evolved through the years from single-phase and three-phase to high-frequency and constant-potential generators. The major goal of such evolution is to improve the efficiency of x-ray production in an effort to reduce the dose delivered to the patient.

The production of x-rays is characterized by the voltage waveform of the x-ray generator. An important characteristic of the voltage waveform is its *ripple*, or the way in which the voltage is supplied to the x-ray tube. The ripple is expressed as a percentage; the ripple is 100% for both single-phase types (half-wave and full-wave), 14% for three-phase, 6-pulse units, 4% for three-phase, 12-pulse units, and < 1 for high-frequency units (Bushong 2013). As the percentage ripple decrease, the generator is said to be more efficient at x-ray production. A ripple of 4% indicates that the x-ray tube voltage never drops below 96% of the maximum value. A ripple of < 1% indicates that the tube voltage is almost constant.

This efficiency implies that the patient dose and hence the exposure technique factors (kVp and mAs) are related to the type of voltage waveform. Three-phase (12-pulse) and high-frequency generators are much more efficient at x-ray production than three-phase (6-pulse) and single-phase x-ray generators. The high-frequency generator, however, produces greater x-ray intensity and greater effective energy compared with single- and three-phase generators (high-frequency generators are now commonplace in not only projection radiographic imaging but also in Computed Tomography (CT)). This means that shorter exposure times (hence mAs) are possible with high-frequency generators.

As noted by Bushong (2013, p. 133):

> *The relationship between x-ray quantity and the type of high-voltage generator provides the basis for another rule of thumb used by radiologic technologists. If a radiographic technique calls for 72 kVp on single-phase equipment, then on three-phase equipment, approximately 64 kVp—a 12% reduction—will produce similar results.*

The above discussion implies that less dose can be delivered to a patient when using high-frequency generators compared to single and three-phase generators. This is one of the main reasons that high-frequency generators have become popular and commonplace in diagnostic radiology.

Filtration

Like the x-ray generator waveform, filtration—or more specifically, x-ray beam filtration—is not under the direct control of the operator. The x-ray beam emerging from the x-ray tube is a heterogeneous beam. This means that the beam consists of low-energy and high-energy photons. Whereas the high-energy photons penetrate the patient to form the image at the image receptor, low-energy photons do not have enough energy to penetrate the patient, and they do not, therefore, play a role in image formation. They are merely absorbed by the tissues, thus increasing the dose to the patient.

These low-energy photons can be selectively removed by inserting metal absorbers (e.g., aluminum) in the beam before they react with the patient. These absorbers are called **filters**, and the absorption or removal of the low-energy photons is referred to as **filtration**.

There are two types of filtration: **inherent** and **added**. The former type of filtration is accomplished by the x-ray tube itself, which consists of the glass or metal envelope and the insulating oil. Added filtration is so named to refer to the addition of a specified thickness of aluminum outside the x-ray tube (close to the tube port). The total filtration can be calculated using the following relationship:

$$\text{Total Filtration} = \text{Inherent Filtration} + \text{Added Filtration}$$

The total filtration in diagnostic radiographic imaging is generally 2.5 Al (e.g., 0.5 mm Al equivalent inherent + 1.0 mm Al added + 1.0 mm Al equivalent of the mirror in the collimator). It is important to note here as well, that other materials can be used as added filters. These include copper and tin as well as rare-earth filters such as gadolinium and holmium. Rare earth filters are commonplace in pediatric imaging.

Filtration is the selective removal of low-energy photons from the radiation beam. It is intended to protect the patient from unnecessary radiation. The result of filtration is a reduction of the intensity (quantity) and an increase in the effective energy of the beam—that is, the beam becomes harder and therefore more penetrating. Specifically, and as early as 1993, Wooton (1993) noted that filtration reduces the patient skin dose, and later, several studies on filtration appeared in the literature. For example, Dance et al. (2000) investigated the effect of anode/filter material and tube potential on contrast, signal-to-noise ratio, and average absorbed dose in mammography. They found that a molybdenum/molybdenum combination resulted in the lowest dose to a 2-cm breast, "but gives the highest dose for thicker breast" (p. 1056). Additionally, they showed that tungsten/rhodium or rhodium/aluminum crude/filter respectively "provide the lowest doses at greater thicknesses" (p. 1056).

In 2008, Moore et al. examined the optimum kVp and filtration for chest examinations using a computed radiography system. Using a phantom with varying amounts of kVp and copper (Cu) filtration, they found that "…a 0.1 mm Cu thickness was found to provide a statistically increase in the contrast-to-noise ratio (CNR) in the diaphragm region with tube potentials of 60 kVp and 80 kVp, without affecting the CNR in the other anatomical regions" (p. 771).

Another interesting study is one by Fetterly (2010), who examined the addition of 0.1 mm Cu filter for a cine imaging system. Fetterly essentially found that "for these clinical systems, use of the 0.1 mm Cu filter resulted in a favorable compromise between reduced skin dose rate and image quality, and increased x-ray tube burden" (2010, p. 624).

Finally, a study on the use of Cu filtration in pediatric digital imaging by Brosi et al. (2011) showed that "Cu filtration reduces the entrance surface dose (ESD), but generally does not reduce the effective dose. Cu filters can help protect radiosensitive superficial organs, such as the mammary glands in AP chest projections" (p. 148).

Collimation and Field Size

The term *collimation* refers to a method of defining the size and shape of the primary x-ray beam so that it covers only the region of anatomical interest. The area covered by the beam falling on the patient is the *field size*.

Devices for limiting the field size have evolved from the aperture diaphragm, cones, and cylinders to the variable aperture collimator (Bushong 2013). The latter has become commonplace and involves two approaches to limiting the beam to the area of interest. One approach is manual collimation, where the leaves of the collimator shutters are directly adjusted by the technologist to the field size and the size of the image receptor used for the examination. The second approach is automatic collimation, a technique referred to as *positive beam limitation* (*PBL*), where the beam is automatically collimated to the size of the image receptor in the Bucky tray. The technologist, however, may override the PBL to ensure that the beam can be collimated to a size smaller than the image receptor size.

The purpose of collimation is to protect the patient from unnecessary radiation by limiting the beam field size to the anatomy of interest. In this manner, the volume of tissue irradiated is reduced. Limiting the field size to the smallest practicable area results in a decrease in the total radiation energy to the patient, because the surface integral exposure (total radiation) is directly proportional to the size of the irradiated area. Collimation also decreases not only the bone marrow and gonadal doses but reduces the genetically significant dose by about 65% (Bushong 2013).

A 2013 study by Fauber and Dempsey on the effect of collimation on patient dose showed that "a significant reduction in patient exposure (27%) resulted when the x-ray field size decreased from

14 × 17 in (35 × 43 cm) to 8 × 17 in (20 × 43 cm). The abdominal tissue located farthest from the focal spot and the central axis received the least amount of exposure. The TLDs [thermoluminescent dosimeters] located closest to the lateral edge of the 8 × 17 in (20 × 43 cm) collimated x-ray beam received the least amount of exposure (> 60% reduction)" (Faubers and Dempsey 2013, p. 159).

Last but not least, collimation is an effective means of assuring dose optimization and hence working within the ALARA philosophy. Collimation must be a part of best practices in diagnostic radiography, including digital radiography.

Electronic Collimation

Electronic collimation is a post-processing technique in digital radiography that uses digital shutters to electronically collimate the image after the patient has been imaged in the x-ray room. Several authors, such as Bomer et al. (2013), Morrison et al. (2011), Zetterberg et al. (2011), and Willis (2009), have reported that technologists fail to effectively collimate manually during image acquisition, since they use electronic collimation when images are viewed and assessed before they are sent to the Picture Archiving and Communications System (PACS). Reduction of the field-of-view by electronic collimation improves image quality that is in contrast is optimized in the area of interest (Bomer et al 2013).

In film-screen radiography, evidence of collimation can simply be checked by looking for the "silver lining" (a white margin about 1 mm wide) around the perimeter of the processed film. "These margins appear bright on the image, as beyond the edges of the collimated beam no x-rays hit the detector" (Bomer et al. 2013, p. 724). Two important points made clear by Bomer et al. (2013) to which technologists should pay careful attention are as follows:

1. "Electronic collimation implicates that the original field size should have been smaller and the child has been exposed to unnecessary radiation.

2. Also by use of electronic collimation, potentially important information may be lost" (p. 723).

Furthermore, Bomer et al. (2013) concluded that:

The ability to electronically collimate an image after acquisition carries the risk of over exposure ……. If the field size has been overestimated, we can use electronic collimation to optimize image quality. However, the original images should always be sent to the PACS, as they may contain critically important information and the patient has a right to all information at all times" (p. 727)

Beam Alignment

Beam alignment refers to the alignment of the radiation field and the light-field of the collimator. If these two fields are not congruent (that is, in perfect alignment), the anatomical region of interest may not be included because of beam "cut-off," and the patient receives unnecessary radiation because of beam "overlap." In a quality control test for congruency, the misalignment must not exceed 2% of the source-to-image receptor distance (SID) (Bushong 2013).

Source-to-Image Receptor Distance/ Source-to-Skin Distance

The SID is the distance from the focal spot of x-ray tube to the image receptor (Figure 7-1). For most radiographic examinations, the SID is usually set at 101 cm (40 in). As the SID (and the source-to-skin [SSD]) decreases, the divergence of the beam increases. This offset has an impact on the concentration of photons on the surface of the patient. A short SID increases the photon concentration, thus increasing the surface exposure to the patient. This is graphically shown in **Figure 7-2**.

In conducting x-ray examinations, the technologist should pay particular attention to the proper use of the correct SID recommended for the particular anatomical area of interest.

It is noted in this regard (finding a balance between image quality and patient dose) that increasing the SID can be considered an optimization technique and useful tool when working

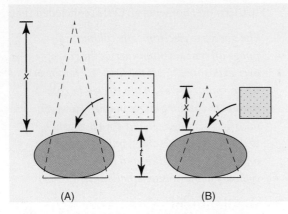

(A)   (B)

Figure 7-2 The concentration of photons (surface exposure) on the patient (A) decreases on the surface of the patient at the long SID, but (B) increases as the SID decreases.

within the ALARA philosophy. A recent study by Joyce et al. (2013) investigated the increase in the SID as an optimization tool in digital cranial radiography. The researchers found that "statistically significant reductions in the effective dose between 19.2% and 23.9% were obtained when the SID was increased from the standard 100 to 150 cm (P ≤ 0.05), and visual grading analysis scores indicate that image quality remained diagnostically acceptable …." (Joyce 2013, p. 180).

Patient Thickness and Density

The dose to the patient also depends on the patient thickness and the density (mass per unit volume). In general, the technologist has no direct control of these variables, except in some cases in which compression may be used to decrease the thickness in an effort to control the amount of scattered radiation reaching the image receptor. As patient thickness and density increase, more radiation is needed for image formation (Bushong 2013) the exposure of course depends on whether a fixed or variable kVp technique is applied in the imaging process. For example, for a technique fixed at 80 kVp, the mAs values of 16, 20, 24, and 30 cm patient thickness are 12, 22, 45, and 120 mAs respectively (Bushong 2013).

X-Ray Table Top

The purpose of the table top is to support the patient during the examination, and therefore, it must be constructed of materials that can withstand the weight of heavy patients. These materials must have a low attenuation characteristic to allow a good proportion of the beam to be transmitted through the table top to reach the image receptor. The ratio of the patient-to-receptor exposure will increase if the table top attenuates a greater fraction of the beam transmitted through the patient (Sprawls 1995). For this reason, materials are carefully chosen in the design of x-ray table tops.

Table tops used in diagnostic imaging are made of carbon-fiber materials because they allow a high transmission of the beam. As a result, the absorb dose to the skin of the patient is reduced. The ICRP (1993) stated that with the use of carbon-fiber table tops, the absorbed dose in the skin of the patient is reduced by 3–15% at 80 kVp.

Anti-Scatter Grids

As shown in Figure 7-1, a grid is placed between the table top and the image receptor. The purpose of the grid is to improve image contrast (in F-S radiography) by absorbing radiation scattered from the patient and preventing it from reaching the image receptor. Grids are carefully designed so that their lead strips allow transmission of the primary beam but prevent most of the scattered radiation from reaching the image receptor.

The characteristics of a grid that have an influence on the radiation dose to the patient are the grid ratio, grid frequency, interspace material, selectivity, and the Bucky factor. The reader should refer to Bushong

(2013) for a detailed description of scattered radiation grid construction, types, and performance.

The *grid ratio* is the ratio of the height of the lead strip to the distance between the strips. Typical grid ratios used in clinical imaging are 8:1, 12:1, and 16:1, with 12:1 being the most commonly used in Bucky mechanisms. As the grid ratio increases, the dose to the patient increases. Furthermore, a moving grid (found in Bucky mechanisms) requires about 15% more radiation than a stationary grid with the same design characteristics (Bushong 2013).

The *grid frequency* is the number of lead strips per centimeter of the grid. The grid frequency is also referred to as the grid lattice or strip density. Grid frequencies range from 24 to 43 lines per cm, although higher strip densities are available. As the grid frequency increases, the relative patient exposure increases, because there is more lead, which absorbs a small proportion of the primary radiation beam.

The *interspace material* of the grid supports the lead strips and provides an equal amount of separation between them. The interspace material is usually aluminum or plastic fiber. While each of these has its advantages, aluminum, with its high atomic number, absorbs more radiation than the plastic fiber, especially when using low kVp techniques. This feature will result in an increase in the patient dose by about 20% (Bushong 2013).

The *Bucky factors* (**B**) (or grid factor, as it is sometimes referred to) affects the dose to the patient. B is defined as the ratio of the incident total radiation striking the grid (primary plus scatter) to the total radiation transmitted through the grid (Wolbarst, 2005). B is related to the grid ratio as well as the kVp. As the grid ratio and kVp increase, B increases. For example, the B for a 12:1 grid is 3.5, 4 and 5 at 70, 90, and 120 kVp respectively. As B increases, patient dose increases proportionally (Bushong 2013).

The *selectivity* of a grid is not usually one of the characteristic features described in radiologic imaging textbooks, yet it is another factor that affects patient dose. Selectivity is defined as the ratio of primary radiation transmission to scattered radiation transmission. Selectivity depends on not only the grid ratio but also on the amount of lead used in the construction of the grid. In general, grids with high selectivity will result in higher patient doses, because of an increase in the thickness of the lead strips.

Sensitivity of the Image Receptor

The *image receptor* or *image detector* captures the radiation transmitted through the patient and is used to create the image. In F-S radiography, the image receptor is the film cassette, while in digital radiography, it is the digital detector. The *image receptor sensitivity* accounts for the amount of radiation needed to produce an image. It is also refined to as the *image receptor speed*. For F-S radiography, it refers to film speed, as well as screen speed. High-speed (fast) systems require much less radiation than low-speed (slow) systems. For digital radiography systems, the term speed does not apply, since the digital detector operates on any speed class.

An equivalent or related characteristic is the *detective quantum efficiency* (*DQE*). The digital detector takes an input exposure and converts it into a useful output image. The DQE is a measure of the efficiency with which the detector performs this task. The DQE for a perfect detector is 1 or 100%. This means that there is no loss of information (Seeram 2011). The nature of the DQE will be described in more detail elsewhere.

Film Processing

For departments that still use F-S imaging, film processing is an integral part in the imaging chain of factors affecting the dose to the patient. Correct processing techniques are mandatory, not only to produce images of optimum quality, but also to reduce dose to the patient by eliminating the need to repeat examinations due to poor film processing.

Repeat Radiographic Examinations

Radiologic technologists should always strive avoid repeating an examination; however, in some instances, there are problems that may lead to the need to perform the examination again. The repeat rates for F-S radiography have been studied and papers published in the literature (David 1994; Statkiewicz-Sherer et al. 2013; and ICRP 1993). The ICRP (1993), for example reported that repeat rates varied from 3% to 15% and that the major causes of repeats were due to patient positioning errors and exposure technique errors.

In digital radiography, the problem of repeating examinations persists, and efforts have been devised to decrease the repeat rates (Willis 2011). Quality control acceptance criterion for repeat rates is that the rate should not exceed 5% (Bushong 2013).

Apart from poor positioning, poor technique selection, and equipment malfunction, other possible causes for repeat examinations include:

- Poor image processing, whether chemical or computer processing
- Collimation errors
- Not including the anatomy of interest
- Incorrect angulation of the tube
- Incorrect centering of the beam on the body part being examined
- Poor or incomplete instructions to the patient
- Not observing the patient during the exposure
- Poor placement of the gonadal shield
- Uneducated and untrained operators
- Incorrect identification of the patient
- Poor selection of the image receptor
- Incorrect interpretation of the requisition (request for an x-ray examination, etc.)

In view of the wide variety of sources of errors, technologists must always be alert when performing radiographic examinations. To minimize errors and optimize the performance of the examination,

technologists should have a carefully planned strategy for conducting the examination. One such strategy might include the following sequence of steps:

1. Obtain and correctly interpret the patient's requisition.
2. Prepare the x-ray room for the particular examination.
3. Correctly identify the patient.
4. Explain the examination to the patient, emphasizing the need to follow all instructions, including the admonition against movement during exposure. Breathing instructions should also be clearly explained as well.
5. Measure the patient correctly, particularly if the exposure technique chart is based on a measurement. If automatic exposure timing is used, the patient size must also be correctly assessed. Note also whether patient pathology might have an effect on the exposure technique.
6. Established and set up the correct exposure technique factors for the particular examination based on the assessment done in Step 5.
7. Position the patient correctly.
8. Check for proper collimation, SID, marker placement, proper placement of the image receptor/detector in the Bucky for non-flat-panel digital radiography.
9. Check that gonadal shielding issued correctly.
10. Observe the patient during the exposure to ensure that they follow instructions.
11. After exposure, process all images recorded check that processing is in proper working order.
12. Check all images for acceptability.
13. If images are acceptable, discuss the patient.
14. Clean up the room and prepare for the next examination.

These steps, if carefully executed, should assist the technologist in conducting the examination in a smooth and orderly fashion to ensure optimization of image quality.

Repeat Rates in Digital Radiography

The analysis of repeat rates in diagnostic radiology is an essential part of a QC program. Repeat analysis is also referred to as **reject analysis** and it is "a time-honored method for assessing and improving quality of imaging operations" (Willis 2011). Reject/Repeat analysis is also important in digital radiography, and the QC elements have been described in detail by Willis (2011).

An interesting study of repeat rates in digital radiography is one by Fintelmann et al. (2012). The researchers examined specifically the repeat rates (RR) of chest images with portable computed radiography (CR) and fixed or installed direct radiography (DR) systems. The results of this study showed that:

> The initial RR of digital chest radiographs was 3.6% (138/3818) for portable CR and 13.3% (476/3575) for installed DR systems. By combining RR measurement with workflow analysis, targets for technical and teaching interventions were identified. The interventions decreased the RR to 1.8% (81/4476) for portable CR and to 8.2% (306/3748) for installed DR... (Fintelmann et al. 2012, p. 148). Furthermore, after a thorough discussion of these results, the researchers concluded that:
>
> .... the RR of direct digital chest radiography [was found] to be significantly higher than that of computed chest radiography. We believe that this is because of the ease with which repeat images can be obtained and discarded, and it suggests the need for ongoing surveillance of RR... (p. 151)

Shielding Radio-Sensitive Organs

Shielding is yet another factor to consider when thinking about optimization of radiation protection in diagnostic imaging. Shielding very radio-sensitive organs such as the gonads, eyes, thyroid, and breasts is especially important because of the risks of stochastic effects and deterministic effects (e.g., cataracts in the eyes). For the gonads, shielding will reduce the gonadal dose. For example, the *correct* use of a 1-mm lead-equivalent shield will reduce the gonadal dose by about 50% for females and about 90%–95% for males (Statkiewicz-Sherer et al. 2013).

Two types of shields have been described in the literature (Bushong 2013; Statkiewicz-Sherer 2013): **contact shields** and **shadow shields**. While contact shields are flat and shaped, shadow shields are designed so that they attach to the x-ray tube by means of a ring. The shadow of the radiopaque sector-like portion of the shield is positioned over the patient's gonads; shadow shields are perhaps best used in examinations where it is important to maintain a sterile field.

Gonadal shielding is intended to protect the gonads from primary radiation, and as such, the thickness of the shield must be at least 0.5-mm lead equivalent. If gonadal shielding is to be effective, placement of the lead shield on the patient must be accurate to ensure protection of the gonads. For males, it is useful to use the symphysis pubis as the external landmark to guide the placement of the shield. For females, the external landmark 2.5 cm medial to the anterior superior iliac spine can be used for accurate placement of the shield to protect the ovaries from radiation.

Shielding of the breasts during certain x-ray examinations has been advocated by some authors (Bushong 2013) due to the extreme radio sensitivity of the glandular tissue. Shielding is suggested especially where the x-ray field is in close proximity to radio-sensitive tissues such as the breasts or gonads (e.g., urinary tract examinations, upper humerus, shoulder, thoracic spine, clavicle, abdomen, and scoliosis examinations in children). Furthermore, there has been some controversy surrounding the use of thyroid shields during mammography, arising from a popular television talk show. In this regard, the American College of Radiology (ACR) and Society of Breast Imaging (2015) has issued the following statement:

> *For annual screening mammography from ages 40–80, the cancer risk from this tiny amount of radiation scattered to the thyroid is incredibly small (less than 1 in 17.1 million women screened). This minimal risk should be balanced with the fact that thyroid shield usage could interfere with optimal positioning and could result in artifacts—shadows that might appear on the mammography image. Both of these factors could reduce the quality of the image and interfere with diagnosis. Therefore, use of a thyroid shield during mammography is not recommended. Patients are urged not to put off or forego necessary breast imaging care…*

It is clear that correct placement of gonadal shields is an important practice for effective optimization of radiation protection. It has been reported in the literature, however, that correct placement is often difficult, and "as a consequence, many images are suboptimal or worse, leading to a loss of diagnostic information that impairs the radiologist's work" (Frantzen et al. 2012). The obvious question that arises is whether the advantage of using gonadal shielding "is still worthwhile in view of its negative consequences" (Frantzen et al. 2012).

An interesting study in this regard is one by Frantzen et al. (2012) entitled *Gonadal shielding in paediatric pelvic radiography: disadvantages prevail over benefit*, published in *Insights Imaging Journal* (see reference listing). The goal of this study was to reevaluate shielding the gonads in children with respect to reducing the radiation risk and loss of diagnostic information. The results showed that:

> For girls, gonadal shields were placed incorrectly in 91% of the radiographs; for boys, in 66%. Without gonadal shielding, the hereditary detriment adjusted risk for girls ranged between 0.1×10^{-6} and 1.3×10^{-6} and for boys between 0.3×10^{-6} and 3.9×10^{-6} dependent on age. With shielding, the reduction in hereditary risk for girls was on average $6 \pm 3\%$ of the total risk of the radiograph, for boys $24 \pm 6\%$. Without gonadal shielding, the effective dose range from 0.008 to 0.098 mSv. (Frantzen 2012, p. 23)

This study was done to address the ICRP's optimization principle—and after a thorough data analysis and discussion of the results, the authors conclude that:

> *With modern optimized x-ray systems, the reduction of the detriment adjusted risk by gonadal shielding is negligibly small. Given the potential consequences of loss of diagnostic information, of retakes, and shielding of automatic exposure-control chambers, gonadal shielding might better be discontinued.* (Frantzen 2012, p. 23)

The above study serves as a good reminder for departments to establish policies around the use of gonadal shielding in pediatric radiography.

Summary of Key Concepts

1. The major exposure components for radiographic systems affecting dose include the x-ray generator, the x-ray tube, x-ray beam filter, the x-ray beam collimator, the x-ray beam area or Field-of-View (FOV) as it is sometimes referred to), patient thickness and density, table top, scattered radiation grid, the image receptor (detector) image processing, source-to-skin in distance (SSD), source-to-image receptor distance (SID) and finally the user (technologists and radiologists) who have direct control of the x-ray beam quantity and quality needed for the examination. The latter refers to the mAs and kVp respectively.

2. *Clinical factors* refer to the overall responsibilities of the individuals involved in exposing patients to radiation. These responsibilities relate not only to the prescription of the x-ray examination but also to the non-technical procedural aspects such as patient care, communications and comfort. The individuals who shoulder the responsibility for determining the nature and extent of a patient's radiologic examination are the referring physician, the radiologist, and the technologist.

3. These responsibilities are often identified and stated in Radiation Safety Codes of most countries.

4. Exposure technique factors are characterized by the tube potential, defined by the kilovolts (kVp), the tube current, defined by the milliamperage (mA), and the exposure time in seconds (s).

5. With low kVp techniques, more doses are deposited in a larger area of the patient because the photons do not have enough energy to penetrate the entire thickness of the patient. Furthermore, with high kVp techniques, fewer doses are deposited in the tissues because the photons have a high enough energy to penetrate the tissues and get to the image receptor.

6. The radiation dose is directly proportional to the mA and doubling the mA doubles the radiation dose to the patient. The same applies to the time (s) of the exposure and the mAs (mA x s)

7. AEC systems ensure that a pre-selected amount of radiation reaches the image receptor, and in this manner provide correct exposures regardless of the problems mentioned above.

8. High-frequency generators deliver fewer doses to the patient compared with single and three-phase generators, and is one of the main reasons why high-frequency generators have become popular and commonplace in diagnostic radiology.

9. Filtration is the selective removal of low-energy photons from the radiation beam and it is intended to protect the patient from unnecessary radiation. The result of filtration is a reduction of the intensity (quantity) and an increase in the effective energy of the beam, that is, the beam becomes harder and therefore more penetrating.

10. The purpose of collimation is to protect the patient from unnecessary radiation by limiting the beam field size to the anatomy of interest. In this manner, the volume of tissue irradiated is reduced. Limiting the field size to the smallest practicable area results in a decrease in the total radiation energy to the patient, because the surface integral exposure (total radiation) is directly proportional to the size of the irradiated area

11. *Beam alignment* refers to the alignment of the radiation field and the light-field of the collimator. If these two fields are not congruent (that is in perfect alignment), the anatomical region of interest may not be included because of beam "cut-off," and the patient receives unnecessary radiation because of beam "overlap."

12. As the SID (and the source-to-skin (SSD)) decreases, the divergence of the beam increases. This offset has an impact on the concentration of photons on the surface of the patient. A short SID increases the photon concentration, thus increasing the surface exposure to the patient.

13. As patient thickness and density increase, more radiation is needed for image formation

14. Table tops used in diagnostic imaging are made of carbon-fiber materials because they allow a high transmission of the beam. As a result, the absorb dose to the skin of the patient is reduced.

(Continues)

15. The characteristics of a grid that have an influence on the radiation dose to the patient are the grid ratio, grid frequency, interspace material, selectivity, and the Bucky factor. As then grid ratio and grid frequency increase, the dose increases. The use of aluminum (high atomic number) as an interspace material, results in more dose to the patient compared with the use of plastic fiber, especially when using low kVp techniques

16. The Bucky Factor (B) is related to the grid ratio as well as the kVp. As the grid ratio and kVp increase, B increases.

17. In general, grids with high selectivity will result in higher patient doses, because of an increase in the thickness of the lead strips.

18. As the sensitivity (relative speed) of an image receptor (detector) increases, the dose to the patient decreases

19. The repeat rate of an examination increases the dose to the patient.

20. Gonadal shielding is intended to protect the gonads from primary radiation, and as such, the thickness of the shield must be at least 0.5 mm lead equivalent. If gonadal shielding is to be effective, placement of the lead shield on the patient must be accurate to ensure protection of the gonads. For males, it is useful to use the symphysis pubis as the external landmark to guide the placement of the shield. For females, the external landmark 2.5 cm medial to the anterior superior iliac spines can be used for accurate placement of the shield to protect the ovaries from radiation.

Discussion Questions

Answer the following questions to check your understanding of the information presented in Chapter 7.

1. Describe the major components affecting the dose for radiography imaging systems.

2. Discuss the overall responsibilities of the physician, technologist, radiologist, and the patient in radiation protection.

3. Identify and discuss 15 technical factors affecting the dose to the patient in radiographic imaging.

References

American College of Radiology and the Society of Breast Imaging (2015). The ACR and Society of Breast Imaging Statement on Radiation Received by the Thyroid from Mammography. (Available at http://www.acr.org/Search?q=Thyroid%20 shields%20in%20mammography; Retrieved April 30, 2015.)

Bomer J, Wiersma-Deijl L, Holscher HC. Electronic collimation and radiation protection in paediatric digital radiography: Revival of the silver lining. *Insight Imaging.* 2013;4:723–727.

Brosi P, Stuessi A, Verdun F. R, Vock P, Wolf R. Copper filtration in pediatric digital x-ray imaging: its impact on image quality and dose. *Radiol Phys Technical.* 2011;4(2):148–155.

Bushong S. *Radiologic Science for Technologists: Physics, Biology and Protection.* St. Louis, MO: Mosby-Elsevier; 2013.

Dance DR, Klang AT, Sandborg M, Skinner CL, Castellano IA, et al. Influence of anode/filter material and tube potential on contrast, signal-to-noise ratio, and average absorbed dose in mammography: A Monte Carlo Study. *Br J Radiol.* 2000;73:1056–1067.

EPA. *EPA-Federal Guidance Report No. 14: Radiation protection guidance for diagnostic and interventional x-ray procedures.* Washington, DC: U.S. Environmental Protection Agency; 2012.

Fauber TL, Dempsey MC. X-ray field size and patient dosimetry. *Radiol Technol.* 201385(2):155–161.

Fetterly KA. Investigation of the practical aspects of an additional 0.1 mm copper x-ray spectral filter for cine acquisition mode imaging in a clinical care setting. *Health Phys.* 2010;99(5):624–630.

Fintelmann F, Pulli B, Abedi-Tari F, Trombley M, Shore MT, et al. Repeat rates in digital chest radiography and strategies for improvement. *J Thorac Imaging.* 2012;27(3):148–151.

Frantzen M, Robben S, Postma AA, Zoetelief J, Wildberger JE, Kemerink GJ. Gonad shielding in paediatric pelvic radiography: Disadvantages prevail over benefit. *Insights Imaging.* 2012;3:23–32.

Health Canada. *Radiation protection in radiology – Large facilities. Safety Code 35.* Ottawa: Ministry of Health; 2008.

International Commission on Radiological Protection (ICRP). Protection of the patient in diagnostic radiology. ICRP Publication 34. *Ann ICRP.* 1973;9(2-3). (Available at http://ani.sagepub.com /site/includefiles/icrp_publications_collection .xhtml; Retrieved August 21, 2015.)

Joyce M, McEntee M, Brennan P, O'Leary D. Reducing dose for digital cranial radiography: The increased source-to-the image-receptor distance approach. *J Med Imaging Radiat Sci.* 2013;44:180–187.

Kaza RK, Platt JF, Goodsitt MM, Al-Hawary MM, Maturen KE, et al. Emerging techniques for dose optimization in abdominal CT. *Radiographics.* 2014;34:4–17.

Moore CS, Beavis AW, Saunderson JR. Investigation of optimum x-ray beam tube voltage and filtration for chest radiography with a computed radiography system. *Br J Radiol.* 2008;81:771–777.

Morrison G, John SD, Goske MJ, et al. Pediatric digital radiography education for radiologic technologists: current state. *Pediatr Radiol.* 2011;41:602–610.

Seeram E. (2011). *Digital radiography: An introduction.* Clifton Park, NJ: Delmar Cengage Learning.

Sierzenski PR, Linton OW, Amis Jr. ES, Courtney DM, Larson PA, Mahesh M, et al. Applications of justification and optimization in medical imaging: Examples of clinical guidance for computed tomography use in emergency medicine. *J Am Coll Radiol.* 2004;11:36–44.

Sprawls P. *Physical principles of medical imaging* (2nd ed.). Decatur, IL: Perry Sprawls and Associates; 1995.

Statkiewicz-Sherer MA, Visconti PJ, Ritenour ER, Haynes K. Radiation protection in medical radiography, 7th ed. St. Louis, MO: Mosby; 2011.

Uffmann M, Schaefer-Prokop C. Digital radiography: The balance between image quality and required radiation dose. *Eur J Radiol.* 2009;72(2):202–208.

Willis CE. Optimizing digital radiography in children. *Eur J Radiol.* 2009;72:266–273.

Willis C. Quality control for digital radiography. In Seeram E, *Digital radiography: An introduction.* Clifton Park, NJ: Delmar Cengage Learning; 2011.

Wolbarst AB, Capasso P, Wyant AR. *Medical Imaging: Essentials for Physicians.* Hoboken, NJ: Wiley-Blackwell; 2013.

Wooton R (Ed.). *Radiation Protection of the Patient.* Cambridge, UK: Cambridge University Press; 1993.

Zetterberg LG, Espeland A. Lumbar spine radiography – Poor collimation practices after implementation of digital technology. *Br J Radiol.* 2011;84(1002):566–569.

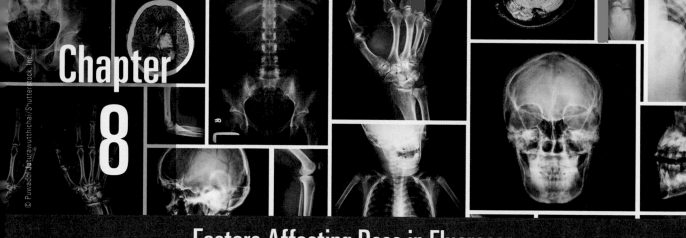

Chapter 8

Factors Affecting Dose in Fluoroscopy

Outline

- Introduction
- Radiation Effects from Fluoroscopic X-Ray Exposure
- Fluoroscopy Systems: Types and Major Components
  - Image intensifier-based fluoroscopic system
  - The flat-panel digital detector-based fluoroscopy system
- Major Dose Factors in Fixed Fluoroscopic Imaging Systems
  - Fluoroscopic exposure factors
  - Fluoroscopic instrumentation factors
- Major Factors in Mobile Fluoroscopy Systems
- C-Arm Computed Tomography Fluoroscopy
- References

Objectives

On completion of this chapter, you should be able to:

1. Describe the typical radiation effects from fluoroscopic exposure.

2. Describe the major components of an image intensifier-based fluoroscopic imaging system.

3. Describe the major components of a flat-panel digital detector-based fluoroscopic system.

4. State the meaning of each of the following:
   - Fluoroscopic exposure factors
   - Fluoroscopic instrumentation factors

5. Discuss how fluoroscopic exposure factors affect dose to the patient.

6. List nine fluoroscopic instrumentation factors and describe how each of them affects the dose to the patient.

7. State the influence of the patient-image intensifier distance (P-IID) in mobile fluoroscopic imaging systems on patient dose.

8. Explain briefly what is meant by a C-arm computed tomography fluoroscopic imaging system.

Introduction

While radiographic imaging systems produce static or stationary images, fluoroscopy is an imaging modality that produces dynamic or moving images acquired and displayed for viewing in real time. The overall goal of conducting fluoroscopy on patients is to study not only the anatomy but also organ movements and the flow of contrast media in hollow anatomical structures, such as blood vessels and the intestines. The purpose of such an examination is to obtain functional information (Bushong 2013; Johnston and Fauber 2012; Wolbarst et al. 2013).

The introduction of fluoroscopy dates back to 1896, soon after the discovery of the x-ray by W.C. Roentgen in 1895. The first fluoroscopy system was developed by Thomas Edison. The evolution of fluoroscopy through the years is marked by several significant technical innovations, which had the ultimate goal of providing the best possible image quality using a lower radiation dose compared with the first direct-viewing fluoroscopic unit. The innovations have resulted in an evolution from analog-based fluoroscopy systems to digital fluoroscopy based on the use of flat-panel digital detectors.

Radiation Effects From Fluoroscopic X-Ray Exposure

In a recent paper on optimization of dose and image quality in fluoroscopy, Jones et al. (2014) present an excellent summary of the literature on "established facts regarding fluoroscopic x-rays." These facts indicate that fluoroscopy has not only caused cancer induction and has seriously injured patients, but has also induced cancers and skin injuries in staff as well. In addition, the authors report that "staffs have died from diseases induced by fluoroscopic x-rays." Furthermore, the authors point out that another established fact is that the risks of exposure of patients in fluoroscopy are not well understood by medical workers. It is also interesting to note that:

In workers, observable radiation effects are commonly caused by long-term accumulation of radiation dose. In patients effects are typically caused by the delivery of high radiation doses in a short period of time, except for potential stochastic effects which are hypothesized as being possible at any dose. Stochastic effects include neoplasm and hereditable genetic effects; although no hereditable human genetic effects have been confirmed by descendants of exposed persons.

Additionally, the authors state that the following potential effects are as follows:

1. *"Short term (weeks to months) debilitating tissue effects; e.g, radiation-induced injury to skin and underlying tissues.*

2. *Long-term (years to decades) debilitating tissue effects; e.g, cataracts, osteonecrosis.*

3. *Long-term stochastic risks; e.g, cancer. Typically, long-term stochastic risks are the primary concern for abdominal and thoracic procedures in small children.*

4. *Short-term cosmetic risks; e.g, depilation".*

(Jones et al. 2014).

The above facts provide the rationale for operators of fluoroscopic equipment to be well versed in the technical factors affecting the dose in fluoroscopy, in an effort to minimize the risks involved. The purpose of this chapter is to describe these technical factors in fluoroscopic imaging systems, including fixed and mobile fluoroscopic systems.

Fluoroscopy Systems: Types and Major Components

There are two types of fluoroscopic imaging systems: (1) Image intensifier-based fluoroscopic systems and (2) Flat-panel digital detector-based fluoroscopic systems.

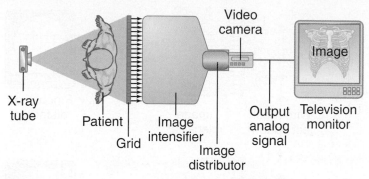

Figure 8-1 Major components of an image intensifier-based fluoroscopy system.
Courtesy of Euclid Seeram.

Image Intensifier-Based Fluoroscopic System

The image intensifier-based fluoroscopic system is shown in **Figure 8-1**. The major components include the x-ray tube, anti-scatter grid, image intensifier tube, image distributor, video camera, analog-to-digital converter (ADC), digital computer, and a television monitor for image display.

The following outlines the overall imaging principles, which lay the foundation for understanding the various factors affecting the dose in /fluoroscopy:

1. The x-ray tube and generator provide the appropriate x-ray beam for both fluoroscopy and radiography. The system operates in the pulsed or continuous fluoroscopic modes. Modern units use high-frequency generators to ensure efficient production of x-rays.

2. A filter is attached to the x-ray tube (not shown in Figure 8-1) for the main purpose of protecting the patient from low-energy x-ray photons. The filter removes these photons from the beam, making it "harder"—that is, the mean energy of the beam increases.

3. X-rays pass through the patient to strike the scattered radiation grid and the image intensifier tube (image detector). The grid removes scattered rays from the patient for the purpose of improving image quality.

4. The image intensifier tube converts x-ray photons to light photons which are captured by the video camera, and the signals from the camera are used to create the fluoroscopic images. The image intensifier tube is specially constructed for the purpose of using less radiation (compared with the direct viewing fluoroscopic used in the very early days) and produces bright images suitable for diagnosis. The conversion of x-ray photons to light photons using the image intensifier is referred to as *image intensification*. The image intensifier tube can also be made to operate in the magnification mode (to enhance the image for viewing and interpretation) by adjusting the field-of-view (FOV), which refers to the size of the input screen upon which the x-ray beam falls during imaging. Sizes can vary from 23 cm, 30–35 cm, and 40 cm FOV (Bushberg et al. 2012).

5. An important feature of the image intensifier-based fluoroscopic system is that it is a closed-circuit x-ray television system. This means that the video camera (Figure 8-1) is coupled to the television monitor via a coaxial cable and control electronics. The video camera can be either a television camera tube or a charge-couple device (CCD). The CCD has replaced the television camera tube in recent fluoroscopic systems.

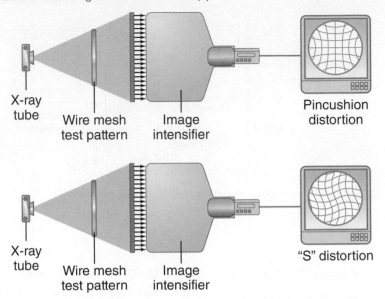

Figure 8-2 Two typical image artifacts characteristic of image intensifier-based fluoroscopy systems.
Courtesy of Euclid Seeram.

The Flat-Panel Digital Detector-Based Fluoroscopy System

The image intensifier-based fluoroscopic system poses several limitations, such as image artifacts, image magnification that increases the dose to the patient, and the degradation of image contrast due to light and electron scattering within the tube. Two of these, pincushion and "S" distortions, are illustrated in **Figure 8-2**. These problems are overcome by the state-of-the-art flat-panel digital detector (FPDD)-based fluoroscopy system.

The major imaging components of a FPDD-based fluoroscopy system are shown in **Figure 8-3**. These include the x-ray tube, scattered radiation grid, the flat-panel digital detector, digital computer, and the television monitor for image display.

The following points are noteworthy, since they are related to dose factors in FPDD-based fluoroscopy:

1. The most significant difference between image intensifier-based fluoroscopy and FPDD-based fluoroscopy is that the FPDD has replaced the image intensifier tube.

2. The FPDD is a dynamic detector, since it can produce dynamic images that can be displayed in real time. There are two types of FPDDs available for digital fluoroscopy: the cesium-iodide, amorphous-silicon, thin-film transistor (CsI a-Si TFT) indirect digital detector, and the amorphous-selenium TFT (a-Se TFT) direct detector. How each of these works is described briefly below:

- **The CsI a-Si TFT indirect detector**. X-ray photons full upon the CsI phosphor, which converts them to light photons. The light photons strike the a-Si TFT and are subsequently converted into electrical signals, which are digitized by an ADC and sent to the computer, which generates images of the examination.

- **The a-Se TFT direct detector**. This is a direct-conversion detector, since it converts

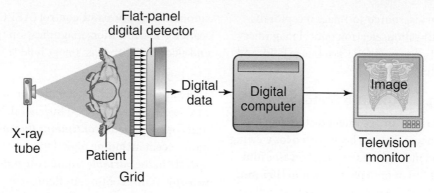

Figure 8-3 Major system components of a flat-panel digital detector-based fluoroscopy system.
Courtesy of Euclid Seeram.

x-rays directly into electrical signals for digitization by the ADC. X-rays fall upon the a-Se TFT and are converted directly into electrical signals. There is no conversion of x-rays to light in this detector.

3. These FPDDs basically utilize three sequences to create a single image in at least 33 ms for fluoroscopy. These sequences include initialization, integration, and readout while initialization prepares the detector electronics for x-ray exposure, integration and readout are intended to collect the detector signal (analog) for digitization and image display.

The characteristics and operating principles of these detectors are described in detail in Seeram (2011), Bushberg et al. (2012), and Bushong (2013).

A second important point about digital fluoroscopy compared with image intensifier-based fluoroscopy is that the tube current "is measured in hundreds of mA instead of less than 5 mA, as in image-intensifying fluoroscopy" (Bushong 2013). Such mA values are notable in radiographic imaging. To address increase in dose from the use of hundreds of mA, the x-ray tube and generator operate in the *pulse-progressive fluoroscopy* mode.

There are several advantages of FPDD-based fluoroscopy compared to image intensifier-based

fluoroscopy. Spahn (2005) noted that these include "high low-contrast resolution; high Detective Quantum Efficiency (DQE) across all dose levels, particularly for a CsI a-Si based flat detector; high dynamic range covering all dose levels from fluoroscopy...." Furthermore, distortions such as pincushion and 'S' distortions are eliminated with the use of FPDD-based fluoroscopy.

The dose factors in fluoroscopy, be it image intensifier-based or FPDD-based fluoroscopy will be described in the next section of this chapter.

Major Dose Factors in Fixed Fluoroscopic Imaging Systems

The term *fixed fluoroscopy* refers to fluoroscopy units installed in the radiology department and cannot be transported to the patient's bedside. This is to distinguish it from *mobile fluoroscopy*, which implies that the unit is small and can be transported to the patient's bedside or to the operating room in the hospital.

The principal factors affecting dose in fixed fluoroscopy units are fluoroscopic exposure technique factors (kVp, mA, and time in seconds) and instrumentation factors. The latter includes factors such as the operational mode, high-level control fluoroscopy, automatic exposure rate control, anti-scatter grids, source-to-image receptor distance (SID), filtration, electron optical magnification and field-of-view (FOV), last image hold, and image recording modes.

Fluoroscopic Exposure Factors

Fluoroscopic exposure technique factors are used to produce images that can be displayed for viewing on a television monitor and recorded on cine film (35-mm roll film) or onto photospot film (105-mm cut film or roll film) if film images are part of the fluoroscopic system. In these situations, images are recorded off the output screen of the image intensifier tube by means of the image distributor light optics system. These fluoroscopic factors are generally low mA and high kVp, with a range of 1–3 mA and 65–120 kVp, depending on the examination. For example, a single-contrast barium enema requires a range of 110–120 kVp, while a range of 50–90 kVp is acceptable for a double-contrast (air-contrast) barium enema (Bushong 2013).

The exposure time in fluoroscopy can range from minutes to hours depending on the examination. In light of these high exposures, it is important for the operator to limit the "beam-on" time (fluoroscopy time) by using *intermittent fluoroscopy* (short bursts of "beam-on" time) rather than continuous fluoroscopy. Additionally, every fluoroscopic unit is equipped with a *cumulative timer* not only to keep track of the fluoroscopic exposure time ("beam-on" time) but also to remind the operator of each 3-minute maximum (for modern units) time period of exposures by producing an audible sound and by interrupting x-ray production at the end of 3 minutes of radiation exposure.

As noted earlier, the x-ray tube in a digital fluoroscopy imaging system operates in the radiographic mode, thus allowing the use of hundreds of mA instead of less than 5 mA characteristic of image intensifier-based fluoroscopy.

Fluoroscopic Instrumentation Factors

These factors refer to equipment factors, including modes of operation, dose level control fluoroscopy,

automatic exposure rate control (AERC), anti-scatter grids, filtration, magnification (geometric and electronic), and last image hold (LIH).

Modes of Operation

There are two modes of operation upon which fluoroscopic systems are based in general. While older units operate used a *continuous fluoroscopy mode*, more recent including digital fluoroscopy systems operate in the *variable frame-rate pulsed fluoroscopy*. While continuous fluoroscopy involves the production of a continuous x-ray beam, pulsed fluoroscopy allows for the x-ray generator to produce x-rays in shorts bursts (pulses) rather than continuously. The *frames per second* (*FPS*) are typically 30, 15, 7.5, and 3.75 FPS. These variable frame rates allow the operator to select the appropriate frame rate for the examination with dose reduction in mind; the higher the FPS, the greater the radiation dose. A frame rate of 7.5 FPS reduces the dose to 25% (7.5/30) (Bushberg et al. 2012).

The main advantage of pulsed fluoroscopy is to reduce the dose to the patient. A study by Smith et al. (2013) that compared the radiation dose between continuous and pulsed fluoroscopy showed that "pulsed fluoroscopy reduced fluoroscopy time by 76% and radiation dose by 64% compared with continuous fluoroscopy." In terms of dose reduction, both the *Image Wisely*® campaign promoting radiation safety in adult medical imaging (www.imagewisely.org) and the *Image Gently*® campaign for pediatric imaging safety (www.imagegently.dnnstaging.com) endorse the use of pulse fluoroscopy. The Image Gently® website features an educational module entitled "Image Gently: Enhancing Radiation Protection During Pediatric Fluoroscopy."

Dose Level Settings

Manufacturers of fluoroscopic imaging systems provide at least three level of *dose settings* within which the system can operate. These settings include low, medium, and high, "with the dose being half or twice the medium level at the low and high settings, respectively" (Mahesh 2008). These levels provide choices to be made when imaging patients for particular examinations. Some systems also feature **high-level control** (HLC) that provides a higher dose note compared with the conventional exposure. The higher dose rate is intended to improve image quality by reducing quantum noise.

The U.S. Food and Drug Administration (FDA) specifies that during normal fluoroscopy, the exposure rate shall not be greater than 100 mGy/min (10 R/min). During HLC fluoroscopy, an exposure rate of up to 200 mGy/min is allowable (Bushong 2013). These exposures rates (entrance dose rates) can be measured according to well-established dosimetry, described in detail by Bushberg et al. (2012).

Automatic Exposure Rate Control

Automatic exposure rate control (AERC) is a relatively new term that has replaced the old term referred to as automatic brightness control (ABC). The purpose of the ABC system was to maintain a constant brightness of the image displayed on the monitor, by adjusting the exposure factors automatically as the x-ray beam moves from a thin to a thick body part.

The AERC system, on the other hand, is intended to keep the signal-to-noise ratio (SNR) of the image constant, by adjusting the exposure factors automatically as patient thickness varies in the beam path (Bushberg et al. 2012). Adjusting mA and kV in this situation is intended to control the dose to the patient. As Bushberg et al. (2012) note, "when the generator responds by increasing the kV, the subject contrast decreases, but the dose to the patient is kept low, because more x-rays penetrate the patient at higher kV. In situations where contrast is crucial (e.g, angiography), the generator can increase the mA instead of the kV; this preserves the subject contrast but at the expense of higher patient dose."

Anti-Scatter Radiation Grids

The purpose of an **anti-scatter radiation grid** is to improve image contrast by absorbing radiation scattered from the patient. The grid is so designed as to let the primary radiation pass through to create the image, but absorbs or removes scattered radiation. The use of an anti-scatter grid during fluoroscopy can increase the radiation dose 2 to 4 times (Bushberg et al. 2012). The degree of increase depends on the construction characteristics of the grid, such as the grid ratio (ratio of the height of the lead strip to the distance between the strips). Ratios used in fluoroscopy are 6:1 to 12:1.

The removal of the grid during fluoroscopy will decrease the dose to the patient and is a recommended practice during pediatric fluoroscopy.

Filtration

The purpose of **filtration** of the x-ray beam in medical imaging (radiography and fluoroscopy) is to protect the patient. The filter removes low-energy photons (which do not penetrate the patient) from the beam, thus increasing the beam's mean energy; the beam becomes "harder" and therefore more penetrating. For fluoroscopy imaging in particular, the skin dose is reduced through the use of metal filters such as copper (Cu), aluminum (Al), or other metals. A study conducted by Nicholson et al. (2000) showed that the skin dose can be reduced by 30%–50% when a 0.1–0.3 mm Cu filter was added during interventional fluoroscopy.

Image Magnification

The purpose of magnifying the image in fluoroscopy is to provide a higher spatial resolution (Bushberg et al. 2012), but at the expense of higher doses to the patient. Image magnification in fluoroscopy can be accomplished in two ways: geometric magnification, and electronic magnification. While the former uses the source-to-object (patient) distance or the image receptor (image intensifier tube)-to-patient distance, the latter is based on the focusing of electrons in the image intensifier tube by the voltages to the electrodes in the image intensifier tube. Collectively, these electrodes are called the **electrostatic lenses** (Bushong 2013). Sometimes, the term **electron optical magnification** is used to refer to electronic magnification.

In *geometric magnification*, as the patient is moved closer to the x-ray tube (for a fixed SID system) a smaller area of the patient to a large area on the image intensifier input screen, and magnification results using the beam geometry with subsequent increase in dose. In systems that do not use a fixed SID (where the x-ray tube and the image intensifier tube can be altered independently) increasing the object-to-receptor distance can also magnify the image. For example, in a fixed SID system (100 cm) when the source-to-patient distance is changed from 80 cm to 40 cm, a magnification factor of 2.50 is obtained and the dose increases by a factor of 4 (Mahesh 2001).

Electronic magnification occurs as follows when using multi-field image intensifier tubes, which allow variation in the FOV (the area of the input screen that the x-ray beam falls upon). For example, a dual-field image intensifier can operate in two modes: one mode will use the full diameter of the input screen, and the other mode, the magnification mode, will use a smaller central portion of the input screen. In the magnification mode, the x-ray beam is first collimated to the central portion of the screen and the voltages to the electrostatic lenses change to ensure that the smaller FOV area falls upon the full size of the output screen. When this occurs, the AERC ensures that the exposure technique factors are automatically increased to maintain the same brightness level of the image on the monitor. This action increases the exposure rate to the patient. For example, going from a FOV of 30 cm to a FOV of 17 cm increases the exposure rate by a factor of 3.1 $(30/17)^2$ (Bushberg et al. 2012). Furthermore, going from a 23-cm FOV (full field) to a magnification of 15 cm and 11 cm FOVs increases the dose by a factor of 2.4 and 4.4, respectively (Mahesh 2001).

For FPDD-based fluoroscopy systems, Bushberg et al. (2012) emphasize that "it is logical that the same approximate dose rate-versus-FOV performance as with image intensifier systems should be used, since that is what users are familiar with."

Last Frame Hold

The term *last frame hold* (Bushberg et al. 2012) has replaced the older term, *last image hold* (**LIH**); modern fluoroscopic imaging systems feature this technique where by an image or images can be held in digital storage and subsequently be displayed for viewing, when the fluoroscopy system is turned off. This technique is viewed as dose reduction strategy, by reducing the total fluoroscopic time of exposure.

Image Recording Techniques

Image recording techniques refer to the use of cassette-loaded spot films, photospot camera spot films, and a cine camera to record a movie of the procedure. Since these systems are obsolete or are becoming obsolete, they will not be described in this text.

Major Factors in Mobile Fluoroscopy Systems

Mobile fluoroscopy simply refers to a fluoroscopic unit that can operate at the patient's bedside. These units are referred to as C-arms and hence the technique is popularly labeled as *C-arm fluoroscopy*. C-Arm fluoroscopy is used in operating rooms general surgery, orthopedics, ambulatory situations, urology, trauma surgery, and in pain management.

C-Arm fluoroscopy units are generally operated with image intensifiers that are smaller than the ones used in fixed fluoroscopy systems. A typical image intensifier tube size is 23-cm (9-inch) input diameter. These units operate under the same technical principles as fixed image intensifier-based fluoroscopy systems, and therefore the same technical factors affecting dose in image intensifier-based fixed fluoroscopy units apply to mobile C-arm fluoroscopy. In summary, these include fluoroscopic exposure technique factors (mA, kV, and beam-on-time), filtration, and LIH.

An important factor affecting the dose in C-Arm fluoroscopy that must be considered by the operator is the *patient-image intensifier distance* (P-IID). The P-IID should be as short as possible to reduce the dose to the patient.

C-Arm Computed Tomography Fluoroscopy

C-Arm computed tomography (C-arm CT) refers to C-arm fluoroscopy systems designed specifically for use in interventional radiology procedures. This system is based on the use of CT principles (described elsewhere) except that the x-ray tube and flat-panel digital detector do not rotate 360° around the patient, but rather 220° around the patient (Bushberg et al. 2012). The data acquired during this 220° rotation is reconstructed using CT image reconstruction algorithms to create images of the procedure. These images lack resolution "because the rotational axis on the C-Arm system is rigid, and the cone beam geometry results in a detection of much higher scatter levels compared to whole body CT systems" (Bushberg et al. 2012). The images are still useful, however, to show details of structures of interest in angiography. Furthermore, the magnitude of the doses from these systems is high (Bushberg et al. 2012).

Summary of Key Concepts

1. Fluoroscopy produces dynamic or moving images acquired and displayed for viewing in real time. The purpose of such an examination is to obtain functional information.

2. The use of very high doses in fluoroscopy has the potential to cause cancer induction and skin injuries in patients and staff as well.

3. There are two types of fluoroscopic imaging systems:
   - Image intensifier-based fluoroscopic system
   - Flat-panel digital detector-based fluoroscopic system

4. The major components of an image intensifier-based system include the x-ray tube and generator, anti-scatter grid, image intensifier tube, image distributor, video camera, analog-to-digital converter (ADC), digital computer, and a television monitor for image display. Each of these components is described in detail.

5. Flat-panel digital detector-based (FPDD-based) fluoroscopy systems overcome the problems of image intensifier-based fluoroscopic systems.

6. The major imaging components of a FPDD-based fluoroscopy system include the x-ray tube, scattered radiation grid, the flat-panel digital detector, digital computer, and the television monitor for image display. Details of each of these components and how they function are described.

7. There are two types of FPDDs available for digital fluoroscopy, described as follows:
   - **The CsI a-Si TFT indirect detector**. X-ray photons full upon the CsI phosphor, which converts them to light photons. The light photons strike the a-Si TFT and are subsequently converted into electrical signals, which are digitized by an ADC and sent to the computer, which generates images of the examination.
   - **The a-Se TFT direct detector**. This is a direct-conversion detector, since it converts x-rays directly into electrical signals for digitization by the ADC. x-rays fall upon the a-Se TFT and are converted directly into electrical signals. There is no conversion of x-rays to light in this detector.

8. A second important point about digital fluoroscopy compared with image intensifier-based fluoroscopy is that hundreds of mA are used instead of less than 5 mA, as in image-intensifier fluoroscopy.

9. To address increase in dose from the use of hundreds of mA, the x-ray tube and generator operate in the pulse-progressive fluoroscopy mode.

(Continues)

10. The major dose factors in fixed fluoroscopy units are fluoroscopic exposure technique factors (kVp, mA, and time in seconds) and instrumentation factors. The latter includes factors such as the operational mode, high-level control (HLC) fluoroscopy, automatic exposure rate control (AERC), anti-scatter grids, source-to-image receptor distance (SID), filtration, electron optical magnification and field-of-view (FOV), last image hold, and image recording modes. These are briefly described.

11. An important factor affecting the dose in C-arm fluoroscopy that must be considered by the operator is the patient-image intensifier distance (P-IID). The P-IID should be as short as possible to reduce the dose to the patient.

12. C-Arm computed tomography (C-arm CT) refers to C-arm fluoroscopy systems designed specifically for use in interventional radiology procedures. This system is based on the use of CT principles except that the x-ray tube and flat-panel digital detector do not rotate 360° around the patient, but rather 220° around the patient.

Discussion Questions

1. Compare and contrast the major components of an image intensifier-based fluoroscopic imaging system and a flat-paned digital fluoroscopic imaging system.

2. Distinguish between fluoroscopic exposure factors and fluoroscopic instrumentation factors affecting the dose in fluoroscopy.

3. Describe the meaning of C-arm fluoroscopy and C-arm CT fluoroscopy.

References

Bushberg JT, Seibert JA, Leidholdt Jr EM, Boone JM. *The Essential Physics of Medical Imaging* (3rd ed.). Philadelphia: Wolters Kluwer/Lippincott Williams & Wilkins; 2012.

Bushong S. *Radiologic Science for Technologist: Physics, Biology and Protection* (10th ed.). St. Louis, MO. Elsevier-Mosby; 2013.

Johnston JN, Fauber TL. *Essentials of Radiographic Physics and Imaging*. St. Louis, MO. Elsevier-Mosby; 2012.

Jones AK, Balter S, Rauch P, Wagner LK. Medical imaging using ionizing radiation: Optimization of the dose and image quality in fluoroscopy. *Med Phys.* 2014;41(1):014301-1-26.

Mahesh M. Fluoroscopy: Patient radiation exposure issues. *Radiographics.* 2001;21:1033–1045.

Nicholson R, Tuffee F, Uthappa MC. Skin sparing in interventional radiology: The effect of copper filtration. *Br J Radiol.* 2000;73:36–42.

Seeram E. *Digital Radiography: An Introduction*. Clifton Park, NY: Delmar-Cengege Learning; 2011.

Smith DL, Heldt JP, Richards GD, Agarwal G, Brisbane WG, Chen CJ, et al. Radiation exposure during continuous and pulsed fluoroscopy. *J. Endourol.* 2013;27(3):384–388.

Spahn M. Flat detectors and their clinical applications. *Eur J Radiol.* 2005;15:1934–1947.

Wang J, Blackburn TJ. x-ray image intensifiers for fluoroscopy. *Radiographics.* 2000;20:1471–1477.

Wolbarst AB, Capasso P, Wyant A. *Medical Imaging: Essentials for Physicians*. Hoboken, NJ: Wiley-Blackwell; 2013.

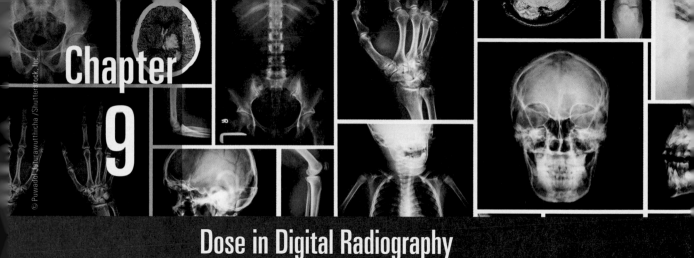

Chapter 9

Dose in Digital Radiography

© Puwadol Jaturawutthicha /Shutterstock, Inc.

Outline

- Introduction
- Film Screen Technology
- The Digital Imaging Era: A New Paradigm
  - Exposure creep
  - Highlighting inappropriate exposures
- Principles of Exposure Indices
  - Scientific criteria for proposed exposure indices
  - Practical criteria for proposed exposure indices
- How Are Exposure Indices Established?
  - What are the options?
  - Exposure indices represent the exposure
  - Previous manufacturers solutions
  - AAPM TG 116 solution

- Deviation Index
  - Why an exposure index?
  - Deviation index action levels
  - IEC publication
  - What can be gained from audits of exposure index?
  - Other factors to consider with the exposure index
- Dose Optimization Research
  - Example of a dose optimization study in computed radiography
- References

Objectives

On completion of this chapter, you should be able to:

1. Discuss briefly the problems associated with film-screen imaging.
2. Identify a significant advantage of using digital radiography to overcome the problems of film-screen radiography.
3. Discuss what is meant by the term "exposure creep."
4. State the meaning of the term "exposure index" and briefly explain its purpose in imaging.
5. Explain how exposure indices are established.

6. Describe the chain of events from exposure of the detector to image presentation.
7. Discuss efforts to standardize the exposure index.
8. State the meaning of the term "deviation index" and identify several action levels following specific deviation indices.
9. Discuss what can be gained from audits of exposure index.
10. Discuss other factors to consider with the exposure index.

Introduction

The Linear No Threshold (LNT) model, which is accepted by most of the radiobiological community, suggests that every dose of radiation delivered to a biological unit carries with it a certain level of risk that is proportional to the amount of radiation. This model underpins the *as low as reasonably achievable* (ALARA) principle with which almost all radiographic, physics, and medical students will be familiar, wherein every time we expose a patient, we try to keep the radiation dose to the lowest amount possible while promoting good diagnostic efficacy. This principle is a fundamental tenet of radiographic and radiologic activity.

Film-Screen Technology

A decade ago, when film-screen technology dominated, adherence to the ALARA principle was arguably easier than it is today. The sensitometric response of film demanded highly accurate exposures, otherwise the densities on the film would be too dark if overexposed or too light if underexposed. **Figure 9-1** demonstrates this where

we have a typical characteristic curve for film, but the range of exposures leaving the patient (log rel E: x axis) that can produce optical densities (blackening on the film: y axis) that were appropriate to the detection of disease or injury by the human eye was limited.

In other words, selection of kVp and mAs had to be finely tuned to achieve the correct level of blackening of the film, and if a radiographer got it wrong, this was immediately apparent on the film (**Figure 9-2, A–C**). This process, while challenging, achieved two things: (1) A high level of radiographic skill ensuring that exposure levels were appropriate to the condition and type of patient presenting; and (2) immediate feedback to the radiographer (and supervisors) as to whether the exposure was optimal or not. While wide-latitude films did increase the range of exposures that could be used to achieve an image of acceptable density, this range remained small.

The predicted response of films to exposures enabled the introduction of a speed classification system, which provided a number for a particular

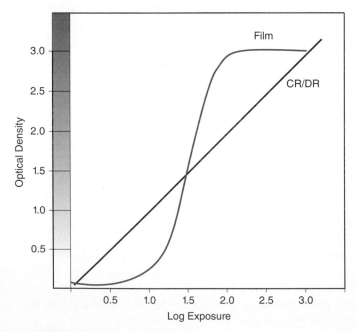

Figure 9-1 Optical density, log relative response curves for film (blue line) and digital receptors (red line).
Courtesy of Patrick C. Brennan.

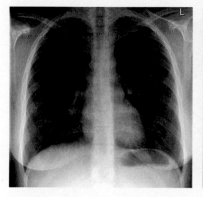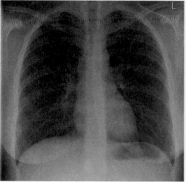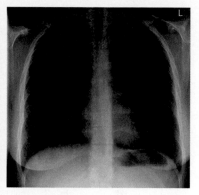

Figure 9-2 Correctly and incorrectly exposed posteroanterior chest. The image on the left is correctly exposed, the remaining two are either under or over exposed.
Courtesy of Patrick C. Brennan.

film for example indicating how responsive or fast the photographic system was to exposures. This classification was widely used in the photographic industry. This number could range from 25–1500, the larger numbers indicating a faster system and thus less required exposure, but also indicating less image sharpness or spatial resolution. Typically in diagnostic radiography, a film-screen speed system of 400× was used (moving from the 200× system widely available in the late 1980s), with slower systems being employed when higher resolution was required such as with extremity exposures (**Figure 9-3**).

The Digital Imaging Era: A New Paradigm

The introduction of digital technology within diagnostic imaging has changed the situation entirely. In Figure 9-1, we can see that when digital receptors are used, such as those employed by computed radiography or flat-panel technologies (red curve), the response to exposures is much more linear and extends over a much greater range. These properties of digital acquisition, coupled with the post-processing capabilities of windowing the image to alter the brightness and contrast, mean that we can no longer rely upon the brightness of an image to inform the radiographer or radiologist if the exposure is correct; indeed, it opens up the opportunity for much more careless selection of kVp and

mAs. An alternative feedback system is required if we are to be able to ensure that patient exposures are not excessive.

In practice, there are some limitations to the exposure range that can be used with digital receptors (**Figure 9-4**).

If the exposure is very, very high, then *saturation* of the receptor will occur resulting in saturation of the image (**Figure 9-5**).

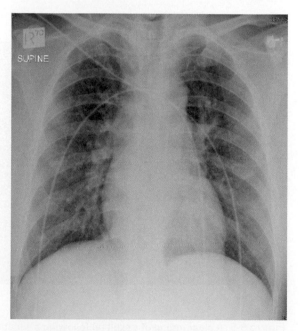

Figure 9-3 An underexposed, digitally acquired PA chest image demonstrating quantum mottle.
Courtesy of Patrick C. Brennan.

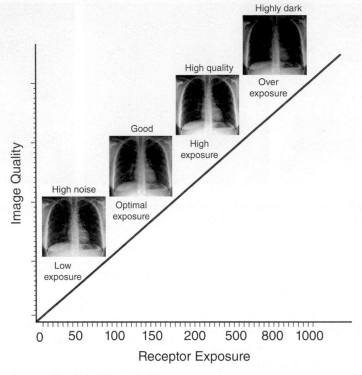

Figure 9-4 The impact of different levels of exposure on image quality using digital receptors.
Courtesy of Patrick C. Brennan.

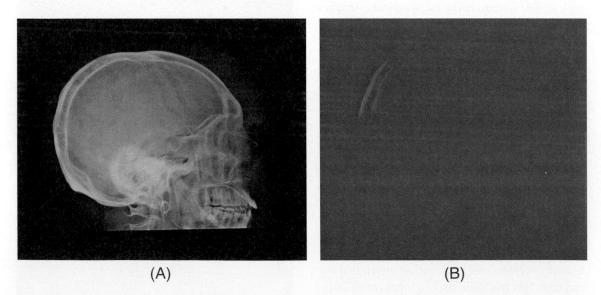

Figure 9-5 A clear image of a skull (a) following a suitable exposure; (b) demonstrates saturation at a very high exposure where all, apart from a very small amount of the cranium, is no longer visible.
Courtesy of Patrick C. Brennan.

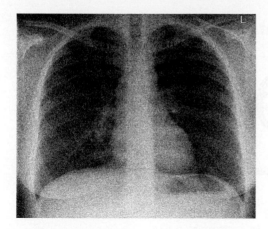

Figure 9-6 An underexposed, digitally acquired PA chest image demonstrating high levels of noise.
Courtesy of Patrick C. Brennan.

If exposures are too low, then the presence of *quantum mottle*, which is a type of noise resulting from too few x-ray photons being available to produce uniform amounts of blackening, increases (**Figure 9-6**). Indeed, noise is now a key image feedback mechanism for informing the radiographer or radiologist if the exposure is appropriate.

With the types of exposures typically employed within x-ray departments, this latter affect (quantum mottle) is much more likely than the former (saturation) and so radiographers when under pressure for example in a busy emergency situation, may be tempted to turn the kVp and mAs upwards to reduce the possibility of quantum mottle.

Exposure Creep

Over time, this temptation to increase the exposure can lead to the well-reported concept of *dose creep*. In theory, this is where radiographers may be used to, for example, selecting 60 kVp and 20 mAs for a typical anteroposterior abdomen exposure. However, under pressure to avoid having to repeat the exposure, and with the knowledge that increased presence of quantum mottle is the most likely cause of an exposure-related repeat, the temptation is to increase the normal exposure to perhaps 60 kVp and 25 mAs. Over time, these settings become the normal exposure factors, and in

time the temptation is to increase this further—and the process of dose creep has commenced. The extent of dose creep since the introduction of digital medical imaging is currently debated (Mothiram et al. 2014; Shepard et al. 2009).

Highlighting Inappropriate Exposures

Whatever the actuality of dose creep, we do have to accept that in the digital era, we no longer have the safeguard of needing accurate exposures to achieve correct image densities, nor the feedback when exposures are not optimal. This must be addressed if patients who are now being irradiated using digital receptors are to be assured that exposures are optimized, and in particular that excessive levels of radiation are not being employed. Exposure indices have been introduced to address this need, and this chapter looks at their development and current status.

Principles of Exposure Indices

Scientific Criteria for Proposed Exposure Indices

In recent years the major manufacturers of digital radiography equipment have introduced various types of exposure index; however, to judge whether the needs of the users of the equipment and their patients have been met, it is worth assembling some criteria on which any proposed indices can be judged. These criteria arise mainly from a document produced by the American Association of Physicists in Medicine (AAPM) Task Group (TG) 116 (**Figure 9-7**), which provides an excellent basis for the latest Exposure Indices recommendations and is summarized in Shepard et al. (2009).

In summary, the criteria suggest that any proposed indicators (that should be available for all radiography systems) should:

- Provide an instant feedback indicating that a reasonable level of radiation has been delivered to the patient for a single examination or exposure;

AAPM REPORT NO. 116

An Exposure Indicator for Digital Radiography

Report of AAPM Task Group 116

July 2009

DISCLAIMER: This publication is based on sources and information believed to be reliable, but the AAPM and the editors disclaim any warranty or liability based on or relating to the contents of this publication.

The AAPM does not endorse any products, manufacturers, or suppliers. Nothing in this publication should be interpreted as implying such endorsement.

Figure 9-7 AAPM Task Group Report: An Exposure Indicator for Digital Radiography.

- Not be based on the brightness of the image (as discussed above), but on a measure of the amount of actual radiation reaching the detector;

- Use an image quality parameter, i.e., noise (quantum mottle), to judge the appropriateness of the radiation levels received by the detector;
- Provide readily accessible data facilitating rigorous quality assurance exercises.

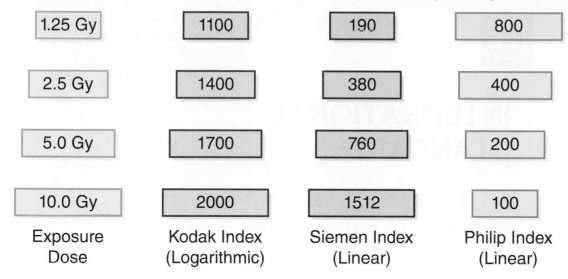

1.25 Gy	1100	190	800
2.5 Gy	1400	380	400
5.0 Gy	1700	760	200
10.0 Gy	2000	1512	100
Exposure Dose	Kodak Index (Logarithmic)	Siemen Index (Linear)	Philip Index (Linear)

Figure 9-8 Exposure index scale used by various manufacturers.
Courtesy of Patrick C. Brennan.

Practical Criteria for Proposed Exposure Indices

Criteria such as the above that provide the scientific basis for Exposure Indices, however, are not enough to ensure effective and widespread implementation of a new idea or innovation. In addition, we must have a system that:

- Is readily understood by the users of the system;
- Is consistent across the different manufacturers;
- Presents values that immediately and intuitively can be understood to represent appropriate, or under and over exposures.

Until the publication of the AAPM TG 116 document, these latter criteria were rarely met by the manufacturer's solutions, leading to a high degree of confusion and under-implementation of EIs (Goske et al. 2011). **Figure 9-8** demonstrates the opportunity for confusion, where: higher EI values could represent higher *or* lower radiation levels; some manufactures presented a linear relationship between exposures and EI values, while others used a logarithmic scale; and little consistency between manufacturers was shown for the actual EI values used and the exposures those values were aiming to represent.

This part of the chapter will now provide a brief summary of the early systems proposed by the manufacturers and will then elaborate upon the AAPM TG 116 solution which aimed to address this opportunity for user confusion. While the AAPM document will provide a substantial source for the material in this chapter, one should acknowledge the contributions of the International Electrotechnical Commission (IEC) International standard IEC 62494-1 (2008)[1] (**Figure 9-9**), which informed particularly the concepts and calibration conditions described by the AAPM.

---

[1]Medical electrical equipment–Exposure index of digital x-ray imaging systems–Part 1: Definitions and requirements for general radiography. (Appareils électromédicaux – Indice d'exposition des systèmes d'imagerie numérique à rayonnement X–Partie 1: Définitions et exigences pour la radiographie générale)

IEC 62494-1

Edition 1.0   2008-08

INTERNATIONAL STANDARD

NORME INTERNATIONALE

Medical electrical equipment – Exposure index of digital X-ray imaging systems –
Part 1: Definitions and requirements for general radiography

**Appareils électromédicaux – Indice d'exposition des systèmes d'imagerie numérique à rayonnement X –
Partie 1: Définitions et exigences pour la radiographie générale**

INTERNATIONAL
ELECTROTECHNICAL
COMMISSION

COMMISSION
ELECTROTECHNIQUE
INTERNATIONALE

PRICE CODE
CODE PRIX   R

ICS 11.040.50

ISBN 2-8318-9944-3

Figure 9-9 International Electrotechnical Commission (IEC) Medical Electrical Equipment-Exposure index of digital x-ray imaging systems: Part 1: Definitions and requirements for general radiography.

How are Exposure Indices Established?

What are the Options?

Since the aim of an exposure index is to provide a value that in some way serves to *represent* the radiation delivered following each diagnostic exposure, there must be some way of monitoring the radiation levels *close to the patient*. One way would be to insert a monitoring device close to, but at the tube side of, the patient; however, this would require input from the radiographer or technologist for each exposure, increasing the time required for each examination and introducing the opportunity for errors and lost data. Another way would be for the manufacturers to place a monitoring device on the detector side of the patient, but this would require extra cost and circuitry along with ongoing maintenance and calibration. Instead, the solution used by the manufacturers and proposed by the AAPM is to utilize an effective monitoring device that is already part of the equipment and is already present every time the patient is exposed: the detector itself (**Figure 9-10**). By cleverly using the value of the pixels within the detector once the radiation has been delivered, an immediate *representation* of the radiation levels delivered is available.

Exposure Indices Represent the Exposure

You will have noticed that I have italicized the words represent and representation in the previous paragraph, and it is worth exploring this for a moment. It is of critical importance to realize that an exposure index is *not a measurement or even representation of radiation levels delivered to the patient. They are not even a measure of radiation levels at the detector.* They are, by utilizing the pixel values following exposures and clever conversion calculations (described below) *a representation of the radiation levels at the surface of the detector* and therefore reflective of the noise level within an image. Remember the aim of the EI: it is not to give an absolute value of patient dose, it is merely to

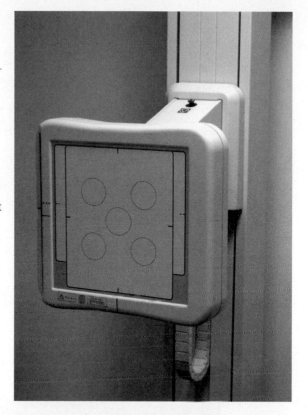

Figure 9-10 A typical arrangement for a digital image receptor system.
Courtesy of Patrick C. Brennan.

provide the user with a value that indicates whether the radiation level delivered has been too high or too low and therefore a metric that allows a relative comparison to be made with some baseline value is what is needed and this is what the EI provides.

Previous Manufacturer Solutions

Carestream Health (Kodak)

Utilizing pixel values to establish an indicator of exposure levels is the principle used in the previous attempts by manufacturers. Carestream Health (formally Kodak), calculates the average values of pixels located in the clinically useful part of the image following patient exposure (**Figure 9-11**).

To do this first it must segment the image using proprietary algorithms so that all pixels within

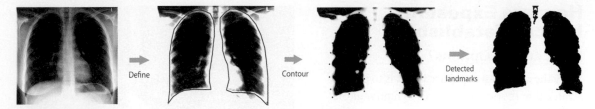

Figure 9-11 Lung segmentation to establish the clinically useful part of the chest radiologic examination.
Courtesy of Patrick C. Brennan.

anatomically regions relevant to a specific examination type are included and all the remaining pixels excluded. This segmentation process is important, otherwise for example we would be including pixel values within the receptor that result from locations not even attenuated by the patient that would be excessively high and certainly in no way would represent the level of quantum mottle within clinically-relevant patient parts. From these pixel values, Carestream Health then suggests particular baseline EI values of around 1700-1900 as a suitably acceptable range and since a *direct logarithmic* scale is employed, an increase in values of 300, represents a doubling of the exposures (**Figure 9-12**).

Siemens

Other manufactures use similar approaches, albeit with subtle segmentation and EI value variations. Siemens, for example, produce an EXI value based on dividing the exposed field into a matrix of 3×3 and then uses the central single section to represent the clinically important part.

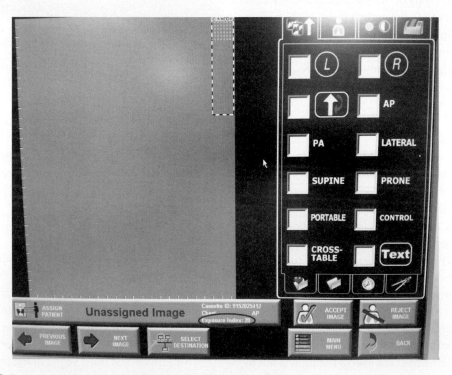

Figure 9-12 Exposure index displayed by Carestream Health.
Courtesy of Patrick C. Brennan.

An EXI value of 380 represents a detector dose of 2.5 µGy, and since a direct linear scale is used, a doubling of an EXI value represents a doubling of detector dose.

Philips Healthcare

Philips Healthcare has produced two types of EI values, with the older one inversely related to dose while the more recent value is directly related to dose (potentially introducing user confusion even within the same manufacturer). Up until DigitalDiagnost 1.2, the selection of pixels relevant for calculating the EI value was linked to the anatomical menu selection, but in more recent versions, this linking has been removed. A more recent system, the DigitalDiagnost DDR system, presents the EI values in discrete, specific steps, e.g., 100, 125, 160, 200, 250, 320, 400, 500, and 630. A change in exposure of more than 25% must occur before the EI value moves from one step to another, meaning that subtle variations in exposure can go unnoticed.

Summary and AAPM TG 116 Aim

As can be seen from the above and from the earlier discussions, the resultant EI value produced is quite unique to each manufacturer, even though the basic methodology used to calculate the value is similar. However, the uniqueness of the resultant value does present opportunity for user confusion and reduces comparisons between exposures to a manufacturer-specific way. The aim of the AAPM solution is to provide a cross-manufacturer solution that is consistent and produces a metric that is instantly recognizable as a detector dose as well as an indication of the deviation from some optimum baseline value.

Aapm Tg 116 Solution

The details relating to the AAPM solution are well described in the executive summary provided by Shepard et al. (2009), *An exposure indicator for digital radiography: AAPM Task Group 116 (Executive Summary)*. Here, we will outline the principles behind the AAPM standard.

Some Principles

Ultimately, the standard being proposed by the AAPM results in the production of two key metrics: An indicated air kerma value at the detector surface, and a deviation index representing how far away this indicated exposure is from an appropriate exposure for a specific body part and projection. To achieve this, the relationship between pixel values and air kerma values at the detector needs in some way to be established. In other words, if the pixel values following a particular exposure are known, the exposure at the detector surface in the form of an air kerma value can be calculated. To achieve this, however, a number of parameters must be considered in more detail. These are:

- The chain of events occurring within the image from exposure of the detector to image presentation;
- The establishment of a relationship between values of specific pixel and a standardized radiation exposure (air kerma at the detector);
- Radiation exposure conditions to achieve the pixel value/air kerma relationship;
- The use of the above relationship to calculate air kerma values at the detector following clinical exposures;
- Other factors affecting the exposure index.

Chain of Events from Exposure of the Detector to Image Presentation

Following patient exposure, the x-ray beam emerging from the body part irradiated interacts with the x-ray detector. This beam consists of a heterogeneous pattern of photon energies and intensities that reflects the attenuation within the patient, resulting in a two dimensional array of pixel values within the detector (**Figure 9-13**).

While the pixel values represent the anatomy and pathology within the examined body part, they do also contain a number of aberrations due to the technology used. These aberrations include zero values when the pixel has been irradiated (dead pixels), values greater than zero when the pixels have not

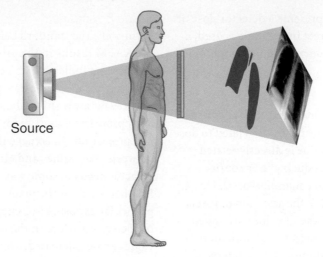

Source

Figure 9-13 Diagram demonstrating the patient and the detector position along with the resultant x-rays pattern and image.
Courtesy of Patrick C. Brennan.

been irradiated (dark current), and changes in the shape of the image (geometric influences). The first step is to correct for these aberrations so that the pixel values better represent the true patient details. Once this is done, the pixel values are known as *for-processing pixels* (and the image is described as the *for-processing image*) and are ready for further processing to present the image to the viewer in a way that maximizes visual interpretation. It is these for-processing pixel values that are relevant to the calculation of exposure indices. It should be acknowledged that there are further processing steps to the images that include adjusting the image densities in a way that is suited to the body part being irradiated, noise reduction, and perceptual linearization—a process to ensure that pixel differences in the darker part of the image are perceived as well as those in brighter regions. After these processing steps, the image is known as the *for-presentation image*.

Relationship Between Specific Pixel Values and a Standardized Radiation Exposure

The key step in the provision of exposure indices is to establish a relationship between the exposure (air kerma) at the detector and the for-processing pixel values. To achieve this, for each digital

imaging system one must first provide a uniform-field (without a patient or phantom) radiation exposure that would typically be used for patient exposures. Since the characteristics of this field can vary depending on features such as the x-ray beam spectra and the geometry of the x-ray beam, relevant details (for example, on the type and quantity of the filtration required) are described in detail within the Shepard et al. (2009) document referred to previously and summarized below.

Once this uniform field is provided, the air kerma at the detector is calculated from an ionization chamber placed in the x-ray beam and the Inverse Square Law, and the relationship between this air kerma and the for-processing pixel values is established. This relationship is detailed for a full range of exposures that is suited to the system being used.

We now have a process whereby a relationship between pixel values and detector dose is established. This means that if the pixel values are evaluated following any exposure, by normalizing or comparing these values to those generated following the standardized exposure, the dose at the receptor can be estimated. *This is the crux of the exposure index.* It is important to note, however, that the relationship between the for-processing pixel values and the detector air kerma may vary depending on the digital radiography system being used and therefore manufacturers are expected to provide details of this relationship to the user as part of the system specifications.

Radiation Exposure Conditions to Achieve the Pixel Value/Air Kerma Relationship

The first step in establishing the above relationship between the standardized exposure and pixel values for each radiographic system is to provide the standardized exposure. The AAPM TG 116 standard has provided information on the spectra and geometry of the x-ray beam that should be employed for this purpose—and while this will be summarized here, the reader should refer to Shepard et al. (2009) for full details.

It is important to note that the procedure detailed below is performed, as an acceptance test when new equipment is being commissioned and at regular intervals thereafter, to ensure that the relationship between the standardized exposure and the pixel values is constantly known so that the EI value presented is a true reflection of the detector dose.

Beam Energy

The standardized exposure should reflect clinical exposure conditions and the first step is to provide a beam with energies typical of those emerging from patient following a clinical exposure. Measurement of beam energies is performed effectively using the metric half-value layer (HVL), which is the thickness of a filter required to reduce the intensity of the radiation by half (**Figure 9-14**) and is usually quoted in terms of mm of aluminum equivalence (mm Al equiv).

It has been shown that if we wish to establish the filter thickness required to equal the level of

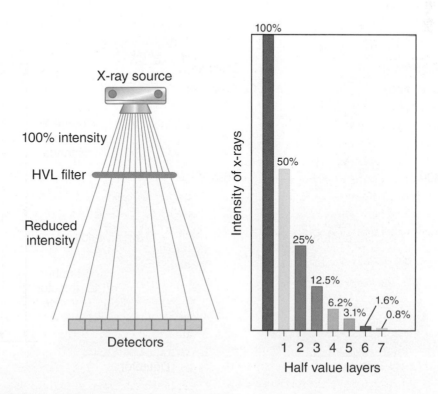

Figure 9-14 The impact of half-value layers on x-ray intensity.
Courtesy of Patrick C. Brennan.

attenuation demonstrated by that of 24 cm of muscle (patient thickness) following a typical exposure, a HVL of approximately 6.8 mm Al is required. This HVL can be achieved using appropriate kVp selection, inherent and added filtration within the x-ray tube, which should exceed 2.5 mm Al equiv (at 70 kVp), plus additional filters that can be made of aluminum, copper or other exotic materials. The precise combinations of kVp and filter thicknesses, along with details on filter materials to be used, are all treated expertly in the AAPM standard; once these combinations are adhered to, the system response should be consistent and close to a 5% tolerance.

Methodology for Performing the Standardized Exposure

The second component required for establishing this standardized exposure is the methodology used to obtain the measurements, of which there are two main stages. This is explained very well in the AAPM document and summarized here:

- The materials demonstrated in **Figure 9-15** are gathered and arranged as shown.
- The x-ray equipment should be tested for exposure (coefficient of variation <0.03) and kVp consistency (±3%) and the ionization chamber must be calibrated. The added filtration is as described above.
- The distance between the x-ray source and the detector should be as large as possible, but certainly greater than 100 cm with the ionization chamber placed at a point exactly midway between the x-ray source and the detector. To achieve this position the distance of the detector from the surface of the detector housing must be known. If a computed radiography system (CR) is being tested, lead should be placed behind the CR plate to minimize

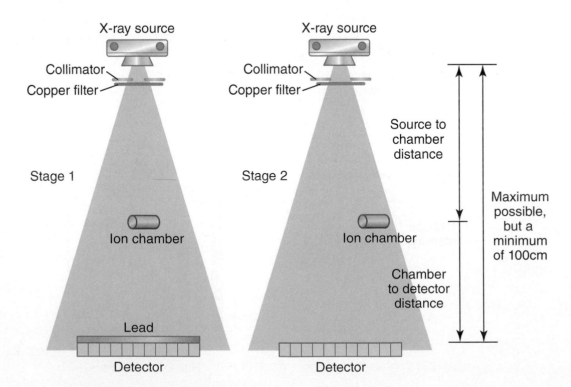

Figure 9-15 The arrangement of equipment for stages 1 and 2 of standardized exposure procedure.
Courtesy of Patrick C. Brennan.

backscatter and a distance greater than 25 cm provided between the CR plate and the supporting surface. The secondary radiation grid should be removed, if possible, and when this is not possible, the relevant attenuation factors should be known. To minimize anode heel affects, the long axis of the detector (if not square) should be placed at right angles to the anode /cathode axis.

Stage 1

The ionization chamber should be placed in the centre of the x-ray beam's cross section and the beam collimated to ensure that all sections of the chamber is exposed, extended to no more than a 2.5-cm perimeter around the chamber. A 0.5-mm copper filter is placed at the collimator surface and lead is positioned over the detector to ensure that the detector is protected from the exposure. The kVp selection and/or filtration is adjusted until a HVL of 6.8-mm Al is achieved and an mAs selected that achieves an exposure at the detector at the midpoint of its response range. An exposure is made, the ionization chamber reading recorded, and using the Inverse Square Law, the air kerma at the detector is calculated.

Stage 2

The exposure conditions established in Stage 1 are employed, but with the following modifications:

- The collimators are adjusted so that the x-ray beam is as large as possible and the detector is completely exposed;
- The chamber is moved in a direction perpendicular to the x-ray as laterally as possible, but within the x-ray beam. Ideally the chamber will be outside the detector's field of view;
- The lead protection placed at the surface of the detector is removed, and an exposure is made.

The air kerma at the detector is finally calculated using the chamber value from stage 2; any correction required for the displaced ionization chamber from the ratio between the chamber values calculated from stage 1 over stage 2; and the

Inverse Square Law. Further corrections, such as correcting for secondary grid attenuation, may be recommended by manufacturers.

At this stage, we have established a process whereby from pixel values we can estimate the detector dose. However, given that the focus of the above is how this is established using a uniform exposure (under specified experimental conditions), some attention must now be given to how we achieve detector dose from *patient or clinical* exposures.

For the exposure indicator to work in clinical practice, we need to be able to estimate the detector dose and its deviation from a baseline value from each patient exposure. Since from the above it can be seen that by the time the x-ray detector is exposed and if the relationship between the pixel values and detector dose is known, calculation of the detector air kerma situation should be straightforward once the pixel values are available following each patient exposure. The calculation of appropriate pixel values is therefore critically important, and careful consideration must be given to *which summary value of the chosen pixel values* should be used and *which region of the clinical image* should be employed to estimate this indicated air kerma value.

Summary Value

In terms of summary value, the AAPM TG 116 document recommends the median value, since this will remove the influence of excessively small or large values that would be more inclined to affect the mean values. Also, to ensure that sufficient numbers of pixels are used to calculate this median value, it is recommended that the image sample size should make up at least 4% of the exposed detector area.

Image Region

With regard to the image region that should be used, this will be dictated by the reason for performing the examination in the first place. It is important to select or segment a region that contains pixels relating to the patient's clinical condition, since the exposure required to visualize soft tissues in the abdomen, for instance, will be different from that required to demonstrate bony structures. For example, if the lumbar spine was chosen to calculate the median pixel value, the included pixels (and the resultant indicated air kerma value) would not represent well the kidney region for a pre-contrast intravenous urographic projection. This is why it has been argued that the for-presentation images (rather than the for-processing image) could be used to determine the segmented region (but not to establish the actual median value), since this would better represent the purpose of the image. Whatever process is used, it is evident that careful selection of the image region is advantageous; however, it should be noted that for some current commercial systems, a region representing the whole attenuated body part is sometimes used.

Deviation Index

Why an Exposure Index?

Having a process that indicates the air kerma at the detector surface is clearly a powerful tool in the optimization of radiographic examinations; however, since the ideal value for a specific examination or condition may vary (e.g., that required

for a consolidated lung compared with a pneumothorax), a system that demonstrates the extent of variation from a target value for a specific patient situation would add considerable value. That is why the AAPM TG 116 recommends that in addition to the indicated air kerma value, a deviation index is also provided. This uses a logarithmic scale where a value of ±1 represents 125% (+) and 80% (–) of the intended exposure.

Deviation Index Action Levels

Deviation index action levels have been recommended by the AAPM TG 116, and these are summarized in **Table 9-1**.

Updating Exposure Index Target Values for Deviation Calculations

Exposure index target values that would facilitate deviation index calculations should be made available to the clinicians by manufacturers; however, it is important to stress that targets should ultimately be determined by each department's radiologists and radiographers. A process for updating tables therefore should be in place so that target values and subsequent deviation indices reflect local expert preferences.

Table 9-1 Action levels following specific deviation indices

Deviation Index action level	Action
−0.5 – +0.5	No action required, target range achieved
Over exposure	
=/>+1.0	Over exposure. Examine image to ensure that saturation of the image over clinically useful regions is not evident
>+3.0	Excessive over exposure. Examine image to ensure that saturation of the image over clinically useful regions is not evident. Initiate corrective action
Under exposure	
<−1.0	Under exposure. Examine image to ensure that quantum mottle of the image over clinically useful regions is not excessive, otherwise repeat the exposure
<−3.0	Repeat the exposure*

* This is the recommendation of the AAPM TG116, but the authors of this text would suggest that the radiographer and/or the radiologist check the image to see whether a repeat exposure is clinically justified.

Courtesy of Patrick C. Brennan.

Important Reminder

Finally, it is worth reiterating that the *exposure index does not describe the incident dose* on the detector for a specific exposure. Instead it is estimating the dose based on a selected number of pixels within the image (see above) and an established relationship between these pixels and the detector air kerma. This is why the AAPM recommend the use of the term *indicated* equivalent air kerma.

IEC Publication

While the focus in this chapter has been on the AAPM TG 116 recommendations, it was mentioned above that these were largely informed by a publication by the International Electrotechnical Commission (IEC), a leading international body that issues standards on electrical, electronic and related technologies. This latter publication, *IEC 62494-1* (IEC 2008) demonstrates significant overlap with the definitions, terminology, principles, and processes described within the AAPM TG 116 document; however, there are distinctions and some of these are summarized here.

1. The IEC document refers to calibration functions and inverse calibration functions, and while this terminology is different from the AAPM TG 116 document, these descriptions relate directly and respectively to the sections above in which the establishment of a relationship between values of specific pixel and a standardized radiation exposure (air kerma at the detector) and the use of this relationship to calculate air kerma values at the detector following clinical exposures are described. In other words, the calibration function expresses the region-of-interest pixel values as a function of the exposure (air kerma at the detector), valid under specific exposure conditions which are described in the section discussing radiation exposure conditions to achieve the pixel value/air kerma relationship. The inverse calibration function simply refers to expression of the detector air kerma as a function of the region-of-interest's pixel values.

2. The AAPM suggests using the median pixel value when establishing the relationship between the pixel values and the detector exposure; however, the IEC proposes that the central tendency of the pixel values may be calculated using the mean, median, mode, or trimmed mean or any other recognized statistical descriptor. While initially this may seem like a major deviation from the AAPM document, one must remember that this is a uniformly exposed (flat) field, and therefore differences between the mean, mode and median should not be excessive.

3. The IEC document proposes that during the calibration process (establishing the relationship between the detector dose and pixel values), that a centrally located region comprising 10% of the uniformly exposed image should be used.

4. While the limitations of using a single-beam energy to establish the relationship between the pixels and the detector dose is considered in the AAPM TG 116 document, this is further emphasized in the IEC publication. Both documents present a graph detailing the varied response of different systems to specific beam energies (**Figure 9-16**).

In summary, while there are differences between the AAPM TG 116 and the IEC documents, and some of these have been outlined above, overall the two documents are complementary and the overall aims and recommended processes are very close to each other.

What Can Be Gained From Audits of Exposure Index?

Storage of exposure indicators presents a good opportunity to retrospectively assess the level of exposure received by cohorts of patients within medical imaging departments, and the AAPM or IEC solution, once adopted by the manufacturers, will facilitate this evaluation across various manufacturers and thus imaging rooms. However, to date there is limited evidence in the medical or

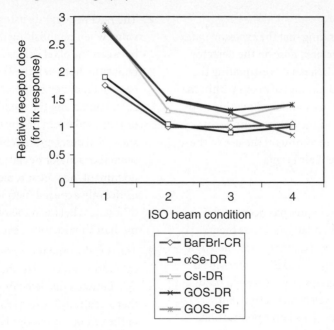

Figure 9-16 Response of different detector systems to specific beam energies (ISO beam conditions).
Courtesy of Patrick C. Brennan.

scientific literature that exposure indices are being analyzed rigorously, but hopefully the introduction of a much more standardized approach such as that being proposed by the AAPM TG 116 will encourage more widespread usage.

An Example of an Audit of Exposure Index Values

It might be worth giving an example of the type of data that can be provided once exposure indices are evaluated effectively. Mothiram et al. (2014) examined 5000 exposure indices over a 6–12 month period across several examinations. Even though the indices examined were not of a standardized form and reflected the traditional manufacturer-based methods, useful information was gleaned. In **Table 9-2**, a number of exposure indices are shown for several manufacturers and include values for chest, abdomen, and pelvis examinations with quartile values provided. The last two columns are probably of most interest, since these demonstrate the proportion of values that were under- and overexposed when compared with the manufacturers' suggested guidelines; it can be seen that these proportions are sometimes substantial.

In the next table (**Table 9-3**), focus was given to the impact of gender on the exposure indices, which showed that for chest and abdomen examinations, statistical differences existed between males and females, suggesting that some inter-gender discrepancies may be present for digital exposures (which had not been described previously).

Detailed treatment of these data by the authors also showed that in addition to the gender issue, significant differences in index values were shown between:

- chest and abdomen examinations taken during normal working hours (9 AM–5 PM) versus those taken outside the normal workday;
- the use and non-use of a grid for chest projections (remembering that, since the exposure index represents exposure at the detector surface, the grid should have minimal impact on the value);
- the presence or absence of an implant or prosthesis for chest projections.

However, possibly even more important than the data themselves, Mothiram and her colleagues (2014) demonstrated the power of retrospective assessment of exposure indices and the wealth of

Table 9-2 Exposure indices for a variety of examinations across several manufacturers (Mothiram et al 2013). The final two columns demonstrate the level of under- or over-exposure values compared with the manufacturers' recommended values

Manufacturer/ examination	Number (n)	Median	First quartile (Q_1)	Third quartile (Q_3)	Exposure % Over	% Under
Siemens digital radiography (DR)						
Chest posterior-anterior	2453	228	195	267	1%	6%
Chest lateral	107	319	278	360	13%	1%
Chest supine	15	226	194	289	0%	0%
Chest lateral decubitus	2	193	142	243	0%	50%
Chest anterior-posterior	4	249	146	270	0%	25%
Abdomen	377	233	205	256	0%	1%
Pelvis	239	467	369	581	67%	0%
Philips DR						
Chest posterior-anterior	213	400	320	400	0%	1%
Chest lateral	15	400	320	400	0%	0%
Chest anterior-posterior	9	400	250	630	11%	11%
Abdomen	26	630	630	630	0%	0%
Pelvis	3	630	500	630	0%	0%
Carestream Health computed radiography (CR)						
Mobile chests	1261	2040	1930	2170	79%	3%
Departmental chests	273	2020	1880	2130	72%	4%
Abdomen	1	1400	1400	1400	0%	100%
Pelvis	2	1650	1510	1790	0%	50%
Total	**5000**				**28%**	**4%**

Mothiram U, Brennan PC, Moran B, Robinson J. Retrospective evaluation of exposure index (EI) values from plain radiographs reveals important considerations for quality improvement. *Journal of Medical Radiation Sciences* 201, 60(4), 2013, pp. 115–122.

information regarding the delivery of radiologic services that could be generated.

Exposure Indices and Diagnostic Reference Levels?

Finally, the author would like to raise what initially may seem like an outrageous question: Could exposure indices ever be used as a diagnostic reference level? When one considers the function of a diagnostic reference level, which ultimately is a value that should guide radiographers and radiologists as to whether the dose being delivered to average-sized patients on a regular basis is at an appropriate level,

its similarity to the aim of an exposure index can be seen. Also, the recordable and accessible nature of an exposure index means that there would be a plethora of data to allow a robust 75th (or any other) percentile value to be calculated. This is unlike the current situation that exists in a number of countries for diagnostic reference levels, whereby the often cumbersome nature of dose measurements in clinical departments makes gathering of sufficient data, particularly for specific examinations, and the subsequent establishment of representative percentile values very difficult.

Having stressed the possibilities, it is equally important to acknowledge that the exposure index

Table 9-3 Exposure index values for each examination type, separated out for each gender (Mothiram et al 2013). Emboldened rows indicate significant differences between genders for specific examinations

Manufacturer/ examination	Gender F=Female; M=male	Number (n)	Median	First quartile (Q₁)	Third quartile (Q₃)	Exposure % Over	% Under	P Value
Siemens digital radiography (DR)								
Chest posterior anterior	**F**	**1207**	**239**	**209**	**275**	**1%**	**3%**	**<0.0001**
	M	**1246**	**216**	**185**	**255**	**1%**	**8%**	
Chest lateral	**F**	**48**	**332**	**285**	**409**	**29%**	**0%**	**0.04**
	M	**59**	**313**	**268**	**343**	**2%**	**2%**	
Chest supine	**F**	**8**	**263**	**218**	**306**	**0%**	**0%**	**0.03**
	M	**7**	**201**	**180**	**227**	**0%**	**0%**	
Chest lateral decubitus	F	2	193	142	243	0%	50%	Numbers too few (nf)
	M	0				0%	0%	
Chest anterior posterior	F	2	269	267	271	0%	0%	nf
	M	2	174	118	230	0%	50%	
Abdomen	**F**	**204**	**227**	**199**	**252**	**0%**	**2%**	**0.001**
	M	**173**	**240**	**212**	**265**	**0%**	**0%**	
Pelvis	F	157	479	384	596	70%	0%	Not significant (ns)
	M	82	447	357	526	62%	0%	
Philips DR								
Chest posterior anterior	**F**	**90**	**400**	**400**	**400**	**0%**	**0%**	**0.01**
	M	**123**	**400**	**320**	**400**	**0%**	**1%**	
Chest lateral	F	3	400	400	400	0%	0%	ns
	M	12	400	320	475	0%	0%	
Chest anterior posterior	F	5	320	225	515	20%	0%	ns
	M	4	630	345	758	0%	25%	
Abdomen	F	17	630	630	630	0%	0%	ns
	M	9	630	630	630	0%	0%	
Pelvis	F	2	565	500	630	0%	0%	nf
	M	1	630	630	630	0%	0%	
Carestream Health computed radiography (CR)								
Mobile chests	F	483	2060	1930	2190	81%	3%	ns
	M	778	2030	1920	2160	78%	3%	
Departmental chests	**F**	**148**	**2055**	**1910**	**2160**	**77%**	**3%**	**0.001**
	M	**125**	**1970**	**1855**	**2080**	**66%**	**5%**	
Abdomen	F	0	1400	1400	1400	0%	0%	nf
	M	1				0%	100%	
Pelvis	F	2	1650	1510	1790	0%	50%	nf
	M	0				0%	0%	
Total		**5000**						

Mothiram U, Brennan PC, Moran B, Robinson J. Retrospective evaluation of exposure index (EI) values from plain radiographs reveals important considerations for quality improvement. *Journal of Medical Radiation sciences* 2014 (in press).

data has been developed specifically for a different function, which means that one must be extremely careful suggesting its efficacy for a different, albeit similar function. Therefore, research looking at issues regarding the ability of exposure indices to serve as diagnostic reference levels will need to be performed, not least exploring the ability of an estimation of a detector dose to represent patient exposures. Nonetheless, the possibility of exploring more widespread applications of exposure indices should not be automatically dismissed.

Other Factors to Consider with the Exposure Index

It should be acknowledged that the exposure index (and the associated deviation index) is not perfect, and on occasion the number presented may not be representative of the air kerma at the detector. There are a number of reasons for this, including the level of collimation used, the presence of materials on or within the patient that may attenuate the x-ray beam excessively, and the beam energy used.

Also, caution must be exercised so that the expectations that we have from the exposure index should not be exaggerated. All this will be discussed below.

Collimation

The production of the exposure index as discussed earlier relies on extracting from the image a certain number of pixels that then can be used to estimate air kerma at the detector. If collimation is excessive, this may mean that insufficient detector area is exposed, and a number of the pixels that are being used to calculate the median value are recording a zero or close to a zero value. This will result in a lower median value than would have occurred with a less collimated beam, thus resulting in a lower and non-representative exposure index.

Attenuating Materials Within the X-Ray Beam

The impact of high-attenuation materials on or within the patient has a similar affect as that with collimation. Gonadal protection (**Figure 9-17**) or metal prostheses such as a hip replacement can

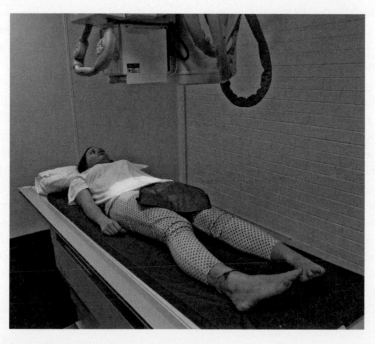

Figure 9-17 Gonadal protection on a patient with hip x-ray.
Courtesy of Patrick C. Brennan.

mean that, for a specific body region, a number of the pixel values are much lower than they would have been for the same examination if these materials were not present, again resulting in a lower-than-normal exposure index. A similar effect may be demonstrated following unusual organ location such as a transplanted kidney in the pelvic region.

This demonstrates the importance of radiographic and/or radiologic examination of the image when deciding on the necessity of a repeat exposure rather than relying solely on the exposure index value.

Beam Energy

The impact of beam energy on the exposure index is a significant one. A basic understanding of the attenuation of x-rays will tell us that as the energy of the x-ray increases or decreases, the amount of radiation incident on the detector surface must decrease or increase if the image noise (median pixel value within the detector) is to remain constant. Although between 55 kVp and 90 kVp this impact has been reported to be small (Van Metter and Yorkston 2006; AAPM TG 116 2009), and the majority of radiographic exposures occur within these peak values, a problem exists for exposures outside this range, such as that which occurs with chest and breast imaging.

With chest imaging, over the last two decades, to reduce image contrast between the lungs and the ribs, heart and mediastinum, there has been a move away from the use of lower kVp values such as 60–75 kVp to peak energies around 120–125 kVp. Clearly this latter value is outside the range stated above, and therefore the AAPM have recommended a separate standard for chest using a HVL around 11.6 mm Al to establish the relationship between the standardized radiation exposure and the pixel values. With breast imaging, where the energies are below the range above, at this time there does not appear to be a proposed solution, although the need for modification of the standardized conditions is

acknowledged by the AAPM. This deficiency needs to be addressed with some urgency when we consider that approximately 1 million screening mammograms alone can take place annually within a typical population of 40 million people.

A Note of Caution

Finally, radiographers and radiologists must be aware that having an exposure index that appears to adhere to the target value following a particular examination doesn't guarantee perfect exposures. It is important to remember that the aim of the exposure index is to represent detector incident dose calculated from pixel values based on the premise that when pixel values are too low, the image will have increased noise, and if too high would suggest excessive patient exposure. *The solution is no more than an estimation.* Therefore, one must be very careful not to rely on indices as a method of judging image quality and justifying repeat exposures. Radiographers and radiologists have highly developed skills and knowledge that facilitates an expert evaluation of image quality, so using an exposure index as a substitute for this process should not occur. For example, the author has a little concern when he sees the AAPM's recommendation that if the deviation value is –3.0, the exposure should be repeated. While it is very likely that there will be excessive noise with such an exposure and that a repeat will be necessary, *the decision for that repeat should be on the basis of image evaluation and not an exposure index.* Also, within the IEC publication (2008), it is proposed that the exposure index "allows the operator to judge if an image was taken at a detector exposure level suitable for the intended level of image quality." The author of this chapter would suggest that while the exposure index provides extremely useful information on the level of exposure employed, judgment of the multi-faceted components of image quality cannot be reduced to a number or a single parameter such as noise.

Summary of Key Concepts

1. **Risks of overexposure with digital technology are greater than film.** These properties of digital acquisition coupled with the post-processing facilities of windowing the image to alter the brightness and contrast mean that we can no longer rely upon the brightness of an image to inform the radiographer or radiologist if the exposure is correct and indeed opens up the opportunity for much more careless selection of kVp and mAs. An alternative feedback system is required if we are to be able to ensure that patient exposures are not excessive.

2. **Need for an effective dose monitoring strategy in digital radiography.** In the digital era, we no longer have the safeguard of needing accurate exposures to achieve correct image densities, nor the feedback when exposures are not optimal. This must be addressed if patients who are now being irradiated using digital receptors are to be assured that exposures are optimized, and in particular that excessive levels of radiation are not being employed. Exposure indices have been introduced to address this need, and this chapter looks at their development and current status.

3. Importance of the AAPM and IEC publications to standardize exposure indices. Providing the scientific basis for exposure indices is not enough to ensure effective and widespread implementation of a new idea or innovation. In addition, we must have a system that is readily understood by the users of the system; is consistent across the different manufacturers; present values that immediately and intuitively can be understood to represent appropriate, or under- and overexposures. Until the publication of the AAPM TG 116 or International Electrotechnical Commission (IEC) International standard IEC 62494-1, these criteria were rarely met by the manufacturer's solutions, leading to a high degree of confusion and under-implementation of EIs.

4. Values presented and factors that can impact upon these values. It should be acknowledged that the exposure index (and the associated deviation index) is not perfect, and on occasion the number presented may not be representative of the air kerma at the detector. There are a number of reasons for this including the level of collimation used, the presence of materials on or within the patient that may attenuate the x-ray beam excessively, and the beam energy used. Also, the expectations that we have from exposure index should not be exaggerated.

Discussion Questions

1. Discuss the increased opportunities for increased radiation doses within digital radiography compared with film/screen technology.

2. Discuss the need for an exposure index and how this measure is achieved.

3. Consider the factors that impact the exposure index.

References

Goske MJ, Charkot E, Herrmann T, John SD, Mills TT, Morrison G, et al. Image Gently: Challenges for radiologic technologist when performing digital radiography in children. *Pediatr Radiol.* 2011;41:611–619.

International Electrotechnical Commission (IEC). International standard IEC 62494-1. Medical electrical equipment – Exposure index of digital x-ray imaging systems –Part 1: Definitions and requirements for general radiography. Appareils électromédicaux – Indice d'exposition des systèmes d'imagerie numérique à rayonnement X – Partie 1: Définitions et exigences pour la radiographie générale. 2008. (Available at http://www.iec.ch; Retrieved August 25, 2015.)

Mothiram U, Brennan PC, Moran B, Robinson J. Retrospective evaluation of exposure index (EI) values from plain radiographs reveals important considerations for quality improvement. *J Med Radiat Sci.* 2013;60(4):115–122.

Neitzel U. *The Exposure Index and Its Standardization.* Hamburg, Germany: Philips Medical Systems, 2006.

Shepard JS, Wang J, Flynn M, Gingold E, Goldman L, Krugh K, et al. AAPM Report No. 116: An Exposure Indicator for Digital Radiography. American Association of Physicists in Medicine. 2009: Report No. 116.

Van Metter R, Yorkston J, Applying a proposed definition for receptor dose to digital projection images. *Proc SPIE.* 2006;6142:426–444.

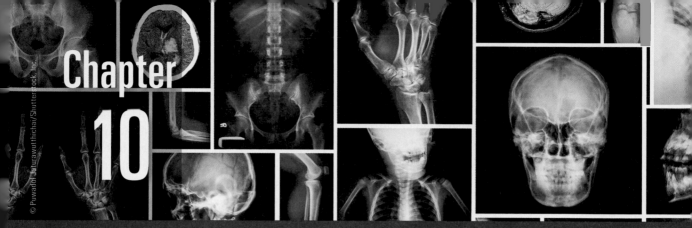

Chapter 10

Radiation Dose in Computed Tomography

Outline

- Introduction
- Early Pioneering Work: Nobel Prize for CT Development
- The CT Process: Basic Principles and Major Components
  - Data flow in a CT scanner
  - Multislice CT technology: the pitch
  - CT image quality characteristics: an overview
- Risks of CT: A Rationale for Dose Reduction and Optimization
- CT Dose Descriptors
  - The computed tomography dose index (CTDI)
  - The dose length product (DLP)
- Factors Affecting Dose in CT
  - Exposure technique factors: mAs and kVp
  - Collimation
  - Pitch
  - Patient centering
  - Automatic tube current modulation (ATCM)
  - Iterative image reconstruction
- Dose-Image Quality Optimization Research in CT
  - An example of a CT dose optimization study
- References

Objectives

On completion of this chapter, you should be able to:

1. State the meaning of the term computed tomography (CT).
2. Identify two pioneers who shared the Nobel Prize in Medicine for their contributions to the development of the CT scanner.
3. Discuss the basic physical principles involved in CT and identify three major components of the CT Technology.
4. Explain the function of each of the three major components of a CT scanner.
5. Define the term "pitch" for multislice CT.
6. Identify three image quality parameters and explain what is meant by each one.
7. Identify the risks of radiation from CT scanning.
8. Describe the characteristic features of the Computed Tomography Dose Index (CTDI) and the Dose Length Product (DLP).
9. Explain how each of the following factors affect the dose in CT:
   - Exposure technique factors
   - Collimation
   - Pitch
   - Patient centering
   - Automatic tube current modulation (ATCM)
   - Iterative image reconstruction
10. Explain what is meant by dose-image quality optimization in CT.

Introduction

Computed tomography (CT) is a sectional digital imaging technique that produces cross sectional digital images of the patient's body. Such images are often referred to as *transaxial* images since they refer to planar sections that are perpendicular to the long axis of the patient. CT uses a digital computer to process and reconstruct x-ray transmission data collected from the patient. It is a multidisciplinary subject based on physics, mathematics, engineering, and computer science.

The purpose of this chapter is to outline nature of the dose in CT scanning. First, a brief description of the CT scanner system components will be briefly described, including CT image quality factors in a nutshell. Secondly, the elements of CT dosimetry and factors affecting the dose in CT will be outlined in an effort to ensure an understanding of how these factors play a role in optimization of the dose-image quality in CT.

Early Pioneering Work: Nobel Prize for CT Development

In the early 1970s, Godfrey Hounsfield (in England) invented the first clinically useful CT scanner using an improved reconstruction algorithm. For this work, Hounsfield received the Nobel Prize in Medicine and Physiology in 1979, a prize which he shared with Allan Cormack, a physicist at Tufts University in Massachusetts. Hounsfield's CT scanner was called the EMI (Electronic and Musical Instruments) scanner, since this was the company where he worked. The EMI scanner was dedicated to imaging the head only. Cormack, on the other hand, developed solutions to the mathematical problems in CT. Later in 1963 and 1964 he published two papers the *Journal of Applied Physics* on the subject, but they received little interest in the scientific community at that time. It was not until Hounsfield began working on the development of the first practical CT scanner that Cormack's work was also viewed as the solution to the mathematical problem in CT. The student should refer to Seeram (2009) for further details of the contribution of these pioneers to the development of CT.

The CT Process: Basic Principles and Major Components

There are three major components in the production of a CT image, as illustrated in **Figure 10-1**. These include data acquisition, image reconstruction, and image display, storage, and communication.

Data acquisition is the systematic collection of x-ray attenuation data from the patient, using an

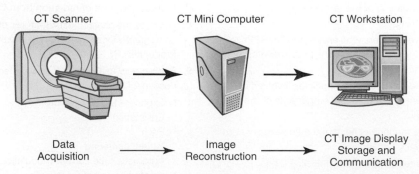

Figure 10-1 Three major system components in the production of a CT image include data acquisition, image reconstruction, and image display, storage, and communication.

Reproduced from: Seeram, E. (2009) *Computed tomography: Physical principles, clinical applications and quality control.* Philadelphia, Saunders: Elsevier. Reproduced by permission.

array of special electronic detectors, coupled to the x-ray tube. The fundamental physical principles of CT are such that during scanning, the x-ray tube and detectors rotate around the patient, and all x-ray attenuation data are sent to the computer for processing. In data acquisition, the x-ray beam passes through the patient and is attenuated according to Lambert-Beer's law:

$$I = I_o e^{-\mu \Delta X}$$

where I is transmitted beam intensity; I_o is original beam intensity; e is Euler's constant; μ is the linear attenuation coefficient; and Δx is the finite thickness of the section. The mathematical problem in CT is to calculate all the attenuation coefficients for all structures shown on the image.

Image reconstruction is a sophisticated process and involves the use special reconstruction algorithms to systematically build up the image using a large number of attenuation measurements obtained at different locations (rotation angles) around the slice to be imaged. **Figure 10-2** illustrates how the attenuation data are converted to integers (0, a positive number, or a negative number) referred to as **CT numbers** using a reconstruction algorithm. These CT numbers are computed using the following relationship:

$$CT\,Number = \frac{\mu_{tissue} - \mu_{water}}{\mu_{water}} \cdot K$$

where K is a manufacturer's scaling factor or contrast factor, and in general, $K = 1000$.

One of the more commonplace algorithms is the *filtered back projection (FBP) algorithm*; however, the iterative reconstruction algorithm has recently become popular in CT scanners. These algorithms are not within the scope of this textbook and the interested student should refer to Seeram (2009) for a description of how these algorithms work.

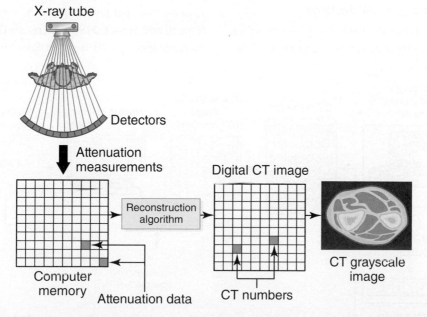

Figure 10-2 In CT scanning, attenuation data are converted to integers (a 0, a positive number or a negative number) referred to as CT numbers using a reconstruction algorithm. The CT numbers are subsequently converted into a gray scale image.

After the image has been reconstructed, it is displayed on a computer monitor for viewing by an observer. At this point, the observer can manipulate the image using special image processing operations to suit his/her viewing needs. Images are subsequently stored on magnetic or optical data carriers and they can be communicated by electronic means to other remote locations using a picture archiving and communications system (PACS).

Data Flow in a CT Scanner

The flow of data in a CT scanner is illustrated in **Figure 10-3** and is as follows:

1. The x-ray tube and detectors (in the CT Gantry) collect x-ray attenuation data from the patient.

2. Detectors measure not only the transmitted photons (transmitted beam) from the patient, but also the intensity of the x-rays from the x-ray tube (reference beam).

3. The transmitted beam and the reference beam are both converted into electrical signals.

4. These electrical signals are then converted into digital data by special digitizers.

5. Data processing involves, first pre-processing, after which the data is referred to as raw data.

6. The raw data are then sent to the array processor for image reconstruction to create the CT image (reconstructed image).

7. The reconstructed image can be display for viewing on a computer monitor, recorded, and stored on magnetic tapes or optical disks. This image can also be sent to the PACS.

8. Further digital image processing can be done on the image via the image processor.

9. The control terminal is usually an operator's control terminal, for complete system control.

Multislice CT Technology: The Pitch

Today, all CT scanners are multislice CT scanners (MSCT). In MSCT, the detector system is a two-dimensional detector array consisting of varying rows, compare to a single-slice CT (SSCT) scanner which has a one-dimensional detector array, and produces one slice per rotation of the x-ray tube and detectors around the patient. An MSCT detector with four rows will collect four slices per revolution. One with 16 rows or 64 rows will collect 16 or 64 slices per revolution of the x-ray tube, respectively. Hence, MSCT increases the volume coverage speed by virtue of its detector design.

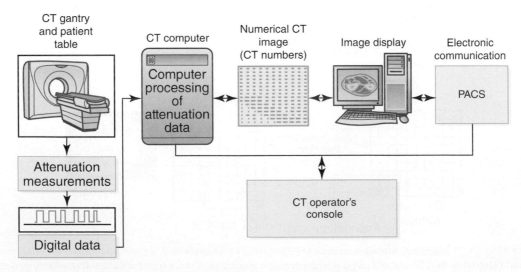

Figure 10-3 The flow of data in a CT scanner. See text for further explanation.

Reproduced from: Seeram, E. (2009) *Computed tomography: Physical principles, clinical applications and quality control.* Philadelphia, Saunders: Elsevier. Reproduced by permission.

There are a number of scanning parameters that are important in MSCT, including the *pitch ratio*, commonly referred to as the pitch (for short), and exposure technique factors including *automatic exposure control* (**AEC**), *slice thickness*, number of slices, and so forth, to be described later in the chapter. Only the pitch will be defined in this section.

The *pitch* (**P**) is defined as the distance the table travels per rotation (*d*) divided by the total collimation (*W*). The *total collimation*, on the other hand, is equal to the number of slices (*M*) times the collimated slice thickness (*S*). Algebraically, the pitch can now be expressed as:

$$P = d \div W \text{ or } P = d \div (M \times S)$$

MSCT uses pitch ratios higher than 1:1 (for example 2:1 and 3:1, etc.) to increase the volume coverage speed; however, increasing the pitch ratio tends to decrease image quality. For a more detailed description of MSCT, the student should refer to Seeram (2009).

CT Image Quality Characteristics: An Overview

There are several characteristics of the CT image that are of significance to the operator and observer for accurate diagnostic interpretation. These characteristics determine the quality of the CT image and include the spatial resolution, contrast resolution, and noise. All three of these are subsequently affected by the dose to the patient. For example, to reduce the noise in an image, the dose must be increased. Factors affecting the dose in CT will be described later in the chapter.

While *spatial resolution*—the ability of the CT scanner to faithfully reproduce the details in an object—depends on geometric factors (such as focal spot size, slice thickness, and pixel size), *contrast resolution* is the ability of the CT system (detector) to show small differences in tissue contrast. *Noise* in CT, on the other hand, is a variation in CT numbers from pixel to pixel in the CT image matrix. Contrast resolution and noise depend on both the

quality (beam energy) and quantity (number of x ray photons) of the x-ray beam. For CT operators, Bushong (2013) provides the following mathematical expression that shows the relationship between dose and image quality:

$$\text{Dose} = k \cdot \frac{\text{Intensity} \times \text{Beam Energy}}{\text{Noise}^2 \times \text{Pixel Size}^3 \times \text{Slice Thickness}}$$

where *k* is a conversion factor. This relationship will be explained later in this chapter.

Risks of CT: A Rationale for Dose Reduction and Optimization

The medical benefits of CT since its introduction in the 1970s are numerous. The technical advances in CT machine design and performance have resulted in a significant increase in its clinical use. However, several studies have shown that the radiation doses in CT are high (Brenner and Hall 2007; Van der Molen et al. 2013), and are "typically in the range of 5–50 mGy to each organ imaged" (Matthews et al. 2013). CT also contributes the highest radiation exposure compared with any other medical imaging modality (Hricak et al. 2011). Additionally, the high doses delivered to patients, particularly pediatric patients, have called attention to the risks of cancer associated with CT scanning (Van der Molen et al. 2013; Matthews et al. 2013; Amis 2011). The risks of radiation exposure fall into two categories: stochastic effects and deterministic effects. *Stochastic effects* are effects in which the probability of the effect occurring depends on the amount of radiation dose—that is, it increases as the dose increases, and there is no threshold dose, as any dose, no matter how small, has the potential to cause harm. Examples of stochastic effects include cancer, leukemia, and genetic effects that may be transmitted to offspring. Stochastic effects are viewed as the risks from exposure to low levels of radiation used in medical imaging, including computed tomography (CT) examinations. *Deterministic effects* are those effects for which the severity of the effect (rather than the probability) increases with increasing radiation dose, and for which there is a threshold dose. Examples of these effects include skin burns, hair loss, tissue damage, and organ dysfunction (Bushong 2013).

The above concerns of the risks have called attention to radiation protection of the patient based on the *as low as reasonably achievable (ALARA)* philosophy. The goal of radiation protection is to prevent deterministic effects by ensuring that doses are kept well below the relevant threshold dose and to minimize the probability of stochastic effects. To accomplish these goals, technologists must have a firm understanding of not only the factors affecting the dose in CT but also the basics of CT dose descriptors, and more important, how to reduce and optimize the dose to the patient without compromising the image quality needed to make a diagnosis.

CT Dose Descriptors

Understanding the nature of CT dose descriptors requires knowledge of several concepts. The first concept to address is the *beam geometry*, a fan-shaped x-ray beam and an array of detectors rotate 360? around the patient to collect attenuation data. The table moves during the scanning process and the x-ray tube traces a spiral or helical beam path around the patient.

As shown in **Figure 10-4**, the width of the x-ray beam is viewed from the side. The collimator near the x-ray source (the width is exaggerated for clarity) determines the beam width. In panel B, an ideal dose distribution along the z-axis is shown. It has a flat top and steep sides and is the same width as the x-ray beam. In panel C, a more realistic bell-shaped dose distribution curve is the distribution typical of most CT scanners.

As noted by Seeram (2009), the dose distribution is given by the function *D(z)* [panel C in the figure above], which describes an arbitrarily shaped dose intensity along the patient axis. In general, the shape of D(z) varies between CT scanners. *D(z) is extremely important to dose in CT, since it is this*

dose distribution that is being measured. To obtain this measurement, different types of phantoms are used (a small one simulates a patient's head and the larger phantom simulates a "body" or torso). An ionization chamber is placed in one of the holes in the phantom, a scan is taken, and a record the amount of charge emitted from the chamber is noted. The chamber can subsequently be moved to the other holes to allow the dose to be determined at different points within the phantom.

To describe the dose in CT, it is important to understand the second concept related to what has been referred to as CT dose descriptors. There are several dose descriptors, including the *volume computed tomography dose index (CTDI)*, the *dose length product (DLP)* and the *effective dose (E)*. Only the first two will be described briefly in this chapter; the effective dose is described at length elsewhere.

The CTDI

The first definition of the CTDI was one developed by the U.S. Food and Drug Administration (FDA) and was therefore labeled $CTDI_{FDA}$ (Boone 2007). This definition proved to be useful for essentially all shapes of dose distribution curves *D(z)* that are emitted by CT scanners. The CTDI therefore is a standardized measure of the radiation output from a CT scanner and is used to compare the radiation output for different CT scanners (McNitt-Gray 2002). With the $CTDI_{FDA}$, however, only 14 sections of 7-mm thickness could be measured, so another dose index, the $CTDI_{100}$, was developed to extend the length of the scan measurement to 100 mm.

The next major change in the CT dose descriptor was the introduction of the weighted CTDI ($CTDI_w$) to account for the average dose in the x-y axis of the patient instead of the z-axis. The $CTDI_w$ is expressed as follows:

$$CTDI_W = (1/3)\,(CTDI_{100})_{center} + (2/3)\,(CTDI_{100})_{periphery}$$

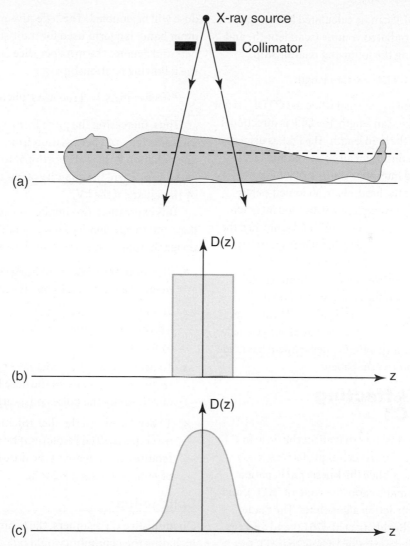

Figure 10-4 The width of the x-ray beam is determined by the collimator near the x-ray tube. An ideal dose distribution along the z-axis has a flat top and steep sides and is the same width as the x-ray beam. A more realistic bell-shaped dose distribution curve, as illustrated here, is typical of most computed tomography (CT) scanners

(From Seeram, E. (2009) *Computed tomography: Physical principles, clinical applications and quality control.* Philadelphia, Saunders: Elsevier. Reproduced by permission)

In order to consider the dose in the z-axis, yet another dose descriptor was developed. This is the $CTDI_{vol}$, which can be calculated using the following relationship for spiral//helical CT imaging:

$$CTDI_{VOL} = CTDI_{W} / PITCH$$

For a pitch of 1, the $CTDI_{vol}$ is equal to the $CTDI_{w}$.

The Dose Length Product

The dose length product (DLP) is yet another dose descriptor used in CT dose studies and reported in the literature and on CT scanners. While the $CTDI_{vol}$ provides a measurement of the exposure per slice of tissue, the DLP provides a measurement of the total amount of exposure for a series of scans. The DLP can be calculated knowing the length of the irradiated volume (scan length) and the CTDI_{vol} using the following relationship:

$$DLP = CTDI_{vol} \times \text{scan length}$$

It is important to note that while the CTDI_{vol} is not dependent on the scan length, the DLP is directional proportional to the scan length. The DLP is displayed on the scanner console for all operators and radiologists to view and interpret. The unit of DLP is mGy-cm. The DLP for the head, chest, abdomen-pelvis examinations, for example, are 930–1300 mGy-cm, 580–650 mGy-cm, and 560–1100 mGy-cm when the CTDI_{w} values are 60, 30, and 36 mGy respectively (Health Canada 2008). These DLP values can be compare those displayed on the CT scanner after the examinations. If the DLP displayed on the CT console is 240 mGy-cm, it is clearly well below the 580–650 mGy-cm value provided by Health Canada. This simply means that the CT department has made every effort to protect the patient.

Factors Affecting Dose in CT

There are several factors that affect the dose in CT, including the exposure technique factors, x-ray beam collimation, slice thickness, pitch, patient centering, automatic exposure control (AEC), and iterative reconstruction algorithms. The reader should refer to Bushberg et al. (2012) and Seeram (2009) for a full description of how these factors affect the dose to the patient.

Exposure Technique Factors: mAs and kVp

Recall the mathematical expression

$$Dose = k \cdot \frac{Intensity \times Beam\,Energy}{Noise^2 \times Pixel\,Size^3 \times Slice\,Thickness}$$

The *intensity* refers to the mAs, the beam energy refers to the kVp, and the noise depends on the mAs and kVp. The dose is directly proportional to the mAs, and therefore if the mAs is doubled, the

dose will be doubled. The "effective mAs," on the other hand, is a term used for multislice CT scanners and denotes the mAs per slice. This is given by the following relationship:

$$Effective\;mAs = True\;mAs/pitch$$

Thus, increasing the pitch from, say, 1 to 2 increases the mAs per rotation from 100 to 200. The radiation dose is proportional to the square of the kVp, where the quantity of photons increases by the square of the kVp.

This expression also implies the following about dose and image quality factors such as the noise, image sharpness (pixel size) and the slice thickness:

1. To reduce the noise in an image by a factor of 2, requires an increase in the dose by a factor of 4.
2. To improve the spatial resolution (pixel size) by a factor of 2, requires an increase in the dose by a factor of 8.
3. To decrease the slice thickness by a factor of 2 requires an increase in the dose by a factor of 2 (keeping the noise constant).
4. To decrease both the slice thickness and the pixel size (spatial resolution) by a factor of 2 requires an increase in the dose by a factor of 16 ($2^3 \times 2 = 2 \times 2 \times 2 \times 2$).

Collimation

On multislice CT scanners, the beam width including the penumbra would fall upon a finite set of detectors depending on the scanner, but the penumbra would not be used to produce the image (because the intensity of the beam at the penumbra regions is less than the intensity at the center of the beam). To address this problem, the beam width (collimation) is increased so that the penumbra extends beyond the active detectors that will receive the central beam intensity.

Pitch

The relationship between the absorbed dose and pitch is as follows:

$$Dose \propto 1\,/\,pitch$$

Patient Centering

Another factor affecting the dose to the patient that is under the control of the technologist is that of patient centering. The patient must be centered in the gantry isocenter for accurate imaging of the anatomy. Inaccurate patient centering (miscentering) degrades the image quality and increases the dose to the patient, especially with the use of automatic exposure control (AEC) in CT (Toth et al. 2007).

Automatic Tube Current Modulation

AEC is now commonplace on CT scanners. AEC uses a technique referred to as *automatic tube current modulation (ATCM)* to optimize the dose to the patient while maintaining constant image quality regardless of the size of the patient in the z-axis, and the attenuation changes in the x-y axis (Toth et al. 2007).

In CT, ATCM refers to the automatic control of the mA in two directions of the patient (the x-y axis and the z-axis) during data acquisition (scanning process) using specific technical procedures that take into consideration not only the patient size but also the attenuation differences of the various tissues. The overall goal of ATCM is to provide consistent image quality despite the size of the patient and the tissue attenuation differences, and to control the dose to the patient (Toth et al. 2007) compared with manual mA selection techniques. For a further description of this technique, the student should refer to Seeram (2009).

While the automatic control of the tube current (mA) in the x-y axis (in-plane) is referred to as angular modulation, changing the tube current automatically in the z-axis (through-plane) is referred to as z-axis modulation or longitudinal modulation. The use of angular-longitudinal modulation can reduce the dose by as much as 52% compared to using only the angular modulation technique (Goodman and Brink 2006).

Iterative Image Reconstruction

As noted earlier, the goal of image reconstruction in CT is to create an image of the x-ray

attenuation measurements through the patient. One popular algorithm, the FBP algorithm, became the workhorse of CT image reconstruction. Two of the major problems with the FBP algorithm, however, are noise (Beister et al. 2012) and streak artifacts (Maldjian and Goldman 2013). The primary advantages of iterative image reconstruction algorithms are to reduce image noise inherent in the FBP algorithm and radiation dose reduction (Fleischmann and Boas 2011; McCollough 2012). Currently, all major CT manufacturers offer iterative reconstruction algorithms (Beister et al. 2012). Examples of these algorithms include:

- Adaptive Iterative Dose Reduction (AIDR – Toshiba Medical Systems)
- Adaptive Statistical Iterative Reconstruction (ASIR – GE Healthcare)
- Image Reconstruction in Image Space (IRIS – Siemens Healthcare)
- Iterative Model Reconstruction (Philips Healthcare)
- Model-Based Iterative Reconstruction (MBIR – GE Healthcare)
- Sinogram-Affirmed Iterative Reconstruction (SAFIRE – Siemens Healthcare)

This chapter will not describe the details of these CT iterative image reconstruction algorithms, but the interested reader may refer to Bushberg et al. 2012, for an excellent description of the basis for these algorithms.

A number of studies have demonstrated reductions in radiation dose using iterative reconstruction that vary from 30% to 50% (Maldjian and Goldman 2013; Kaza et al. 2014). For example, Verona et al. 2011) have shown a reduction in pediatric dose by 33% using ASIR algorithm. Furthermore, Coakley et al. (2011) and McCollough et al. (2009) showed that for CT abdominal examinations, dose reductions of approximately 65% can be achieved using ASIR and IRIS.

Dose-Image Quality Optimization Research in CT

Radiation dose-image quality optimization involves the determination of the lowest dose levels to be used in a CT examination that would not compromise the diagnostic quality of the image. These studies are based on the scientific method, which includes the following steps in the investigation of the problem: statement of the problem, literature review, design of the methodology to find a solution to the problem, data collection, analysis and interpretation of the data, and finally, dissemination of the findings of the research study (Cresswell 2008).

To determine optimal image quality, McCollough et al. (2012) stress that "… both quantitative metrics (e.g., noise) and observer performance are involved. A simplified approach to achieving the optimal image quality is to require a specific noise level for a specific diagnostic task." Of course, the noise level is influenced by the radiation dose.

An Example of CT Dose Optimization Study

There have been several studies published in the literature using the dose-image quality optimization paradigm in CT; however, it is not within the scope of this chapter to examine all of them. Only one example will be given here in brief, and this is a study by conducted by Christie et al. (2013) using iterative reconstruction. The goal of this study was to compare the images obtained with FBP algorithm with those obtained using an iterative reconstruction (IR) algorithm, and a new CT detector (Stellar® detector). Images were obtained at different exposure settings and reconstructed using both the FBP algorithm and the iterative algorithm and the new detector. DLPs were recorded and all images evaluated subjectively by radiologists. The data was also subjected to statistical analysis. Christie et al. (2013) concluded that the results "showed that an average dose reduction between 27% and 70% for the new Stellar® detector, which is equivalent to using IR instead of FBP."

SUMMARY OF KEY CONCEPTS

1. This chapter addressed the basic physical principles and the factors affecting the dose in CT.

2. Godfrey Hounsfield (in England) and Allan Cormack, a physicist at Tufts University in Massachusetts, shared the 1979 Nobel Prize in Medicine and Physiology for significant work in making the CT scanner a clinically useful tool in medicine.

3. There are three major components in the production of a CT image: data acquisition, image reconstruction, and image display, storage, and communication. While *data acquisition* refers to the systematic collection of x-ray attenuation data from the patient, using an array of special electronic detectors, coupled to the x-ray tube, *image reconstruction* uses special reconstruction algorithms to systematically build up the image using a large number of attenuation measurements obtained at different locations (rotation angles) around the slice to be imaged. These attenuation measurements are used to calculate CT numbers.

4. These CT numbers are computed using the following relationship:

   $$CT\,Number = \frac{\mu_{tissue} - \mu_{water}}{\mu_{water}} \cdot K$$

   where K is a manufacturer's scaling factor or contrast factor; in general, $K = 1000$.

5. Today, all CT scanners are multislice CT scanners (MSCT), in which case the detector system is a two-dimensional detector array consisting of varying rows, compare to a single-slice CT (SSCT) scanner which has a one-dimensional detector array, and produces one slice per rotation of the x-ray tube and detectors around the patient. An MSCT detector with 4-rows will collect four slices per revolution. One with 16 rows or 64 rows will collect 16 or 64 slices per revolution of the x-ray tube, respectively.

6. The *pitch* (P) is defined as the distance the table travels per rotation (d)/total collimation (W). The total collimation is equal to the number of slices (M) times the collimated slice thickness (S). Algebraically, the pitch can now be expressed as:

$$P = d \div W \text{ or } P = d \div (M \times S)$$

7. The quality of the CT image is determined by the spatial resolution, contrast resolution, and noise. All three of these are subsequently affected by the dose to the patient.

8. *Spatial resolution* is the ability of the CT scanner to faithfully reproduce the details in an object depends on geometric factors (such as focal spot size, slice thickness, and pixel size, for example). *Contrast resolution* is the ability of the CT system (detector) to show small differences in tissue contrast. *Noise* in CT is a variation in CT numbers from pixel to pixel in the CT image matrix.

9. The relationship between dose and image quality is given by the relationship:

$$Dose = k \cdot \frac{\text{Intensity} \times \text{BeamEnergy}}{\text{Noise}^2 \times \text{PixelSize}^3 \times \text{SliceThickness}}$$

where *k* is a conversion factor.

10. The dose descriptors *volume computed tomography dose index* (CTDI$_{vol}$) and the *dose length product* (DLP) are described briefly.

11. The CTDI$_{vol}$ can be calculated using the following relationship for spiral/helical CT imaging:

$$CTDI_{vol} = CTDI_w/Pitch$$

12. The DLP can be calculated knowing the length of the irradiated volume (scan length) and the CTDI$_{vol}$ using the following relationship:

$$DLP = CTDI_{vol} \times \text{scan length}$$

13. Several factors affect the dose in CT, including exposure technique factors, x-ray beam collimation, slice thickness, pitch, patient centering, automatic exposure control (AEC), and iterative reconstruction algorithms.

14. The following relationships between dose and image quality factors such as the noise, image sharpness (pixel size) and the slice thickness can be stated:
   - To reduce the noise in an image by a factor of 2, requires an increase in the dose by a factor of 4
   - To improve the spatial resolution (pixel size) by a factor of 2, requires an increase in the dose by a factor of 8
   - To decrease the slice thickness by a factor of 2, requires an increase in the dose by a factor of 2 (keeping the noise constant)
   - To decrease both the slice thickness and the pixel size (spatial resolution) by a factory of 2 requires an increase in the dose by a factor of 16 ($2^3 \times 2 = 2 \times 2 \times 2 \times 2$)

15. Dose is inversely proportional to pitch.

16. ATCM provides consistent image quality despite the size of the patient and the tissue attenuation differences, and to control the dose to the patient via automatic control of the tube current (mA) in the x-y axis (in-plane) referred to as angular modulation, and changing the tube current automatically in the z-axis (through-plane) referred to as z-axis modulation or longitudinal modulation.

17. Dose-image quality optimization involves the determination of the lowest dose levels to be used in a CT examination that would not compromise the diagnostic quality of the image.

210 CHAPTER 10 Radiation Dose in Computed Tomography

Discussion Questions

1. Describe the three major equipment components of a CT scanner.

2. Discuss the basics physics of attenuation and explain what are CT numbers and how they are obtained.

3. Discuss five technical factors affecting dose in CT.

References

Amis Jr. ES. CT radiation dose: Trending in the right direction. *Radiology*. 2011;261(1):5–8.

Beister M, Kolditz D, Kalender, WA. Iterative reconstruction methods in x-ray CT. *Physica Medica*. 2012;28:94–108.

Boone, JM. The trouble with the $CTDI_{100}$. *MediPhysics*. 2007;34:1364–1371.

Bushong S. *Radiologic Science for Technologists* (10th Ed.). Philadelphia: Mosby-Elsevier; 2013.

Brenner DJ, Hall EJ. Computed tomography: An increasing source of radiation exposure. *N Engl J Med*. 2007;357:2277–2284.

Christie A, Heverhagen J, Ozdoba C, Weisstanner C, Ulzheimer S, Ebner L. CT dose and image quality in the last three scanner generations. *World J Radiol*. 2013;5(11):421–429.

Coakley FV, Gould R, Yeh BM, Arenson RL. CT radiation dose: What can you do right now in your practice? *Am J Roentgenol*. 2011;196:619–625.

Cressell JW. *Educational Research: Planning, Conducting, and Evaluating Quantitative and Qualitative Research*. Upper Saddle River, NJ: Pearson; 2008.

Fleischmann D, Boas FE. Computed tomography: Old ideas and new technology. *Eur Radiol*. 2011;21:510–517.

Goodman TR, Brink JA. Adult CT: Controlling dose and image quality. In *Categorical Course in Diagnostic Radiology Physics: From Invisible to Visible—The Science and Practice of X-ray Imaging and Radiation Dose Optimization*. Chicago: Radiological Society of North America; 2006: 157–165.

Hricak, H, Brenner DJ, Adelstein SJ, Frush DP, et al. Managing radiation use in medical imaging: A multifaceted challenge. *Radiology*. 2011;258(3):889–905.

Kaza RK, Platt JF, Goodsitt MM, Al-Hawary MM, Maturen KE, et al. Emerging techniques for dose optimization in abdominal CT. *Radiographics*. 2014;34:4–17.

Maldjian PD, Goldman AR. Reducing radiation dose in body CT: Primer on dose metrics and key CT technical parameters. *Am J Roentgenol*. 2013;200:741–747.

Matthews JD, Forsythe AV, Brady Z, Butler MW, Goergen S, Byrnes GB, et al. Cancer risk in 680,000 people exposed to computed tomography scans in childhood or adolescence: Data linkage study of 11 million Australians. *Br Med J*. 2013;346:1–18.

McCollough CH, Chen GH, Kalender W, Leng S, Samei E, Taquchi K, et al. Achieving routine submillisievert CT scanning. *Radiology*. 2012;264(2):567–580.

McCollough CH, Primak AN, Braun N, Kofler J, Yu L, Christner J. Strategies for reducing radiation dose in CT. *Radiol Clin North Am*. 2009;47:27–40.

McNitt-Gray MF. Radiation dose in CT. *Radiographics*. 2002;22:1541–1553.

Seeram E. *Computed Tomography: Physical Principles, Clinical Applications and Quality Control*. Philadelphia: Saunders Elsevier; 2009.

Toth T, Ge Z, Daly MP. The influence of patient centering on CT dose and image noise. *Med Phys*. 2007;34:3091–3101.

Van der Molen AJ, Stoop P, Prokop M, Geleijns J. A national survey on radiation dose in CT in The Netherlands. *Insights Imaging*. 2013; 4:383–390.

Verona GA, Ceschiu RC, Clayton BL, Sutcavage T, Tadross SS, Panigrahy A. Reducing abdominal CT radiation dose with the adaptive statistical iterative reconstruction technique in children. *Pediatr Radiol*. 2011;41:1174–1182.

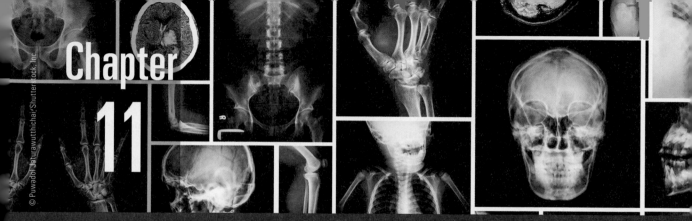

Chapter 11

Image Quality Assessment Tools for Dose Optimization in Digital Radiography

Outline

- Introduction
- Radiation Dose Quantities
- Image Quality in Digital Radiography
  - What is image quality?
  - Assessment of image quality
- Visual Grading of Normal Anatomy
  - Visual grading analysis
  - Dose optimization research
  - Example of a dose optimization study in computed radiography
- References

Objectives

On completion of this chapter, you should be able to:

1. State the International Commission on Radiological Protection (ICRP) principle of optimization.
2. Explain what is meant by the *as low as reasonably achievable* (ALARA) philosophy.
3. State the meaning of the term "image quality."
4. Define each of the following:
   - Spatial resolution
   - Contrast resolution
   - Noise
   - Detective quantum efficiency

5. Discuss the assessment of image quality in terms of objective physical measures and subjective observer performance methods.
6. Explain briefly the nature of visual grading of normal anatomy using the visual grading analysis (VGA) method.
7. State the fundamental elements of dose optimization research.

Introduction

A common theme emphasized in this text is the International Commission on Radiological Protection (ICRP) framework for radiation protection, which includes three fundamental principles: *justification*, *optimization*, and *dose limitation*. The principle of dose optimization is where the technologist may play an important and significant role in radiation protection of patients. In review, this principle states that doses delivered to patients during the imaging examination should always be kept *as low as reasonably achievable (ALARA)*. Technologists and radiologists must always work within this ALARA philosophy.

The ICRP also defines two general categories of optimization, and these include the equipment design and function category, and the techniques used during routine daily practice (Matthews and Brennan 2009). For optimization using the equipment design and function category, the notion of *quality assurance (QA)* and *quality control (QC)* are important considerations, among others. The category of techniques used in routine daily practice includes a wide range of factors affecting patient dose, and this should be an important consideration of optimization of radiation protection in diagnostic radiology.

The ALARA philosophy dictates that doses be kept as low as reasonably achievable without compromising the quality of the image needed to make a diagnosis. Therefore, in order to actively participate in dose optimization practice and research, it is essential that technologists have a firm understanding of not only the factors affecting dose to the patient, but also image quality factors. Furthermore, optimization research in medical imaging involves various methodologies to demonstrate dose reduction without the loss of image quality.

The purpose of this chapter is to present an overview of image quality assessment tools for radiation dose optimization in digital radiography. Specifically, the focus will be image quality descriptors for digital radiography, and the methods of image quality assessment, including objective physical measures and observer performance methods. Of the observer performance methods, the visual grading analysis (VGA) of normal anatomy will be highlighted. The chapter will conclude with a suggested objective approach to carrying out a dose-image quality optimization study.

Radiation Dose Quantities

There are three radiation exposure and dose quantities and their associated units that are important here. These include radiation exposure, absorbed dose, and effective dose.

Radiation exposure refers to radiation travelling through air, and represents the amount of ionization-induced charge produced in a unit mass of air at a particular part of the x-ray or gamma beam. The Système International (SI) unit of exposure is the coulomb per kilogram (C/kg or Ckg^{-1}); an older unit, less commonly used now, is the roentgen (R). *Radiation absorbed dose* refers to radiation travelling though a medium. It is the amount of energy absorbed within an object, such as a person. The SI unit of absorbed dose is the gray (Gy), and the older unit is the rad. The third radiation quantity that is of importance in this text is the *effective dose*, which is a quantity relating exposure to risk of injury. The SI unit of effective dose is the sievert (Sv) and the old unit is the rem. In diagnostic radiology, much smaller units such as millicoulombs mC/kg (0.001 C/kg), mGy (0.001 Gy), and mSv (0.001 Sv) are commonplace.

Image Quality in Digital Radiography

The technical factors affecting dose in digital radiography were described in detail elsewhere, but it is important to note that one of the problems in digital radiography is that of ***dose creep***, that is, "the risk of increasing patient dose, possibly without being aware of it ... or an increase in exposure over time when using digital systems with manual tube settings" (Uffmann and Schaefer-Prokop 2009). For technologists using digital radiography systems, this is a significant problem, and therefore a clear understanding of the dose-image quality relationship is important. Since dose and image quality go hand-in-hand with optimization of radiation protection, it is important to first understand what is meant by the term ***image quality*** and the parameters used to describe image quality. Furthermore, it is worthwhile to consider how image quality can be assessed when conducting studies in dose-image quality optimization of the digital radiography system.

What is Image Quality?

In their description of *image quality*, Bushberg et al. (2012) clearly state that:

> *The image quality on a medical image is related not to how pretty it looks but rather to how well it conveys anatomical or functional information to the interpreting physician such that an accurate diagnosis can be made. Indeed, radiological images acquired ionizing radiation can almost always be made much prettier simply by turning up the radiation levels used, but the radiation dose to the patient then becomes an important concern. Diagnostic medical images therefore require a number of important tradeoffs in which image quality is not necessarily **maximized** but rather is **optimized** to perform the specific diagnostic task for which the exam was ordered.*

Image quality includes four gold standards by which images are assessed. These include what

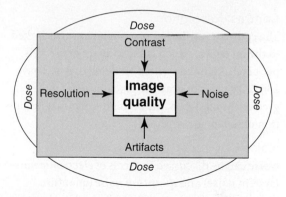

Figure 11-1 The image quality quartet includes the characteristics of resolution, contrast, noise, and artifacts, all influenced by the radiation dose.

Reproduced from Wolbarst et al. *Medical Imaging: Essentials for Physicians.* 2013. Hoboken, NJ, Wiley-Blackwell. Reproduced by permission.

Wolbarst et al. (2013) refer to as the ***image quality quartet*** shown in **Figure 11-1**. The image quality parameters include resolution, contrast, noise, and artifacts. Furthermore, these factors are influenced by the dose used in the examination.

The image quality descriptors for a digital image include spatial resolution (detail), contrast resolution, noise, quantum detective efficiency (DQE), and artifacts (Seibert 2006; Rowlands 2002). Four of these five, namely spatial resolution, contrast resolution, noise, and the detective quantum efficiency (DQE), will be described briefly.

Spatial Resolution

The ***spatial resolution*** of a digital image is related to the size of the pixels in the image matrix. The smaller the pixel size is, the better the spatial resolution of the image will be. The pixel size (PS) is equal to the field of view (FOV)/matrix size. Thus, for the same FOV, the greater the matrix size is, the smaller the pixels will be, and the better the image sharpness is as well.

Contrast Resolution

The *contrast resolution* of a digital image is linked to the bit depth, which is the range of gray levels per pixel. An image with a bit depth of 8 will have 256 (2^8) shades of gray per pixel. In general the greater the bit depth, the better the contrast resolution of the image.

Noise

Noise can be discussed in terms of *electronic noise* (system noise) and *quantum noise* (quantum mottle). The quantum noise is determined by the number of x-ray photons (often referred to as the signal, S) falling upon the detector to create the image. While low-exposure technique factors (kVp and mAs) will produce few photons at the detector (less signal and more noise, N), higher-exposure technique factors will generate more photons at the detector (more signal and less noise). The former will result in a noisy or "grainy" image that is generally poor quality, and the latter will produce a better image at the expense of increased dose to the patient. The noise increases as the detector exposure decreases.

Detective Quantum Efficiency (DQE)

The final descriptor of digital image quality is the *detective quantum efficiency*, or DQE. The DQE refers to the notion that detector converts the input exposure (incident quanta) into a useful output image. The DQE is a measure of the efficiency and fidelity with which the detector can perform this task. Note that the DQE also takes into consideration not only the *signal-to-noise ratio (SNR)* but also the system noise, and therefore includes a measure of the amount of noise added.

The DQE for a perfect digital detector is 1, or 100%. This means that there is no loss of information. The DQE indicates the detector performance in terms of output image quality and input radiation exposure used.

Assessment of Image Quality

Image quality assessment is often a difficult process and includes the notion of quantitative *objective physical measures* as well as *subjective observer performance* when evaluating images in a clinical environment (Båth 2010).

There are a number of methods for evaluating image quality in diagnostic imaging depending on the level of ambition and the investigation technique used. For example, if the level of ambition is low, the investigation technique may involve the use of radiographic exposure technique, then the measurement procedure used may focus on equipment characteristics and exposure parameters (Tapiovaara 2008). If the level of ambition is high, however, the investigation technique may involve the use of images of patients, and the measurement procedure used will focus more sophisticated methods such as receiver operating characteristics (ROC) analysis or ROC-related methods, and visual grading analysis (VGA) as well as image criteria (IC) analysis (Tapiovaara 2008). In between low and high, other techniques may be used; for example, if primary physical characteristics are of interest or overall system performance is investigated, then the measurement procedure will be focused on contrast, spatial resolution, noise, and signal-to-noise ratio (SNR); and DQE, image quality index (IQ), and contrast-detail resolution, respectively (Tapiovaara 2008).

There are two general categories of image quality assessment, namely, objective physical measures and observer performance methods.

Objective Physical Measures

Objective physical measures include those that characterize the primary physical characteristics of the digital imaging system and the overall performance of the imaging system. These characteristics and performance measures include the Modulation

Transfer Function (MTF), the SNR, the Wiener Spectrum (WS, also known as the Noise Power Spectrum [NPS]), and the DQE. It is not within the scope of this chapter to describe details of how the MTF, SNR, WS, and DQE are obtained. The interested student should refer to Bushberg et al. (2012) for a detailed discussion of each of these physical parameters.

While these objective physical measures are essential and useful tools in describing the performance of the imaging system in terms of image quality, Tapiovaara (2008) emphasizes that in examining the acceptability of clinical images, subjective evaluation may be useful. The human observers in diagnostic radiology who play an important role in examining the acceptability of the clinical image are the technologist, whose primary role is to assess the visibility of anatomical structures, and the radiologist, whose primary role is image interpretation. The viewing task in this situation is lesion identification (Smedby and Fredrikson 2010; Bushberg et al. 2012)

Observer Performance Methods

Observer performance methods fall into two categories, depending on the nature of the primary viewing task. If the task of the observer is lesion detection in the image, then the method used would be *the receiver operating characteristics (ROC) analysis*. If the viewing task is the visualization of anatomical structures, then the method used would be *visual grading analysis* (VGA) (Båth 2010; Tapiovaara 2008; Smedby and Fredrikson 2010).

This chapter will concentrate on elements relating to the assessment of the visibility of anatomical structures in an image, and therefore the ROC paradigm will not be reviewed here in any detail; however, the following comment by Tingberg et al. (2005) is noteworthy:

The most widely used is the …. ROC method. The task for the observers in an ROC study is to decide whether a given image contains a pathological structure or not. A grading is given according to a scale (a five-level scale is frequently used) stating the decision of the observer and also the level of confidence of his or her decision.

For more details on the ROC, the interested reader should refer to Chakraborty (2005), and Thompson et al. (2013).

Visual Grading of Normal Anatomy

Visual grading of normal anatomy is a well-established, valid, popular, and simple method of subjectively assessing image quality based on the visibility and reproduction of anatomical structures.

Visual Grading Analysis

The visual grading analysis (VGA) is described briefly by Tingberg et al. (2005) as follows:

In … VGA, the quality of an image or a particular part of an image is compared with a reference image and a grading is given depending on whether the quality of the image is better or worse than the reference image … An advantage of these methods is that contrary to the ROC-related methods, it is the normal anatomy present in almost every patient image which is used for the evaluation of image quality … the use of the VGA is motivated by the assumption that the level of visibility of anatomical and pathological structures are connected, so that if the visibility of normal anatomy is increased, for example by the use of a different diagnostic technique, then the visibility of pathological structures is also increased.

For more details of the VGA, the interested reader should refer to Tingberg et al. (2005).

To avoid any bias due to the subjectivity involved in using the VGA method, formal criteria known as the *European Guidelines on Quality Criteria for Diagnostic Radiographic Images* are used with the VGA analysis of images (Geijer and Persliden 2005). These guidelines were published by the Commission of European Communities (CEC) in 1996 for all diagnostic radiographic images. For every examination, the criteria are organized around diagnostic requirements, criteria for radiation dose to the patient, and examples of good radiographic technique. Specifically, diagnostic requirements relate to the image criteria, which define the degree of visibility of certain anatomical structures. The European guidelines (CEC 1996) define the visual grading of anatomical structures, using four terms: *visualization*, *reproduction*, *visually sharp reproduction*, and *important image details*. While *visualization* means that characteristic features are detectable but details are not fully reproduced, e.g., features are just visible, *reproduction* means that details of anatomical structures are visible, but not necessarily clearly defined; that is, detail is emerging. The term *visually sharp reproduction* means that anatomical details are clearly defined and details are clear. Finally, the term *important image details* define the minimum and limiting dimensions in the image at which specific or abnormal anatomical details should be recognized (CEC 1996). Furthermore, the CEC guidelines recommend the absorbed dose in air (entrance surface dose) for each examination. For example, the CEC recommends an absorbed dose of 10 mGy for the AP pelvis and the AP lumbar spine.

Methods of Visual Grading

Two common methods of visual grading of the visibility of anatomical structures include *image criteria (IC) scoring* and VGA. The IC scoring method requires the observer to assess the image and decide if the image criteria have been met or not met; subsequently, an IC score is obtained. The other approach to grading the visibility of anatomical structures is to use a multi-step scale. This is the basis of the VGA method, and it adds a little more accuracy to the image quality assessment.

VGA used in conjunction with the European quality criteria has become an established tool with high validity in optimization studies in digital radiography (Båth 2010). The VGA approach requires the observer to assess image quality based on his/her opinion about the visualization and reproduction of defined anatomical structures using an absolute or a relative rating scale. In the absolute approach, the observer rates (or scores) his/her opinion about the visibility of the anatomical structures using a scale consisting of at least four steps from 1 to 4—e.g., the structure in the image is: 1 – not visible; 2 – poorly reproduced; 3 – adequately reproduced; or 4 – very well reproduced. In the relative approach, the observer grades (rates) the visibility of each defined anatomical structure using a scale consisting of at least five steps from –2 to +2—e.g., the reproduction of the structure in the image is –2 = much worse than; –1 = worse than; 0 = the same as; +1 = better than; or +2 = much better than the reproduction of the corresponding structure in the reference image. Finally, absolute and relative scores are obtained using specific formulae, as described by Tingberg (2000) and Geijer and Persliden (2005).

Dose Optimization Research

Several examples of optimization research during daily operation of the digital imaging system have been described by Matthews and Brennan (2009) and more recently by Seeram et al. (2013) specifically for CR imaging. In 2005, a special issue of *Radiation Protection Dosimetry* was dedicated to optimization strategies in medical x-ray imaging for radiography, fluoroscopy (including digital radiography and fluoroscopy), mammography, and computed tomography (CT). The studies presented in this issue showed that there are important requirements for optimization research:

- Ensure that the dose to the patient is "safe";
- Determine the level of image quality required for a particular examination;
- Reduce the dose in such a manner so as not to compromise the image quality.

To meet the above fundamental requirements, specific approaches are needed to (1) determine the level of image quality—that is, the ability to differentiate between images that are normal and abnormal (Tingberg and Sjöström 2005), and (2) address the perceptions and evaluation of image quality using human observers, keeping in mind the nature of the detection task. In this regard, various observer performance tests, such as the ROC methodology and the VGA can be used. The task of lesion (pathology) detection would require a different observer performance test than, say, the task of detecting normal anatomical structures.

Example of a Dose Optimization Study in Computed Radiography

A dose optimization study was conducted by Seeram (2013) to investigate the optimization of the mAs and associated exposure indicator of a Fuji computed radiography (CR) imaging system as a radiation dose management strategy in the implementation of the ALARA principle.

The methodology involved (1) measuring the entrance skin dose (ESD) free-in-air to an anthropomorphic phantom model of the pelvis and lumbar spine, using the vendor's recommended exposure settings (kVp and mAs) and dose values above and below the vendor's values (reference dose) for each of the body parts; and (2) obtaining 54 images (27 for each of the AP pelvis and AP lumbar spine) using the dose values mentioned above, and recording the corresponding exposure indicators (EIs) of the Fuji CR system, which is referred to as a sensitivity ("S") value.

The ESD data set was used to examine the correlation between dose and mAs and between dose and EI. The images were assessed in a two-phase process: First, 7 expert observers evaluated image quality based on the appearance of image noise (quantum mottle) for the purpose of establishing an optimized mAs/EI value. Second, observers compared test images (images recorded with doses above and below the vendor's recommended values) with the reference images using the well-established VGA procedure. This procedure is based on the reproduction and visualization of defined anatomical structures.

The results of this study showed a strong, positive, linear relationship between (1) dose and mAs; (2) mAs and inverse EI; and (3) dose and inverse EI for both the AP pelvis and AP lumbar spine. The optimized mAs/EI procedure showed that compared to the reference mAs/EI of 25/86 for the AP pelvis and 50/88 for the AP lumbar spine, 16 mAs with an associated EI of 136 for the AP pelvis and 20 mAs and an associated EI of 220 for the AP lumbar spine were selected by all observers as optimized values. The VGA procedure showed that while the optimized 16 mAs/EI = 136 for the AP pelvis did not compromise image quality, the optimized 20 mAs/EI = 220 for the AP lumbar spine compromised image quality. Further analysis of the VGA scores (VGAS) showed that for the AP lumbar spine, it was deemed that 32 mAs/EI = 139 were optimized values where image quality was not compromised, compared to the vendor's recommended values. The selection of the optimized mAs of 16 and 32 for the AP pelvis and AP lumbar spine, respectively, resulted in a dose reduction of 36% compared to the vendor's recommended mAs (dose) values, without compromising image quality.

The conclusions drawn from this research are that (1) the mAs and its associated EIs can be used as radiation dose management strategy for implementing the ALARA (as low as reasonably achievable) philosophy in routine daily practice of CR imaging, and (2) the dose can be reduced by 36% for both body parts studied in this research, compared to the vendor's recommended exposure technique factors.

SUMMARY OF KEY CONCEPTS

1. This chapter presented an overview of image quality assessment tools for radiation dose optimization in digital radiography, focussing on image quality descriptors for digital radiography, and the objective physical and observer performance methods for the assessment of image.

2. Image quality descriptors for a digital image include spatial resolution (detail), contrast resolution, noise, detective quantum efficiency (DQE), and artifacts.

3. While spatial resolution relates to the size of the pixels in the image matrix (the smaller the pixel size the better the spatial resolution of the image), contrast resolution is linked to the bit depth, (the range of gray levels per pixel.). An image with a bit depth of 8 will have 256 (2^8) shades of gray per pixel. In general, the greater the bit depth, the better the contrast resolution of the image.

4. Quantum noise is determined by the number of x-ray photons falling upon the detector to create the image.

5. The DQE is a measure of the efficiency and fidelity with which the detector can perform this task.

6. Image quality can be assessed using quantitative *objective physical measures* as well as *subjective observer performance*.

7. Objective physical measures characterize the primary physical characteristics of the digital imaging system, and the overall performance of the imaging system. These characteristics and performance measures include the Modulation Transfer Function (MTF), the Signal-to-Noise Ratio (SNR), the Wiener Spectrum (WS), also known as the Noise Power Spectrum (NPS), and the DQE.

8. In subjective evaluation, human observers play an important role in examining the acceptability of the clinical image. These include the technologist, whose primary role is to assess the visibility of anatomical structures, and the radiologist, whose primary role is image interpretation.

9. Observer performance methods fall into two categories depending on the nature of the primary viewing task. If the task of the observer is lesion detection in the image, then method used would be the Receiver Operating Characteristics (ROC) analysis. If the viewing task the visualization of anatomical structures then the method used would be Visual Grading Analysis (VGA) analysis.

10. As described by Tingberg (2005), "In .... VGA, the quality of an image or a particular part of an image is compared with a reference image and a grading is given depending on whether the quality of the image is better or worse than the reference image." The VGA approach requires the observer to assess image quality based on his/her opinion about the visualization and reproduction of defined anatomical structures using an absolute or a relative rating scale.

11. Optimization research entails at least procedures to ensure that the dose to the patient is "safe," to determine the level of image quality required for a particular examination, and reducing the dose in such a manner so as not to compromise the image quality.

Discussion Questions

1. Discuss the ICRP principle of optimization, and explain the acronym ALARA.

2. Explain the four descriptors of image quality.

3. Discuss the assessment of image quality in terms of objective physical measures and subjective observer performance methods.

4. Explain briefly the nature of visual grading of normal anatomy using the visual grading analysis (VGA) method.

References

Båth M. Evaluating imaging systems: Practical applications. *Radiat Prot Dosimetry.* 2010;139(1–3):26–36.

Bushberg J, Seibert AJ, Leidholdt M, Boone JM. *The Essential Physics of Medical Imaging.* (3rd Ed.) Philadelphia: Lippincott Williams & Wilkins; 2011.

Chakraborty DP. Recent advances in observer performance methodology: Jackknife free-response ROC (JAFROC). *Radiat Prot Dosimetry.* 2005;114(1–3):26–31.

Commission of the European Communities (CEC). *European guidelines on quality criteria for diagnostic radiographic images.* EUR 16260 EN. Brussels: CEC; 1996.

Geijer H, Persliden J. Varied tube potential with constant effective dose at lumbar spine radiography using a flat-panel digital detector. *Radiat Prot Dosimetry.* 2005;114(1–3):240–245.

Matthews K, Brennan PC. Optimisation of x-ray examinations: General principles and an Irish perspective. *Radiography.* 2009;15(3):262–268.

Rowlands JA. The physics of computed radiography. *Phys Med Biol.* 2002;47(23):R123–R126.

Seeram E. Optimization of the Exposure Index of a CR System as a Radiation Dose Management Strategy. PhD Dissertation, Medical Radiation Sciences, School of Health Sciences, Faculty of Science, Charles Sturt University, Australia; 2013.

Seibert JA. Computed radiography/digital radiography: Adult. In *Categorical Course in Diagnostic Radiology Physics: From Invisible to Visible—The Science and Practice of X-ray Imaging and Radiation Dose Optimization.* Chicago: Radiological Society of North America; 2006: 57–71.

Smedby O, Fredrikson M. Visual grading regression: Analysing data from visual grading experiments with regression models. *Br J Radiol.* 2010;83(993):767–775.

Tapiovaara MJ. Review of relationships between physical measurements and user evaluation of image quality *Radiat Prot Dosimetry.* 2008;129(1-3):244–248.

Thompson JD, Manning DJ, Hogg P. The value of observer performance studies in dose optimization: A focus on free-response receiver operating characteristic methods. *J Nucl Med Technol.* 2013;41:57–64.

Tingberg AM. Quantifying the quality of medical x-ray images: An evaluation based on normal anatomy for lumbar spine and chest radiography. *Doctoral dissertation.* Department of Radiation Physics. Lund University, Malmo; 2000.

Tingberg A, Båth M, Håkansson M, Medin J, Besjakov J, Sandborg M, et al. Evaluation of image quality of lumbar spine images: A comparison between FFE and VGA. In Mattsson S. Optimization strategies in medical imaging. *Radiat Prot Dosimetry.* 2005;114(1–3):53–61.

Tingberg A, Sjöström D. Optimisation of image plate radiography with respect to tube voltage. *Radiat Prot Dosimetry.* 2005;114(1–3):286–293.

Uffmann M, Schaefer-Prokop C. Digital radiography: The balance between image quality and required radiation dose. *Eur J Radiol.* 2007;72(2):202–208.

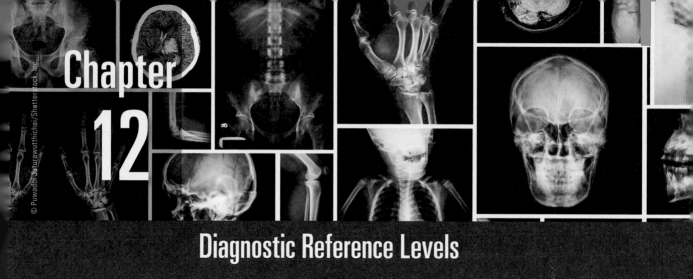

© Puwadol Jaturawutthichai/Shutterstock, Inc.

Chapter 12

Diagnostic Reference Levels

Outline

- Introduction
- Patient Dose Variations
  - Historical perspective
  - Patient dose variations today
- What Are Diagnostic Reference Levels?
  - DRLs: an overview
  - DRLs: a definition
  - What are diagnostic reference levels *not*?
- Why Is It Important to Implement DRLs?
  - Legal or regulatory requirement

- Societal benefits
- Improved awareness of radiation doses
- Have DRLs reduced doses?
- Establishment of Diagnostic Reference Levels
  - The survey to establish current dose levels
  - Calculation of DRL values
  - Pediatric DRL values
  - Diagnostic reference levels: a global activity
  - Practical considerations when gathering the data
- References

Objectives

On completion of this chapter, you should be able to:

1. Define the DRL and discuss its essential characteristics.
2. Discuss what DRLs are not.
3. State the most important reason to implement DRLs and identify other compelling arguments supporting DRL adoption.
4. Discuss whether the use of DRLs has resulted in dose reduction.

5. Identify and discuss the steps in establishing DRLs.
6. State examples of DRI values for pediatric imaging procedures.
7. Discuss the nature of global activities surrounding the use of DRLs.

Introduction

Each radiographer and radiologist is reminded of the *as low as reasonably achievable* (*ALARA*) principle every time a patient is exposed. It is accepted within diagnostic imaging circles that each x-ray diagnostic exposure carries with it a certain level of risk, with that risk being proportional to the amount of radiation. Therefore, the exposure should be kept as low as reasonably achievable, consistent with an image of acceptable diagnostic efficacy. This principle forms the basis of all radiation protection material contained within radiography, medical physics, and medical curricula.

Patient Dose Variations

Historical Perspective

It seems surprising that in many studies, large fluctuations in patient exposures are observed for the same type of examination, apparently depending on the source of the radiation. For example, in the early work of the UK-based National Radiological Protection Board, in partnership with the Institute of Physical Sciences in Medicine and the College of Radiographers, large variations in mean hospital entrance surface doses (ESD) can be seen for even an examination as common as a chest posteroanterior (PA) projections (NRPB 1992) (**Figure 12-1**).

When one looks at the maximum to minimum patient ESD ratio for the same examination type in that publication, this was over 40:1 (**Table 12-1**).

While the variations were less for other common investigations, there were still reasonably large discrepancies for abdomen, lumbar spine, pelvic, and skull examinations. Large variations have also been reported by the United Nations Scientific Committee on the Effects of Atomic Radiation (UNSCEAR) and by the authors of the US-based Nationwide Exposure X-ray Trends (NEXT) program of research.

Patient Dose Variations Today

It may be tempting to suggest that all these data were produced some time ago and that significant variations would not exist now, particularly with the introduction of digital technology; however, the latest publication on diagnostic x-ray exposures by the NRPB's successor in the UK, the Health Protection Agency, would suggest otherwise (HPA 2012). The data contained within this document demonstrated maximum to minimum mean room ESDs of 10:1 or greater for several examinations, with this ratio being greater than 50:1 for

Table 12-1 Patient entrance surface dose variations

Radiograph		Entrance surface dose (mGy)				
		Minimum	1st Quartile	Median	3rd Quartile	Maximum
Abdomen	AP	0.71	4.69	6.68	10.5	62.4
Chest	PA	0.03	0.13	0.18	0.26	1.43
	Lat	0.14	0.49	0.99	1.46	10.6
Lumbar spine	AP	0.03	5.85	7.88	11.2	59.1
	Lat	2.38	12.7	19.7	30.1	108
	LSJ	7.4	24	34.5	50.2	131
Pelvis	AP	0.85	4.19	5.67	7.46	31.6
Skull	AP	0.73	2.97	4.04	4.87	13.8
	PA	1.82	3.26	4.25	5.49	13.1
	Lat	0.36	1.42	2.19	2.85	9.09

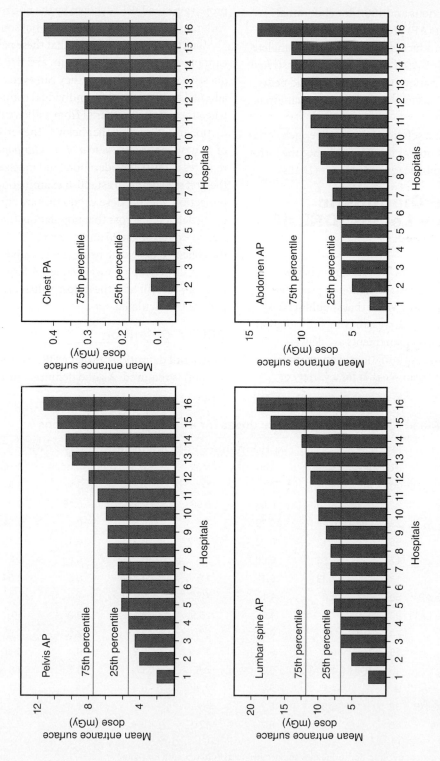

Figure 12-1 Distribution of entrance surface radiation doses are shown for four examination types across several Irish hospitals. The horizontal lines indicate 25th and 75th percentile values.

Courtesy of Patrick C. Brennan.

chest PA projections and 100:1 for abdominal anteroposterior (AP) projections (**Table 12-2**).

Dose area product measurements for complete examinations such as barium meals demonstrated even greater variations (**Table 12-3**), as did pediatric examinations for age-standardized children (**Table 12-4**).

The need for a solution to minimize such variations is as great now as it ever was; hence the introduction of diagnostic reference levels (DRLs).

What are Diagnostic Reference Levels (DRLs)?

DRLs: An Overview

A specific definition for DRLs is given below, but put simply, this is an examination or projection-specific radiation dose value that should serve as an upper level to which we can compare radiation levels that imaging departments are delivering for diagnostic examinations. For example, in Figure 12-1, we can see that for a variety of projections the DRL is shown by the horizontal line, with most centers below this value, but some above.

The challenge, however, is that these values cannot be plucked out of thin air, and it is even questionable as to whether they can even be adopted by or adapted for individual countries when the data are gathered from a different jurisdiction (discussed further below). The setting up of values that *are useful to a particular population* requires careful consideration (and much effort); the first step being to establish examination- or projection-specific dose values that are currently being delivered across that population; the second step to establish useful and relevant DRLs from the collected dose data using, for example, the 75th percentile of hospital mean values. A large focus of this chapter will how these dose values are sourced and DRLs calculated.

DRLs: A Definition

First, a full definition of what a DRL is (and what it is not) is required. A good definition of a DRL can

Table 12-2 Mean room entrance surface doses for a variety of examinations

Radiograph	Number		Room mean ESD distribution (Gy.cm²)				
	Hospitals	Mean	Min	Max	1st Quartile	Median	3rd Quartile
Abdomen AP	70	3.6	0.1	11	2.4	3.2	4.4
Chest AP	9	0.16	0.03	0.56	0.1	0.15	0.2
Chest LAT	23	0.48	0.22	1.26	0.3	0.4	0.54
Chest PA	95	0.12	0.02	1.1	0.1	0.11	0.15
Knee AP	17	0.26	0.09	0.9	0.17	0.24	0.3
Knee LAT	13	0.33	0.1	1.9	0.2	0.3	0.34
Lumbar spine AP	80	4.6	1.1	12.6	2.9	3.9	5.7
Lumbar spine LAT	80	7.9	1.5	26.9	5.3	6.9	10
Pelvis AP	84	3.2	0.8	8.3	2.2	2.8	3.9
Shoulder AP	15	0.4	0.1	1	0.3	0.4	0.46
Skull AP/PA	10	1.8	0.3	3.5	1.6	1.7	1.8
Skull LAT	9	1.1	0.7	2.3	0.9	1	1.1
Thoracic spine AP	38	2.9	0.7	16	1.7	2.4	3.3
Thoracic spine LAT	40	5.2	0.7	17	2.8	4.1	7.2

NRBP 2012 © Crown copyright. Reproduced with permission of Public Health England.

Table 12-3 Dose area product measurement for some completed examination

Examination	Number			Room mean DAP distribution (Gy.cm^2)					
	Hospitals	Rooms	Patients	Mean	Min	Max	1st Quartile	Median	3rd Quartile
Abdomen	14	42	8127	4.3	0.3	38	1.8	3.1	4.4
Barium Enema	73	152	20555	16	1.4	99	7.6	13	21
Barium Meal	38	74	1116	9	0.1	76	3.9	6.5	11.8
Barium Swallow	66	130	9710	7	1.1	167	3	4.7	7.5
Chest	11	35	11484	0.7	0.01	7.4	0.07	0.1	0.3
Coronary Angiography	53	140	36087	25	8	87	16	23	31
Fistulography	13	24	530	7	0.1	28	2.4	5	7.7
IVU	18	22	1531	11.5	1.5	26	7.4	12	14
Lumbar Spine	10	29	1745	5	0.6	35	2	3	6
Nephrostography	19	36	522	6	0.1	25	2.5	4	8.7
Sinography	15	25	124	4.3	0.6	12	1.2	2.7	7.2
T Tube Cholangiography	14	32	301	4	0.2	16	2.1	3.4	4.9

* Mean patient weight range 75-85 kg

NRBP 2012 © Crown copyright. Reproduced with permission of Public Health England.

Table 12-4 Pediatric dose area product measurements

Examination	Standard age (years)	Adjusted room DAP/examination (Gy.cm^2)				
		Minimum	1st Quartile	Median	3rd Quartile	Maximum
Barium meal (370 patients)	0	0.014	0.04	0.14	0.13	0.87
	1	0.06	0.1	0.32	0.21	1.94
	5	0.004	0.1	0.4	0.24	2.7
	10	0.03	0.13	0.54	0.65	1.8
	15	0.18	0.39	1.36	2	4
Barium swallow (190 patients)	0	0.009	0.03	0.27	0.21	1.5
	1	0.05	0.12	0.31	0.39	1.2
	5	0.08	0.19	0.88	0.46	12.8
	10	0.19	0.55	1.47	1.8	6.2
	15	0.19	0.45	2.79	3	17.4
MCU (1776 patients)	0	0.0005	0.02	0.19	0.12	3.95
	1	0.003	0.1	0.57	0.32	16.7
	5	0.016	0.1	0.65	0.34	10.1
	10	0.008	0.18	0.43	0.44	1.4
	15	0.003	0.11	1.69	0.89	13.2

NRPB 2012© Crown copyright. Reproduced with permission of Public Health England.

be found within the European Council's Directive 97/43/Euratom (1997), which is very similar to the DRL description given by the International Commission of Radiological Protection (ICRP). On page 2 of the EC document, it states that DRLs are:

> *Dose levels in medical radiodiagnostic practices or, in the case of radio-pharmaceuticals, levels of activity, for typical examinations for groups of standard-sized patients or standard phantoms for broadly defined types of equipment. These levels are expected not to be exceeded for standard procedures when good and normal practice regarding diagnostic and technical performance is applied.*

It is clear from this two-sentence definition that DRLs apply to all radiographic diagnostic procedures as well as nuclear medicine examinations. It is, however, a loaded definition: The first sentence contains *four* crucially important clauses, and each of these should be examined in turn. Here, we present the quote again, this time with the key phrases marked for consideration in sequence:

> *Dose levels in* [1] **medical radiodiagnostic practices** *or, in the case of radio-pharmaceuticals, levels of activity, for* [2] **typical examinations for** [3] **groups of standard-sized patients or standard phantoms** *for* [4] **broadly defined types of equipment**. *These levels are expected not to be exceeded for standard procedures when good and normal practice regarding diagnostic and technical performance is applied.*

Clause No. 1: Medical Radiodiagnostic Practices

The first boldfaced phrase of the definition emphasizes that DRLs apply only to *medical diagnostic practices* and therefore they should not be used in other contexts such as radiation therapy. It does raise the question as to whether interventional x-ray practices such as coronary angioplasty should have DRLs, but due to the

potentially high radiation dose involved with interventional procedures, recent workers have established and employed DRLs successfully (2009). However, due to the wide variation in dose encountered with interventional procedures, often relating to the complexity of the examination, other workers have suggested that reference levels need to be established that take into consideration the examination complexity, and normalize the dose data according to that complexity (Balter et al. 2008; IAEA 2009).

Clause No. 2: Typical Examinations

The second boldfaced phrase of the definition specifies that DRLs are relevant only to *typical examinations*. This means that if a patient has to undergo an unusual or additional projection or examination to provide the required clinical information, then a DRL may be exceeded. In other words, a DRL should never restrict an examination when more diagnostic information is required.

Clause No. 3: Groups of Standard-Sized Patients or Standard Phantoms

The description, *standard-sized patients*, means that if the patient is larger than normal, than it is perfectly fine for an exposure to result in a dose that exceeds the stated DRL for a specific examination. Of course, this raises a question: What is a "standard-sized" patient? The NRPB (1992) in looking at the establishment of DRLs decided that for a UK population, the mean weight of a patient group to be used to establish DRLs should be within 5 kg of 70 kg, and patients much lighter or heavier than 60 kg or 80 kg should be excluded from DRL calculations. This does not mean that 70 kg would be suitable for all populations across the globe; for example, in Southeast Asia, the average patient size might be considerably less. Such ethnic-based weight variations does mean that DRLs, which should be relevant to individuals in specific populations, will vary between countries regions of the world, and therefore DRL harmonization across countries (as sometimes recommended) should be treated with some degree of caution.

The other important part of the clause highlighted above is that it suggests that phantoms might be used instead of patients to establish DRL values. One of the main difficulties in establishing DRLs is to obtain dose values from sufficient numbers of patients so that representative data can be gathered for specific examinations or projections from which DRLs can be calculated. In fact, the enormity of this issue is one of the main reasons why DRLs have often been implemented slowly in many countries, particularly for examinations that are performed on a less frequent basis. Phantoms, particularly of the anthropomorphic type (**Figure 12-2**) can clearly serve as a solution for this difficulty; however, the question as to how representative this phantom is of patients being imaged in a particular room or center must be answered.

Also, this approach does not provide information on the dose variations that can occur across a group of patients (even of the same size). In practice to date, most work establishing DRLs in radiography have employed patients in their calculations, while in computed tomography (CT) phantoms particularly of the Computed Tomography Dose Index (CTDI) type (**Figure 12-3**) have often been used.

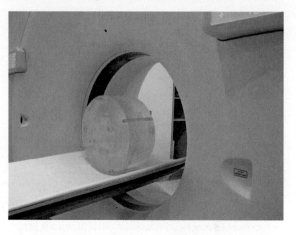

Figure 12-3 Phantom within a CT unit.
Courtesy of Patrick C. Brennan.

Clause No. 4: For Broadly Defined Types of Equipment

This final clause suggests that DRLs, when established, are not specific to individual manufacturers or equipment models. It should not matter if standard-sized patients are being examined in rooms containing Siemens Luminos Agile equipment with radiographic and fluoroscopic capability or a Philips Digital Diagnost facility for solely radiographic procedures; if the examination is the same, the adherence to a national or even hospital-based DRL is expected regardless of which specific model of equipment is being used. In fact, one of the very powerful uses of DRLs is to identify old or faulty equipment that is consistently producing excessively high exposures and therefore offer justification for the need to budget for an update or replacement of existing infrastructure.

These four clauses within the first sentence of the definition place DRLs in context and highlight that they are relevant only for specific circumstances. The second half of the definition simply emphasizes that these values should not be exceeded wherever radiographers or radiologists are employing good skills and using good equipment—the latter highlighting the importance of regular and thorough quality assurance.

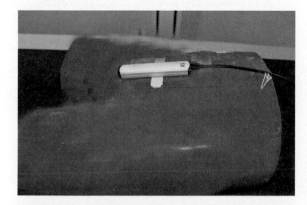

Figure 12-2 An anthropomorphic phantom being x-rayed. Please note the solid state dosimeter on the surface of the phantom.
Courtesy of Patrick C. Brennan.

What are Diagnostic Reference Levels *Not*?

While it may be implicit from the above, it is probably important to explicitly state what DRLs are *not*. They are not any of the following:

Dose limits. It is a common misinterpretation that a DRL is a dose limit. *It is not*. The DRL is simply a guidance value; however, if exposures within an imaging center result in doses that regularly exceed this limit for a particular examination, then the center should introduce corrective action. Also, if a patient who is large or who needs supplementary, unusual, or even repeat exposures to obtain the required clinical information, then the necessary exposures should take place regardless of the dose that is being delivered.

Relevant to radiation therapy. As stated above, DRLs are *only* to be used for diagnostic examinations employing ionizing radiation.

Universal values. Once DRLs have been established in a particular country or region, one should not assume that they can or should be automatically employed in another jurisdiction. Some of the best data have been obtained through a number of very well-planned, -coordinated, and -performed studies within the UK, but these values were established from measurements of individuals *in the UK using UK protocols and procedures*. These may not be necessary relevant, for example, in Southeast Asia or parts of Latin America, where individuals are generally smaller, or in certain parts of Africa, where equipment being used may be substantially older. For example, work done by this author when establishing DRL values for use in Ireland demonstrated that the calculated 75th percentile for AP lumbar spine examinations in Ireland was 40% lower that the DRL being recommended in the UK. Interestingly, the Council of European Communities in the 1990s appeared to adopt the UK DRL values, but whether these were actually relevant to all of the 28 member states of the European Union is unclear.

Static values. This is an important point to stress and will be discussed more below. In summary, once one has established DRLs at a particular value for specific examinations, there is then a guidance value (and some pressure) for diagnostic imaging centers to try and adhere to these values, particularly those centers regularly giving higher doses. Therefore, in time one would expect that the overall population dose would gradually decrease, and updated DRLs would be required reflecting these lower doses. Indeed when one looks at the progression of DRLs in the UK—where there have been four major radiologic dose reviews—each time, the DRL has reduced incrementally, with doses in the latest 2010 review (Hart et al. 2012) being typically less than DRLs calculated from data gathered in the 1980s (IPSM, NRPB, COR 1992). The need for regular updating of DRLs has been stressed by the ICRP.

Values to be implemented without appropriate consideration of image quality. The most important part of any diagnostic examination is to provide the required clinical information, and *DRLs must never limit that provision*. While one wishes to demonstrate that radiation risks within a particular center are low, the drive towards lower doses must not introduce image aberrations such as image noise to an extent where important anatomic and pathologic information relevant for a specific clinical condition is obscured (highlighting the importance of clearly stated clinical objectives on the examination request form). Therefore, in centers where there is a large focus to adhere to DRLs, radiologists and radiographers should monitor image quality closely to ensure diagnostic efficacy is maintained.

Why is It Important to Implement DRLs?

The most important reason to establish DRLs has already been highlighted above: It is difficult to justify large variations in patient doses for the same examination (and same clinical purpose) for patients of the same or similar size. There are, however, other compelling arguments supporting DRL adoption, including legal and societal responsibilities along with an increasing awareness of radiation dose levels being delivered in medical imaging.

Legal or Regulatory Requirements

The legal situation is clear in a number of countries, where it is expected that DRLs should be implemented. For example, in the previously mentioned directive 97/43/Euratom (1997), it was made clear that European Member States should establish DRLs. This requirement was ratified in a number of country-specific statutory instruments such as the Ionising Radiation (Medical Exposure) Regulations 2000 (UK) and Statutory Instrument 478 of 2002 (Ireland). Regulatory documents in other countries have similar obligations, such as the United States' National Council on Radiation Protection and Measurements' report, *Reference Levels and Achievable Doses in Medical and Dental Imaging: Recommendations for the United States*; Health Canada's *Safety Code 35 - Safety procedures for the installation, use and control of x-ray equipment in large medical radiological facilities*; and the Australian Radiation Protection and Nuclear Safety Agency's Code of Practice *Radiation Protection in the Medical Applications of Ionising Radiation*. Where such legal and regulatory requirements exist, DRLs are mandatory.

Societal Benefits

From a societal perspective, the higher doses involved with certain examinations, such as those involving CT and interventional procedures, have highlighted the need to minimize excessive exposures in radiology. This issue is very well considered in the excellent paper of Hall and Brenner (2008) and is further discussed elsewhere in this text. The authors describe that there has been a 20-fold and 12-fold increase respectively in the use of CT in the US and UK, respectively, with higher individual patient radiation dose due to higher doses per examination and more examinations per person. Putting this into context, in 1980, there were approximately 2 million CT examinations in the US alone, compared with 69 million scans in 2007, with this number continuing to increase. In societies such as the US with so many examinations taking place, radiological diagnostic exposure has become a major public health issue, particularly when it can be shown that radiation doses from diagnostic radiology may be reaching levels associated with excess risk of cancer. The responsibility that radiographers and radiologists have to the many people undergoing these examinations and to health systems to minimize the societal burden of induced cancers, through effective implementation of DRLs or otherwise, therefore is not insignificant.

Improved Awareness of Radiation Doses

Awareness demonstrated by radiologists and radiographers of radiation levels being delivering to their patients should increase with active and effective implementation of DRLs. It is the experience of the authors of this text that imaging personnel have not been completely aware of the levels of exposures associated with individual examinations. If, for example, a mother comes in asking about the risk of a particular procedure to her child (which she has every right to do), this question cannot be effectively answered without a good knowledge of doses being delivered. This type of situation is unusual in medical practice, since if a GP prescribes a particular drug, it is a reasonable expectation that the patient will receive detailed information regarding the dosage and potential side effects. With public awareness of radiation hazards increasing, particularly after well-publicized nuclear accidents such as at the Fukushima Daiichi power plant following the Tōhoku earthquake and tsunami, the likelihood is that relatively straightforward questions regarding radiation dose and associated risks will be increasingly presented.

Have DRLs Reduced Doses?

Finally, it should be asked whether there is direct evidence proving that DRLs have achieved any of the above benefits—or even more simply, whether there is data clearly demonstrating that DRLs have been responsible for reducing doses in radiology. The most likely answer to both questions is probably *no*, since the impact of DRLs is extremely hard to measure. For example, one can suggest (as has been done above) that the introduction and implementation of DRLs in the UK over the last two decades has coincided with a gradual but substantial reduction in medical imaging radiation levels over the same time period. But this association does not prove that DRLs were the causal agent, and it may be argued that better education, improved awareness of radiation risk, introduction of new legislation, and so on may have been at least contributing factors—which is most likely true. It can also be argued that more research is required showing the effects of DRLs, however with a number of public health issues such as breast screening, it is hard to choose a methodology that would prove beyond all doubt to all people that this public health intervention was responsible for specific benefits. Dissenters will always be present stressing how other confounding agents are more important than the intervention, yet few of us would doubt the hugely important impact of mammographic screening on women's health, for example. In other words, if we wait for hard, direct evidence that DRLs have made a major impact on radiation doses, we may be waiting a long time, and perhaps we should be focusing instead on the arguments presented above and the strong associations we can find in the literature.

Establishment of Diagnostic Reference Values

At this stage, the argument for DRLs has been presented, so if we accept that they are useful and should be established, how is this achieved within a particular population? The important point that has been stressed a number of times is that these values need to be *representative of, and relevant to* the population and circumstances that present in a particular state or country. Without taking population into account, the values obtained may be unrealistically low and therefore unachievable for medical centers to adhere to, or they are so high as to be ineffective. *The first step therefore is to introduce an effective radiation dose survey to gather sufficient data about the doses currently being delivered.* The next stage of this section of the chapter will focus on *how the DRL is established once the data has been gathered.* The focus will be on establishing DRLs at a national level; however, the issue of *local* diagnostic reference levels will be considered later on in the chapter. Also, the bulk of the discussion below is based on adult exposures, although factors relevant to pediatric examinations will be considered.

The Survey to Establish Current Dose Levels

To identify the DRL, you must first identify what doses are being given in practice via survey. The first key element of performing the survey is to establish a multidisciplinary team, which should ideally consist of radiologists, radiographers, medical physicists, epidemiologists/statisticians, and other relevant personnel. Once the team is established, to ensure that dose data gathered is truly of the highest importance to and is representative of a particular population, careful consideration must be given to a number of key elements:

- types of examinations
- diagnostic centers
- patients (or phantoms)
- dose-measuring/recording methodologies
- accessory data gathered
- survey frequency

It should be acknowledged from the start that, as in any effective scientific study, the appropriateness of resultant mean or percentile values relies on effective sampling strategies. However, obtaining perfect sample sizes and profiles from human participants is extremely difficult (for a variety of reasons), and even the best DRL data to date suffer from this limitation. Therefore, whatever specific methodology is employed, this may be open to criticism from the statistical purist; however, the gathering of as much dose data as possible and using that data efficiently must be promoted and encouraged so that x-ray examinations can be optimized. Furthermore, a pragmatic approach must prevail, since without question the above challenges will not facilitate the perfect methodology and there will be a number of challenges the DRL team must steer through.

Types of Examinations

Legislation or Codes of Practice to date have not singled out specific examinations, and therefore, it may be argued that all radiologic examinations using ionizing radiation should have DRLs. In practice this is not possible, and DRLs would never be established if this was the expectation. Indeed Health Canada's *Safety Code 35* (2008) talks about establishing DRLs "where the number of patients undergoing the procedures is sufficiently high." Therefore, the team must decide which examinations should be prioritized based on the maximum collective benefit to the population from which the data is being gathered. Examination of two key factors should assist with this prioritization: frequency of examination and radiation dose per examination. However, such information may not always be available for a particular population and must be sought from elsewhere. In Ireland, for example, when a similar survey was being performed, there was a paucity of data on examination frequency—so the team there relied on yet another excellent NRPB document (2002), which presented numbers of individuals undergoing specific examinations (**Table 12-5**) in the UK with a population of around 60 million. From the table it can be seen that, solely on the basis of annual examination frequency, dental, chest, mammographic and abdomen examinations are the ones exceeding 1 million.

However, since radiation doses vary substantially between examination types, prioritizing examinations solely on frequency may not yield the maximum benefit for a population; to present overall benefit in a more comprehensive way, *collective*

Table 12-5 Examinations within the UK ordered according to the frequency of examinations

Type of Examination	Number of Examinations
X-RAY	
Teeth(intraoral)	9,562,500
Chest	8,286,520
Mammography	1,726,303
Abdomen (plain film)	1,217,192
Pelvis	919,740
Hip	885,489
Cervical spine	858,547
Lumbar spine	824,763
Colon	359,436
Lumbar sacral joint	338,901
Thoracic spine	281,215
Angiocardiography	162,871
Intravaneous urogram	162,502
Esophagus	123,751
Cardiovascular interventional	121,810
Peripheral angiography	116,903
Stomach and duodeum	98,581
Bladder and urethra	82,941
Biliary system	67,627
Bilary and urinary interventional	47,968
Small intestine	41,089
Abdominal angiography	12,711
Cerebral angiography	11,999
Aortohraphy	11,161
COMPUTED TOMOGRAPHY	
CT head	618,391
CT abdomen	297,244
CT chest	192,885
CT pelvis	139,722
CT spine	63,183
CT neck	24,332
CT interventional	13,184

NRBP 2002© Crown copyright. Reproduced with permission of Public Health England.

dose should be calculated by multiplying examination frequency by dose per examination. Procedures can then be reordered accordingly (**Table 12-6**) and one can immediately see how examinations such as those involving CT, interventional procedures, and some common plain-film examinations such as abdomen, lumbar spine, and pelvis could be prioritized, and this is reflected in the evidence to date.

Conversely, it is interesting to note that while mammography has one of the highest frequencies and presents with substantial collective doses, there is not as much patient DRL data as with other examinations. Finally it should stressed that Tables 12-5 and 12-6 using information published in 2002, are included here only for an example of numbers that may be used to prioritize examinations when data are unavailable for the population under investigation. They should not necessarily be used as a definitive list of examination frequency or collective dose, as (1) values change with time (the numbers of IVUs for example may be much less now than in 2002) and (2) UK values may not be relevant to the country in which DRLs are being established.

Hospital Number and Type

Once the examinations have been established, the next step is to consider how many hospitals and what type of centers should be included. As we are trying to obtain data that would be representative of the whole population within the country, therefore, as with any research study or survey, one would like the sample size to be sufficiently large and contain centers that represent specific subpopulations. Such subpopulations ideally would include the full range of center types where x-ray examinations are performed: (1) urban and rural; (2) large and small centers; (3) primary, secondary or tertiary; (4) adult and pediatric (when pediatric values are being calculated).

In practice, however obtaining such beautifully representative data is often very difficult. Busy clinicians are required to provide details on dose values and other patient and center information back to the coordinating center on a regular basis (see below). This is always a critically important

Table 12-6 Examinations within the UK ordered according to the level of collective dose being delivered

Examinations	Collective Dose (SV/person)
XRAY	
Colon	2587.9
Angiocardiography	1076.4
Cardiovascular interventional	903.9
Abdomen (plain film)	852.0
Lumbar spine	824.8
Pelvis	643.8
Mammography	466.3
Intravaneous urogram	390.0
Peripheral angiography	361.5
Hip	321.2
Abdominal angiography	285.0
Biliary system	270.3
Stomach and duodeum	256.3
Bilary and urinary interventional	235.1
Thoracic spine	196.9
Esophagus	185.6
Chest	165.8
Small intestine	154.2
Aortohraphy	122.6
Bladder and urethra	102.5
Lumbar sacral joint	92.2
Cervical spine	60.1
Cerebral angiography	48.0
Teeth(intraoral)	47.8
COMPUTED TOMOGRAPHY	
CT abdomen	2972.4
CT chest	1543.1
CT pelvis	1397.2
CT head	1236.8
CT spine	252.7
CT interventional	131.8
CT neck	60.8

NRBP 2002 © Crown copyright. Reproduced with permission of Public Health England.

challenge. The team will therefore have to consider the best method for its particular situation. It may be that in a particular country with a small population and an excellent radiologic network, implementation of the survey across the whole country is easily possible; however, in other countries with larger populations and a less cohesive network, a greater sampling approach may be required. It is interesting to note that in the UK, the first DRLs that were proposed were based on a random sample of 20 hospitals (in a population where 800+ relevant centers exist), and the subsequent 75th percentile calculations were considered sufficiently robust to be proposed as EU-wide DRLs. In Ireland, 16 of a potential 43 centers were randomly sampled demonstrating a different sampling rate.

Patient Number and Size, and Phantoms

As with hospital numbers representing a particular jurisdiction, the measurements obtained for a particular examination from patients from a particular room or center must be sufficiently large to ensure that summary data are representative of all patients. In the initial documents of the NRPB (1992), it was suggested that a minimum of 10 patients per examination per room would be sufficient as long as the mean size of the patient sample remained within 5 kg of 70 kg and that no individual patient weight was less than 50 kg or greater than 90 kg. A number of subsequent studies attempted to comply with these guidelines; however, it was observed that adherence to even these fairly broad criteria was difficult. Therefore, the criteria were further examined using statistical methods in the NRPB 2000 review (NRPB 2002) and on the basis of resultant data, the following selection procedure was recommended and implemented in the 2000 (2002), 2005 (2007), and 2010 (2012) reviews: "*the mean weight of patients included in a sample for a particular examination in a particular room should be within 5 kg of 70 kg or if the patient weights are unknown, a minimum of 10 patients per sample should be included.*" There was no differentiation between genders. Obviously, for dental examinations, size is not an issue.

Gathering enough patients for all prioritized examinations, even with the latest (more relaxed) inclusion criteria can prove difficult, so phantom measurements have been proposed as an alternative presenting the advantages that a number of measurements for a series of examination types can be obtained rapidly, measurements can be made at any time of the day so the workflow is not affected and that a single individual could be responsible for obtaining all measurements. However, the difficulties with phantoms are significant and include the following:

- The impact of the survey on image quality cannot be fully assessed.
- The variation in radiations doses within a particular room cannot be fully explored.
- Appropriate phantoms will not available in all sites included in the study for all examinations to be investigated. This may therefore require the transporting of heavy phantoms from hospital to hospital, which in a geographically large country like Australia may be problematic.
- The same type of phantom would have to be used across all hospitals if the resultant radiation doses are to be comparable.
- The exposure factors selected for a phantom may not necessarily reflect those used with a heterogeneous collection of patients.
- Fairly sophisticated and hence expensive phantoms will be required (to ensure that a minimum level of image quality has been achieved) rather than slabs of homogenous material such as acrylic.

Nonetheless, phantom measurements can be used effectively as shown by variety of reference levels published by the NCRP in 2012 (NCRP 2012), and following the ongoing Nationwide Evaluation of X-ray Trends (NEXT) surveys (see below).

Methods of Dose Measurement/Recording

Methods of dosimetry are treated in detail elsewhere; therefore, in this section, dosimetric approaches used to establish DRLs are simply summarized.

Entrance Surface Dose Measurements

The majority of DRL studies to date focusing on radiographic or fluoroscopic examinations have used either ESD or DAP measurements to record the radiation dose being delivered. ESD measurements usually involve placing at least one thermoluminescent dosemeter (TLD) (**Figure 12-4**) on the patient surface facing the x-ray tube in the center of the x-ray beam and produce a value in mGy.

Even though each TLD must be calibrated, they are prone to error and have sizeable measurement uncertainty; however, they do have the advantage of directly measuring the radiation dose entering the patient while including backscattered radiation. Their biggest limitation is that they require considerable radiographer time, expertise, and effort, since individual placement for each projection for each patient is necessary and appropriate storage and record keeping before and after the examination must be in place. Not surprisingly therefore, missed or faulty measurements are not uncommon. Since TLDs must be placed carefully in a projection-specific way, they can only be used for single projections and several will be necessary for an examination requiring several exposures such as a lumbar spine procedure. They cannot be used where the patient is moving during the exposure such as in fluoroscopy.

DAP Measurement

DAP measurements, on the other hand, can be used for complete examinations even when the patient is moving while being exposed. DAP values are obtained by way of an ionization chamber

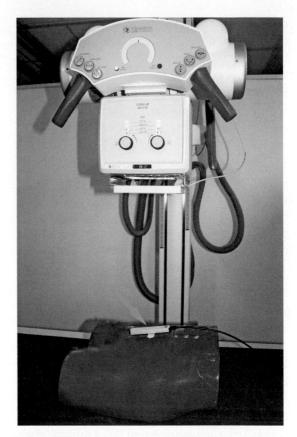

Figure 12-5 The position of the DAP meter is shown at the lower part of the collimation device.
Courtesy of Patrick C. Brennan.

(**Figure 12-5** and **12-6**) at the x-ray tube, which records the radiation level being emitted by the tube and multiplies the dose by the area of the

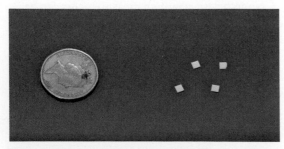

Figure 12-4 Lithium fluoride, manganese doped TLDs.
Courtesy of Patrick C. Brennan.

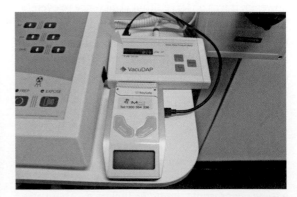

Figure 12-6 Read out of the DAP meter is shown to the right of the console.
Courtesy of Patrick C. Brennan.

x-ray beam resulting in the dose area product value such as 50 Gy-cm². It offers the significant advantage of requiring much less human intervention, since apart from setting up the device in the first place, patient specific arrangement is not required, and since the advent of the DICOM standard, it will be likely that the radiation dose will generally be automatically included within the examination records, although in some instances recording must be done manually. Such a reduction in human effort means that measurements are much more likely to happen with a potentially reduced error rate. Also, they are the only effective mainstream dosimetric method for fluoroscopic procedures. The main downside with the DAP option is that they measure the dose emitted from the tube, which is not the same as that being received by the patient due to the Inverse Square Law and other factors, and backscatter from the patient is not recorded. In addition, an ionization chamber must be in place to record the exposures, which while mandatory in some jurisdictions such as the European Union, are not necessarily required elsewhere. Naturally the DAP meter must be calibrated regularly to ensure that appropriate recordings are being presented.

As mentioned above, both ESD and TLD methods are used, and in the latest UK review, the measurement numbers show a reasonably close balance between the two methods.

Free-in-Air Measurements

There is another method occasionally used for establishing DRL values known as **free-in-air measurements** that relies on calculations rather than patient- or phantom-specific measurements. This produces **entrance surface air kerma (ESAK)** values (without the patient), obtained at the center of the x-ray beam using a calibrated electronic dosemeter (**Figures 12-7** and **12-8**).

However, without appropriate correction factors, free-in-air measurements cannot be performed for procedures requiring an automatic exposure control (AEC) device, since during the measurement procedure appropriate patient

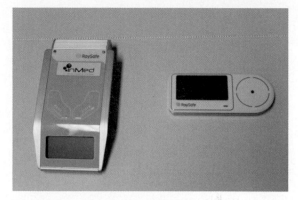

Figure 12-7 Electronic dose meters.
Courtesy of Patrick C. Brennan.

attenuation will not have occurred and therefore the radiation dose (at the x-ray tube) needed to terminate the exposure will be unrealistically low. However, correction procedures have been described elsewhere (2012) to facilitate the use of free-in-air measurements and broadly involve

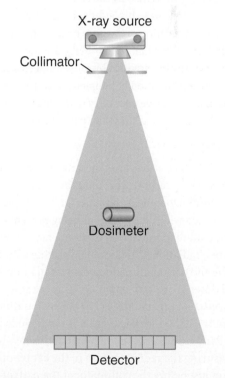

Figure 12-8 Position of the dose meter for air kerma measurements.
Courtesy of Patrick C. Brennan.

calibration measurements using an ionization chamber at a variety of kVp and mAs values at a distance corresponding with the focus detector distance. The radiation dose delivered per unit mAs is then recorded, and this is used to calculate specific projection entrance surface air kerma values using patient examination-specific exposure details such as focus detector and focus skin distances along with the kVp and mAs being employed. A back-scatter factor is also included.

CT Examinations

The above methods are focused on radiographic and fluoroscopic examinations. Other procedures require specific consideration, such as CT, dental, and mammographic exposures. With CT measurements involving patients, two dosimetric quantities can be employed: $CTDI_{vol}$, which represents the average weighted dose in mGy averaged along the length of the scan; dose length product (DLP), which is simply the $CTDI_{vol}$ multiplied by the length of the scan, the unit being Gy-cm—this latter value giving a more complete indication of the dose being delivered for a whole examination. Both $CTDI_{vol}$ and DLP should automatically be provided by most modern scanners once the examination is complete; however, for earlier machines, it may be necessary to use the CTDI phantom (**Figure 12-3**) rather than patient measurements.

Dental Examinations

Dental examinations are generally divided into two types: intra-oral procedures and panoramic exposures. Dose measurements for both types are performed without the patient being present using typical adult (or pediatric) exposure factors. For the former, radiation is measured by placing a dosimeter at the end of the collimator as shown in **Figure 12-9** and doses are recorded in mGy. This is known as the ***patient entrance dose (PED)***, which is different from the ESD since backscatter is not included.

Panoramic exposure measurements involve measuring the radiation dose in the center of the beam just before the collimator at the patient exit and multiplying this by the width of the x-ray beam (at the same location) to produce the dose-width

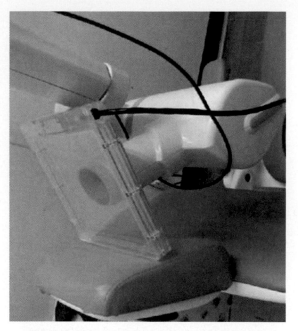

Figure 12-9 An intraoral dental x-ray machine with an ionisation chamber positioned at the end of the collimator.

2012 by Korean Academy of Oral and Maxillofacial Radiology.

product (DWP) in mGy-mm. Otherwise the DAP can be determined in mGy-cm^2, either by multiplying the DWP by the beam height or by alternatively (and more simply) using a DAP meter.

Mammography

Dose measurements in breast imaging are quite complex. It is difficult to calculate doses to patients directly since placing a TLD directly on the patient breast, particularly for the beam energies employed, is likely to result in an image artifact. ***Mean glandular dose (MGD)*** is the metric that best describes radiation dose to the breast and this requires a variety of information including tube output, half-value layer (HVL) (the level of filtration required to reduce the x-ray intensity by 50%), tube current exposure time product, source-to-detector distance, and thickness of the compressed breast. The MGD is then calculated using the well-accepted method of Dance et al. (2000):

$$MGD = Kgcs$$

where MGD is mean glandular dose, K is air kerma at the upper surface of the breast, g corresponds to a glandularity of 50%, c is a correction factor based on differences from a 50% glandularity and based on patient age and compressed patient thickness, and s is a correction factor for any non-molybdenum anode/molybdenum filter combination. K is calculated as follows:

$$K = O_d P_{It}(d_{sd}/(d_{sd} - T))^2$$

where O_d is tube output at the level of the detector, P_{It} is tube current exposure time product, d_{sd} is source detector distance, and T is the thickness of compressed breast.

Accessory Data Gathered

The key aim of the survey is ultimately to gather enough high-quality data so that DRLs can be calculated; however, it also provides the opportunity to present immensely helpful information and feedback to the participating hospitals that may help reduce the radiation dose. It is arguably not sufficient to simply present to Hospital A the national DRL for an abdomen examination and say that in its Room X, the dose generally delivered is above this value without suggesting potential corrective action that would bring the dose in line with other centers. Therefore, in addition to the dose data, the survey team should gather detailed information on technologies and techniques employed facilitating hospital- or room-specific remedies that will enable adherence to DRL values.

These accessory data falls broadly into two main categories, the first relating specifically to each individual examination, the second pertinent to the room in which the examination was performed. For the examination, information (wherever possible) is gathered on the projection, date and location of the procedure, the patient gender age and size, along with all the exposure information such as kVp, mAs, source detector distance, use of AEC, focal spot size, fluoroscopic time and difficulty of the examination (with the latter two particularly pertinent to fluoroscopic examinations) (**Figure 12-10**). In terms of the room, details are collated on the

generator, x-ray tube, anti-scatter grid, AEC, examination table and the detector (**Figure 12-11**).

At the end of the survey, it is then possible to compare radiation doses delivered across the centers with the equipment or techniques used and perform fairly simple statistical approaches (such as a stepwise regression) that identify the main causal agents for high doses or dose variations. Armed with this information, the survey team can then go back to the individual centers with not just the relevant dose data, but highly specific and valuable suggestions on how radiation doses can be reduced. Such approaches have been used previously, where factors such as fluoroscopic time, level of filtration and use of a secondary radiation grid were shown to be key elements for barium enema and meal examinations dose variations (2003).

Survey Frequency

As stressed above several times, DRLs are not a static quantity. As technologies, procedures and even the level of compliance with DRL values change, so too will the relevance of the proposed DRL value. Therefore, each examination-specific DRL should be seen as something that requires regular updating to reflect changing practice. There is no set interval for performing dose surveys; however, in the UK, since the mid to late 1980s these have been performed on a five-yearly basis.

Calculation of DRL Values

If the survey in a particular country has been performed well, adhering to the recommendations described above, there should be enough dose data to facilitate the calculation of DRL values. In general, for each projection or examination, mean hospital room values are calculated and sometimes demonstrated graphically, as seen in **Figure 12-12**, and the 75th percentile across these values is calculated. The 75th percentile is easily calculated using the most rudimentary of statistical packages and generally means that approximately three-quarters of the hospital rooms are below this value and one-quarter above it, clearly indicating which hospital rooms need to

1 - Measurements of entrance surface dose per radiograph

(a) For each patient

Date: ....   Hospital: ....

X-ray room: ....

Patient data   Sex: ....   Weight: ....

[No.   ]   Age: ....   Height: ....

Examination data

Type of examination: ....

[If chest – reason for referral ....]

Radiographic data

Radiograph 1   **Radiograph 2**

Projection: ....   Projection: ....

FFD (cm): ....   FFD (cm): ....

Applied potential (kV): ....   Applied potential (kV): ....

Exposure setting (mA s): ....   Exposure setting (mA s): ....

AEC used: YES/NO   AEC used: YES/NO

Film size (cm x cm): ....   Film size (cm x cm): ....

Focal spot size (mm): ....   Focal spot size (mm): ....

Film density OK: YES/NO   Film density OK: YES/NO

- -

ATTACH TLD HERE   ATTACH TLD HERE

- -

Entrance surface dose .... mGy   Entrance surface dose .... mGy

Radiograph 3   **Radiograph 4**

Projection: ....   Projection: ....

FFD (cm): ....   FFD (cm): ....

Applied potential (kV): ....   Applied potential (kV): ....

Exposure setting (mA s): ....   Exposure setting (mA s): ....

AEC used: YES/NO   AEC used: YES/NO

Film size (cm x cm): ....   Film size (cm x cm): ....

Focal spot size (mm): ....   Focal spot size (mm): ....

Film density OK: YES/NO   Film density OK: YES/NO

- -

ATTACH TLD HERE   ATTACH TLD HERE

- -

Entrance surface dose .... mGy   Entrance surface dose .... mGy

---

Figure 12-10 Form allowing details on the examination to be recorded

1(b) For each X-ray room

Date: ....   Hospital: ....

  X-ray room: ....

Equipment data
X-ray generator   Make: ....

                             Type: ....

                             Waveform: ....

X-ray tube   Make: ....

                             Type: ....

                             Target angle: ....

                             Total filtration: ...., mm Al

Anti-scatter grid   Grid ratio: ....

                             Strips/cm: ....

                             Stationary or moving: ....

                             Carbon fibre covers: YES/NO

Automatic exposure control (AEC)   YES/NO

Table top   Material: ....

                             Al equivalence: .... mm Al

Film   Make and type: ....

Intensifying screen   Make and type: ....

Film/screen   Speed class: ....

Cassette   Carbon fibre front: YES/NO

Figure 12-11 Form allowing the recording of the examination room details.
NRPB 1992 Crown © Reproduced with permission of Public Health England

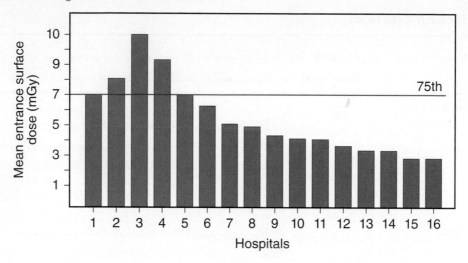

Figure 12-12 Entrance surface radiation doses for a specific examination is shown for 16 hospitals. A horizontal line indicates the 75th percentile value.

Courtesy of Patrick C. Brennan.

implement some level of corrective action to bring their dose values below the DRL.

It is important to note that while the 75th percentile is not a universal choice and alternative metrics such as the mean have been proposed, in the main, the 75th percentile of hospital room mean values is selected as the DRL. So why the 75th percentile? One must remember that for DRLs to work in a particular jurisdiction, they need to be adopted by the relevant hospitals and therefore should be reasonably achievable. **Figure 12-13** shows the frequency of hospitals at specific radiation doses. If the mean or even median values were chosen (blue and red vertical line respectively in Figure 12-13) one can see that around 50% of hospitals would be above the red vertical line, meaning that corrective action would be required in up to half of all hospitals surveyed.

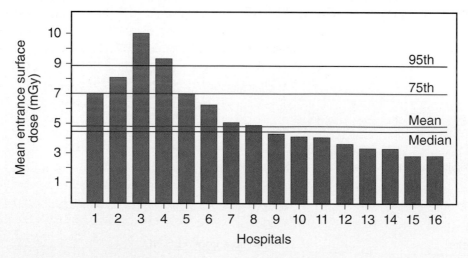

Figure 12-13 Entrance surface radiation doses for a specific examination is shown for 16 hospitals. A red, blue and black line indicates median, mean, 75th percentile value respectively.

Courtesy of Patrick C. Brennan.

This would be excessive, would be difficult to be accepted in so many hospitals and would arguably impose a very stringent and difficult to achieve DRL for many centers. Such an excessive value may also trigger excessive reduction in doses at the expense of diagnostic efficacy. If however the 75th percentile is chosen (green line, Figure 12-13), this means that only one-quarter of hospitals are above this value, presenting a much more acceptable situation. An even higher percentile value such as the 90th or 95th (black line Figure 12-13) may present an even more accepted value; however, if one looks at to dose distributions in Figure 12-13, which is fairly typical of the evidence to date, a normal distribution is not evident, but rather a negative skew with a large tail towards the higher doses. This highlights that there are still a reasonable number of centers delivering doses above the mean value by several factors, highlighting the need to provide a DRL stricter than that provided by a 95th percentile. Clearly, therefore, there must be a balance between being overly strict and excessively lenient, and this is why the 75th percentile is generally chosen. Arguably, as more and more hospitals adhere to DRLs and the DRL values are driven downwards, then the large positive tails may decrease and percentiles above the 75th level may be possible, but so far after 20 years of DRLs in the UK, this has not happened.

Pediatric DRL Values

The focus so far has been on the establishment of adult DRL values; however, the need to establish values for pediatric examinations is obvious, with children having radio sensitivities that are up to 10 times higher than adults. While some data are available for children, these are much scarcer than adults due to the added complexities associated with children around patient size and examination types. Regarding size, it is clear that one cannot have a single DRL value for abdomen exposures accommodating both newborn babies and 15-year-old adolescents, and therefore age-specific values are required. The NRPB (2000) along with other workers have decided that five

standard sizes could be identified around the age categories of 0, 1, 5, 10, and 15 years. While not all children belong to these 5 ages, the NRPB has developed a beam energy-dependent normalization system based on the thicknesses of the child being measured and the standard child, and therefore doses for all individual children can be normalized to the nearest standard age category. The system allows for the inclusion of all children being measured and therefore facilitates good numbers of individuals for each category. Nonetheless, it can be seen that unlike the single value required for adults, 5 separate DRL values are needed for a single examination type, resulting in significant data collection.

The other issue is around prioritizing examination types. While some diagnostic procedures are performed across all children sizes such as chest and abdomen exposures, others are carried out more frequently for specific age categories. For example, micturating cystograms are fairly common procedures for the younger child, but these are rarely performed on adolescents. Prioritizing examinations for DRL establishment therefore needs to consider such age-specific variations.

It is clear therefore that determining pediatric DRL values demonstrates a higher level of complexity and difficulty compared with adult values. Unsurprisingly, there is less pediatric data compared with adult data, even though the need is arguably greater than adults. Nonetheless, some good data has been published. A sampling of the DRL status for a number of countries for both adult and pediatric examinations is shown in **Table 12-7**.

Diagnostic Reference Levels: A Global Activity

This chapter has included information from a variety of sources, but much of the data and techniques presented originate from the UK, not surprisingly since much of the original data and DRL methodologies originated there. However, it is important to also acknowledge a series of DRL-based surveys from a variety of other European

Table 12-7 An indication of the number of examinations with diagnostic reference values in a number of countries

Country	Type	Number of DRLs
Australia	CT (Adult 15+ years)	6
	CT (Paediatric)	6
France	Conventional X-rays (Adult)	9
	Conventional X-rays (Paediatric)	9
	CT (Adults)	4
	Nuclear medicine	4
Germany	Conventional X-rays (Adult)	12
	Flouroscopy (Adult)	5
	CT (Adult)	7
	Interventional procedure (Adult)	2
	Conventional X-rays (Paediatric)	6
	Flouroscopy (Paediatric)	1
	Nuclear medicine	17
Greece	Mammography - Nuclear medicine	12
	CT	7
Italy	Conventional X-rays (Adult)	7
	Conventional X-rays (Infant)	4
	Mammography	1
	CT (Adult)	4
	Nuclear medicine	48
Sweden	Conventional X-rays (Adult)	6
	CT (Adult)	4
	Nuclear medicine	19
Switzerland	Conventional X-rays (Adult)	9
	Mammography	1
	Interventional procedure (Adult)	12
	CT (Adult)	8
	CT (Infant)	4
	Nuclear medicine	47
United Kingdom	Conventional X-rays (Adult)	13
	Flouroscopy (Adult)	15
	CT (Adult)	12
	Interventional procedure (Adult)	5
	Interventional procedure (Paediatric)	3
	CT (Paediatric)	2
	Nuclear medicine	96
The United States of America	Conventional X-rays (Adult)	3
	Conventional X-rays (Paediatric)	2
	Flouroscopy	4
	CT (Adult)	3
	CT (Paediatric)	2
	Dental	5

countries, Australia, and the United States; the DRL status in some of these countries is summarized in Table 12-7. For example, in the US the Nationwide Evaluation of X-ray Trends (NEXT) resulting from a partnership between the US Food and Drug Administration and the Conference of Radiation Control Program Directors (CRCPD) has been responsible for a series of invaluable surveys. Each survey was sizeable and involved 300 US clinical centers that volunteered and were randomly selected, gathering data similar to that already described above. This effective federal-state initiative is supported by the active input from radiation control personnel within 45 states who have agreed to conduct the surveys. To date, data have been gathered for many examination types, including chest, spine, abdomen, mammography, fluoroscopy, CT, dental, and pediatric exams. In the early days, the focus was simply on exposure factors selected for a standard-sized patient; however, following the advent of automatic exposure devices, economic and transportable phantoms were developed for the examinations described, meaning that phantom exposures were the dominant source of data. Consideration has been given to assessment of image quality, often overlooked by other radiation dose surveys and currently the focus is on the impact of digital technology.

Practical Considerations When Gathering The Data

The bottom line when planning this survey is that pragmatism must prevail, and an approach suitable for a particular environment that will yield the most useful data should be implemented. This text cannot present a precise formula suited to all situations, and whatever sampling method is used, the amount of data gathered will vary significantly across centers and examinations. This is why the team should involve an experienced statistician/epidemiologist to plan the work in the first place and evaluate the information gathered in the most effective but scientifically valid way.

From a personal perspective, the authors of this text have been involved in gathering data for DRL calculations for many years. Without repeating what has already been said, we suggest the following additional pieces of advice that may help teams setting out to obtain data from clinical centers and facilitate establishment of DRLs:

1. Involve hospitals where good contacts exist (this may obviously affect a random sampling approach). It is hugely important to have a clinical coordinator in the hospital who is known to the survey team and can be relied upon to implement the study, encourage local involvement and collate and forward data to the team.

2. Start in a limited number of centers with a few high-priority examination types so that the gathering of data is efficiently managed.

Even if data produced at the start of the initiative is limited in volume, it is much better to initially gather good-quality data from a number of sites and get the concept of DRLs well accepted rather than have too few data spread across many centers. One must always remember that DRL implementation must employ a long-term strategy due to the dynamic nature of radiation doses, and therefore starting small and building up a DRL network over time may be the appropriate approach. Certainly this has worked very effectively in the UK where, as stated previously, data were gathered from 20 hospitals on 5 examination types resulting in proposed DRL levels in 1992 for chest, abdomen, pelvis, skull and lumbar spine examinations. Two decades on, the latest Health Protection Agency (UK) publication on x-ray procedure radiation doses contained data derived from 165,000 ESD values for single exposures and 185,000 and 221,000 dose area products (DAP) for single and complete examinations respectively, across 54 adult and pediatric procedures from 320 hospitals (25% of the total population). The power of starting small to allow the concept of DRLs to be embraced within the imaging community, but coupled with a longer-term strategy is advised.

3. Regular communication is essential. Well before the survey is being implemented, the plan to establish DRLs must be presented at as many national and local meetings as possible. This should then be followed up with visits, if possible, to each center involved in collecting data to present the rationale and plan for the survey, and describe the role that each radiographer, medical physicist, and radiologist should play. It is important to note that all clinical staff will need to embrace the study if the maximum amount of data is to be gathered and that checks are performed to ensure that image quality is not compromised. The clinical coordinator

from the center's current staff should be appointed (ideally there needs to be one of these in each center). Once the survey is underway, at least weekly conversations should be held between the team and the clinical coordinator with regular feedback on how the study is going.

4. Limited period of time for gathering data. This may be a controversial suggestion, but in an initial data gathering stage, it may incentivize the local staff if they know they are only required to gather data over a period of 2–4 weeks, for example, rather than indefinitely. Once these data is gathered, analyzed and preliminary percentile values established, clinicians may become more familiar with DRLs, leading to a longer term on-going strategy for data collection.

5. Make sure you have the money. Unfortunately to accommodate travel to centers, dose measurements, coordination of the study, etc., some funds will be required. This can always be a stumbling block, but without some financial support, it is likely that the scope of the survey will be limited.

6. Create or coordinate with a national regulatory/advisory body or network to implement values. This is entirely necessary if DRL values that have been generated from the survey are to be adopted and effectively implemented across a country. Without this arrangement, the fear is that all this work will simply be a very useful academic exercise, and will not reach its ultimate goal of systematically reducing radiation doses. In the UK, for example, though the work of the National Radiological Protection Board and later the Health Protection Agency in active collaboration with radiologic, radiography and medical physics personnel, DRLs have been effectively adopted over the last two decades across the country. This is unlike a series of Irish DRL surveys coordinated from University College Dublin involving good numbers of diagnostic centers. These resulted in proposed DRL values, which were published in several leading academic journals from 2000 to 2008 (Johnston et al. 2000; Carroll et al. 2003a, 2003b; D'Helft et al. 2008) but unfortunately in the absence of a national regulatory or advisory body with a specific responsibility for DRLs, implementation of national reference values for the relevant examinations did not occur.

Summary of Key Concepts

1. **Variations that exist in radiation doses for the same examination.** It has been shown in many studies that large fluctuations in patient exposures for the same type of examination are observed, apparently depending on the source of the radiation. For example, in the early work of the UK-based National Radiological Protection Board, in partnership with the Institute of Physical Sciences in Medicine and the College of Radiographers, large variations in mean hospital entrance surface doses (ESD) can be seen for even an examination as common as a chest posteroanterior projection.

2. **What DRLs are—and what they are not.** A good definition of a DRL can be found within the European Council's Directive *97/43/Euratom on health protection of individuals against the dangers of ionizing radiation in relation to medical exposure, and repealing Directive 84/466/Euratom* (1997), which is very similar to the DRL description given by the International Commission of Radiological Protection (ICRP). They are not dose limits.

3. **Why DRLs are an important dose monitoring measure.** The most important reason to establish DRLs is that it difficult to justify large variations in patient doses for the same examination (and same clinical purpose) for patients of the same or similar size. There are however other compelling arguments supporting DRL adoption including legal and societal responsibilities along with an increasing awareness of radiation dose levels being delivered in medical imaging.

4. **Key considerations that are required when setting up DRLs.** The first key element of performing the survey is to establish a multidisciplinary team that should ideally consist of radiologists, radiographers, medical physicists, epidemiologists/statisticians and other relevant personnel. Once the team is established, to ensure that dose data gathered is truly of the highest importance to, and are representative of a particular population, careful consideration must be given to a number of key elements: types of examinations; diagnostic centers; patients (or phantoms); dose-measuring/recording methodologies; accessory data gathered; survey frequency.

5. **How DRL values are calculated.** If a dose-survey in a particular region or locality has been performed well, there should be enough dose data to facilitate the calculation of DRL values. In general, for each projection or examination, mean hospital room values are calculated and sometimes demonstrated graphically and a percentile value (often the 75th percentile) across these values is calculated.

6. **Practical difficulties that are encountered when DRLs are being established.** When planning DRLs pragmatism must prevail and an approach suitable for a particular environment that will yield the most useful data should be implemented. This text cannot present a precise formula suited to all and whatever sampling method is used the amount of data gathered will vary significantly across centers and examinations.

Discussion Questions

1. Discuss the need for DRLs.

2. Discuss what DRLS are not.

3. Discuss the process for setting up DRLs and consider the difficulties potentially encountered when trying to set up DRLs.

References

Australian Radiation Protection and Nuclear Safety Agency. *Radiation Protection in the Medical Applications of Ionizing Radiation.* Victoria NSW: ARPANSA; 2008. (Available at http://www.arpansa.gov.au/publications/codes/rps14.cfm; Retrieved August 18, 2015.)

Balter D, Miller L, Vano E, Ortiz Lopez P, Bernardi G, Cotelo E, Faulkner K, Nowotny R, Padovani R, Ramirez A. A pilot study exploring the possibility of establishing guidance levels in x-ray directed interventional procedures. *Med Phys.* 2008;35:673–680.

Brennan PC, Johnston D. Irish x-ray departments demonstrate varying levels of adherence to European guidelines on good radiographic technique. *Br J Radiol.* 2002;75:243–248.

Carroll EM, Brennan PC. Investigation into patient doses for intravenous urography and proposed Irish diagnostic reference levels. *Eur Radiol.* 2003a;13:1529–1533.

Carroll EM, Brennan PC. Radiation doses for barium enema and barium meal examinations in Ireland: potential diagnostic reference levels. *Br J Radiol.* 2003b;76:393–397.

Dance DR, Skinner CL, Young KC, Beckett JR, Kotre CJ. Additional factors for the estimation of mean glandular breast dose using the UK mammography dosimetry protocol. *Phys Med Biol.* 2000;45:3225–3240.

D'Helft CJ, Brennan PC, McGee AM, McFadden SL, Hughes CM, Winder JR, Rainford LA. Potential Irish dose reference levels for cardiac interventional examinations. *Br J Radiol.* 2009;976:296–302.

European Commission. On health protection of individuals against the dangers of ionizing radiation in relation to medical exposure and repealing directive 84/466/EURATOM. European Council Directive 97/43/EURATOM; 1997.

Hall EJ, Brenner DJ. Cancer risks from diagnostic radiology. *Br J Radiol.* 2008;81:362–378.

Hart D, Hillier MC, Shrimpton PC. *Doses to patients from radiographic and fluoroscopic X-ray imaging procedures in the UK – 2010 Review. CRCE-034*: Chilton, UK: Health Protection Agency-Center for Radiation, Chemical and Environmental Hazards; 2012.

Hart D, Wall BF. *Radiation exposure of the UK population from medical and dental x-ray examinations. NRPB – W4/* National Radiological Protection Board; 2002.

Hart D, Wall BF, Shrimpton PC, Bungay DR, Dance DR. *NRPB-R318-Reference Doses and Patient Size in Pediatric Radiology.* National Radiological Protection Board; 2000.

Health Canada. *Radiation protection in radiology – Large facilities: Safety code 35.* Ottawa: Government of Canada; 2008. (Available at: http://www.hc-sc.gc.ca/ewh-semt/pubs/radiation/safety-code_35-securite/index-eng.php; Retrieved August 20, 2015.)

Institute of Physical Sciences in Medicine, National Radiological Protection Board, College of Radiographers. *National protocol for patient dose measurements in diagnostic radiology.* Chilton, UK: National Radiological Protection Board; 1992.

International Atomic Energy Agency. Establishing guidance levels in x-ray guided medical interventional procedures: A pilot study. Safety Report Series No. 59; Vienna, 2009.

Johnston DA, Brennan PC. Reference dose levels for patients undergoing common diagnostic x-ray examinations in Irish hospitals. Br J Radiol. 2000;73:396–402.

NCRP. NCRP Report No. 172: *Reference Levels and Achievable Doses in Medical and Dental Imaging: Recommendations for the United States.* Bethesda, MD: NCRP; 2012.

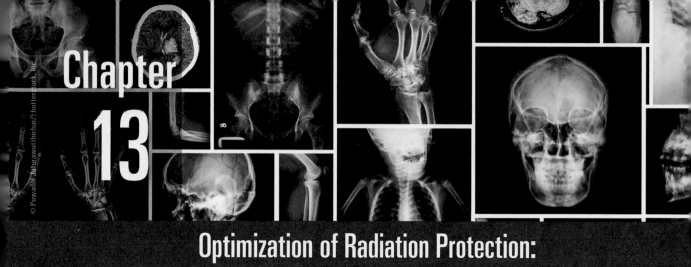

Chapter 13

Optimization of Radiation Protection: Regulatory and Guidance Recommendations

Outline

- Introduction
- Radiation Protection Reports
- Optimization of Radiation Protection
  - Education and training
  - Equipment specifications
  - Personnel practices
  - Shielding
- Equipment Design and Performance Recommendations
  - Radiographic equipment: general recommendations

- Radiographic equipment: specific recommendations
- Fluoroscopic equipment
- Mobile radiographic equipment
- Recommendations for Personnel Practices
  - Protection of personnel
  - Protection of patients
  - Recommendations for radiography in pregnancy
- Recommendations for Quality Assurance
- References

Objectives

On completion of this chapter, you should be able to:

1. Identify selected radiation protection reports relating to regulatory and advisory recommendations.
2. Describe four ways by which optimization of radiation protection can be accomplished.
3. Discuss the general and specific design and performance recommendations for radiographic equipment.
4. Discuss the general design and performance recommendations for fluoroscopic radiographic equipment.

5. Discuss the general design and performance recommendations for mobile radiographic equipment.
6. Describe the fundamental recommendations for the protection of patients and personnel.
7. Explain the recommendations for radiography of the pregnant patient and pregnant worker.
8. State the recommendation for quality assurance in diagnostic radiology.

Introduction

Optimization of radiation protection requires that the operator of ionizing radiation-emitting equipment not only understand the framework of radiation protection and the technical factors affecting the dose to the patient, but have a firm understanding of the influence of mandatory requirements of the design and performance of imaging equipment as well as advisory recommendations on the safe use of the equipment and procedures used to image patients. These guidelines and recommendations are also focused on how to protect personnel and members of the public from unnecessary radiation exposure.

In terms of regulation and guidance to ensure optimization of radiation protection, there are two major groups that play active roles, namely *regulatory agencies* and *advisory bodies*, which are specific to each country. With respect to regulation, Bushberg et al. (2012) state that:

> A number of regulatory agencies have jurisdiction over various aspects of the use of radiation in medicine. The regulation promulgated under their authority carry the force of law. These agencies can inspect facilities and records, levy fines, suspend activities, and issue and revoke radiation use authorizations.

For example, when manufacturers build x-ray equipment (for use in the United States), they must confirm to various regulations on the design and performance aspects, imposed by the U.S. Food and Drug Administration (FDA). Additionally, the FDA also publishes what they refer to as "guidance documents" on the use of x-ray machines, specifically including the term *Code of Federal Regulations* (CFR). For example, CFR Title 21: Part 1020 deals with "performance standards for ionizing radiation emitting products" and includes Sections 31 and 32 dealing mainly with performance standards for radiography and fluoroscopy respectively.

Advisory bodies, on the other hand, include both international and national authorities that provide recommendations on radiation protection. While these recommendations are not regulations and "do not carry the force of law, they are usually the origin of most of regulations adopted by regulatory agencies and are widely recognized as 'standards of good practice.' Most of these recommendations are voluntarily adopted by the medical community even in the absence of a specific legal requirement" (Bushberg et al. 2012). Examples of such bodies are the *International Commission on Radiological Protection (ICRP)* and the *National Council on Radiation Protection and Measurements (NCRP)*, a U.S. body. Another U.S. agency that provides radiation protection guidance is the Environmental Protection Agency (EPA). The EPA, most notably the Administrator, serves "to advise the President with respect to radiation matters, directly or indirectly affecting health, including guidance for all Federal agencies in the formulation of radiation standards and in the establishment and execution of programs of cooperation with States" (EPA 2012a).

With the plethora of recent technological developments in medical imaging, the EPA has made available a Federal Guidance Report (FGR), *FGR No 14: Radiation Protection Guidance for Diagnostic and International X-Ray Procedures* (EPA 2012b). In particular, FGR No. 14 includes topics that were not included in the older FGR No. 9, its initial guideline issued in 1976: reference levels, dose optimization, newer dose metrics, and guidance on technologies that were not in widespread use in 1976, such as positron emission tomography (PET) and CT.

Radiation Protection Reports

Various radiation protection agencies produce reports that address specifically the guidelines and recommendations for radiation protection in medical x-ray imaging; these reports are comprehensive and are prepared by experts in the field of radiation protection. Students and technologists alike should consult the reports, not only to become aware of them, but also to get a glimpse of the wording of the actual statements of the various guidelines and recommendations.

In this chapter, selected regulatory and guidance recommendations will be highlighted, including short direct quotes (so as not to detract from the original) from the following:

1. FDA. Code of Federal Regulations Title 21: Part 1020 – *Performance Standards for Ionizing Radiation Emitting Products.* Section 1020.31 Radiographic Equipment and Section 1020.32 Fluoroscopic Equipment. U.S. Food and Drug Administration; 2011; Revised April 1, 2015.

2. NCRP Report 102 – *Medical X-Ray, Electron Beam and Gamma Ray Protection for Energies up to 50 MeV: Equipment Design, Performance and Use.* NCRP; 1989.

3. *Safety Code 35: Radiation Protection in Radiology – Large Facilities. Safety Procedures for the Installation, Use and Control of X-Ray Equipment in Large Medical Radiological Facilities.* Health Canada; 2008.

While most countries adopt current radiation protection standards and practices recommended by the International Commission on Radiological Protection (ICRP), others develop their own recommendations in cooperation with the ICRP and other national radiation protection organizations (described in detail elsewhere).

Optimization of Radiation Protection

Optimization of radiation protection is a broad term used in this book to refer to various methods and techniques used to vary the factors affecting dose in diagnostic x-ray imaging in an effort to immunize the radiation dose to patients, personnel, and members of the public. These methods and technologies are influenced by regulatory and advisory bodies.

Optimization of radiation protection can be accomplished in several ways; however, this chapter addresses, in general, those radiation protection recommendations relating to education and training, equipment design and performance, personnel practices, and shielding considerations.

It is not within the scope of this chapter to examine the details of all of the recommendations, and therefore students and technologists should refer to recommendations specific to their countries and regions for a more complete picture.

Education and Training

Several decades ago, the ICRP (1982) in Publication 33 stated that:

> *No person shall operate radiological equipment without adequate technical competence, or perform radiological procedures without adequate knowledge of the physical properties and harmful effects of ionizing radiation.*

Subsequently, in Publication 113, *Education and Training in Radiological Protection for Diagnostic and Interventional Procedures,* the ICRP (2009) emphasized the value of education and training in radiation protection of patient, personnel, and members of the public.

The ICRP recommendations on education and training are supported by national organizations such as the NCRP and the Radiation Protection Bureau–Health Canada. In addition, various professional radiologic technology organizations, such as the American Society of Radiologic Technologists (ASRT), and the Canadian Association of Medical Radiation Technologists (CAMRT), have a significant role to play in the training and certification of technologists in an effort to ensure that they meet minimum standards for the clinical practice of radiography. These minimum standards are clearly defined in radiography curricula and allow students to pursue studies in basic physics, radiation physics, instrumentation, anatomy and physiology, patient care and communications, radiographic technique and patient positioning, image evaluation, pathology, radiobiology, and radiation protection. Following years of education and clinical experience, students then take national certification examinations. Successful completion of these examinations indicates that individuals are now capable of working competently in the radiology department.

Equipment Specifications

Equipment specifications refer to the design and performance of diagnostic x-ray equipment used in the radiology department. These requirements are under the influence of regulatory agencies. For example, the USFDA plays a significant role in regulating the manufacture of equipment under the Radiation Control Health and Safety Act of 1968. Furthermore, the FDA also establishes performance standards for x-ray equipment. In Canada, on the other hand, equipment specifications must meet the requirements of two Acts: the Food and Drugs Act (under Medical Devices Regulations), which addresses the safety and usefulness of the equipment; and the Radiation Emitting Devices Act (under the Radiation Emitting Regulations), which deals with the design and performance issues relating to safety. The manufacturer has the responsibility to ensure that the equipment meets the requirements of these regulations.

The topic of dose reduction by equipment design and performance will be described in the next section of this chapter.

Personnel Practices

A significant aspect of dose reduction is based on the skills and knowledge of the technologist performing the examination. Such performance must always focus on the "as low as reasonably achievable" (ALARA) philosophy, including regulatory and advisory recommendations. Technologists must always strive to achieve excellence in radiation protection by putting into practice those recommendations for dose reduction. These recommendations will be described later in the chapter.

In addition, this topic is reflected in the Code of Ethics of various professional associations. For example, the ASRT Code of Ethics, Principle 7, states that:

> *The radiologic technologist utilizes equipment and accessories, employs techniques and procedures, performs services in accordance with an accepted standard of practice and demonstrates expertise in limiting the radiation exposure to the patient, self and other members of the health care team.*

Shielding

Shielding is a significant principal action of radiation protection recommended by all regulatory and advisory bodies on radiation protection. Shielding is yet another means of reducing the dose of absorbable radiation, and other texts are solely dedicated to **protective shielding** in diagnostic radiology. Protective shielding addresses topics such as categories of shielding, protective barriers, factors affecting barrier thickness, and determination of barrier thickness and materials for shielding.

Specific-area shielding, on the other hand, refers to the use of lead shields to protect radio sensitive organs such as the gonads and breasts.

Equipment Design and Performance Recommendations

The recommendations and guidelines for equipment specifications **design and performance** are intended to protect not only the patient but also the technologist during the course of the examination. These recommendations have been developed for radiography, fluoroscopy, mammography, and computed tomography (CT). It is not within the scope of this chapter to address all of these recommendations, and therefore only the more commonplace ones of importance in routine daily use, for radiography and fluoroscopy will be briefly reviewed in this section. CT is reviewed in chapter 10.

Radiographic Equipment: General Recommendations

The general recommendations for equipment design include the use of warning signs, labels, indicator lights, and meters; mechanical stability; exposure control, filtration, indication of exposure, use of exposure technique factors; and x-ray tube shielding, to mention but a few.

Equipment should be designed so that the operator has a clear view of all warning signs, labels, and meters on the control console. The location of the x-ray tube focal spot must also be clearly indicated on the x-ray tube housing. Filtration must be marked on the tube head and the minimum permanent inherent filtration must be indicated. Furthermore, there are specific requirements for the total permanent filtration, to be stated subsequently.

Other general recommendations of importance to the technologist relate to exposure control and x-ray tube shielding. **Exposure control** refers to the exposure switch and timer, which are used to start and stop the exposure to the patient. For radiography and fluoroscopy, the exposure switch must be of a "dead-man" type, which means that the operator must apply continuous pressure to activate and deliver the exposure.

For fixed radiographic equipment, the position of the exposure switch is such that the operator must be in the control booth during the exposure. X-ray tube shielding recommendations are intended to address leakage radiation from the x-ray tube. The NCRP (1989) recommends that the leakage radiation measured at 1 m from the tube not exceed 0.1 centigray (cGy) per hour.

Radiographic Equipment: Specific Recommendations

In addition to the general recommendations, there are specific recommendations vital to the practice of radiation protection. The FDA, in CRR Title 21 Section 1020.31 (2015) present 13 performance standards, such as, for example, control and indication of technique factors, timers, reproducibility, linearity, field limitation and alignment, positive beam limitation (PBL), and so on. The reader should consult this document for details relating to the above standards.

Collimation and Beam Alignment

CFR Title 21 (FDA 2011) several recommendations with respect to collimation and beam alignment as follows:

- *For variable field limitation — A means for stepless adjustment of the size of the field shall be provided. Each dimension of the minimum field size at an SID of 100 centimeters (cm) shall be equal to or less than 5 cm…*
- *For visual definition (1) … The total misalignment of the edges of the visually defined field with the respective edges of the x-ray field along either the length or width of the visually defined field shall not exceed 2 percent of the distance from the source to the center of the visually defined field when the surface upon which it appears is perpendicular to the axis of the x-ray beam.*

With respect to field indication and alignment, CFR Title 21 (FDA 2011) states that:

- *Means shall be provided to indicate when the axis of the x-ray beam is perpendicular to the plane of the image receptor, to align the center of the x-ray field with respect to the center of the image receptor to within 2 percent of the SID and to indicate the SID to within 2 percent…*
- *The beam-limiting device shall numerically indicate the field size in the plane of the image receptor to which it is adjusted.*

For systems with automatic collimation or **positive beam limitation** (PBL), CFR Title 21 (FDA 2011) recommends that the technologist should not be able to make an exposure if the x-ray field size is greater than the size of the image receptor by >3% of the source-to-image receptor distance (SID). An override system must be provided to allow the operator to collimate to the size of the image receptor or smaller.

Leakage radiation from the collimator is just as important as leakage from the x-ray tube, and in this regard, the recommendation is that the collimator must offer the same degree of shielding as that of the x-ray tube housing.

Filtration

The purpose of filtration is to protect the patient by absorbing low-energy photons, which do not penetrate the patient. The recommendations are very specific for diagnostic x-ray beams, depending on the kVp used. For example, the minimum total filtration in the useful beam must be as follows (NCRP 1989):

- 0.5 mm aluminum (Al) when the x-ray tube is operated below 50 kVp
- 1.5 mm Al, when the tube is operated in between 50 kVp to 70 kVp
- 2.5 mm Al, when the tube is operated above 70 kVp

These filters must be permanently mounted onto the tube housing or collimator.

Source-to-Skin Distance (SSD)

The **source-to-skin distance (SSD)** in radiography influences the dose to the patient, and as such, the NCRP (1989) recommends that "the SSD *shall not* be less than 30 cm (12 in) and *should not* be less than 38 cm (15 in)." As the SSD decreases, the dose increases, since there is an increase in the concentration of photons per unit area on the patient.

The NCRP (1989) also recommended that for table-top radiography, the SID should not be less than 100 cm (40 in), and for upright chest radiography, the SID should not be less than 180 cm (72 in).

Exposure Reproducibility

When the same exposure technique factors are used repeatedly, the output radiation intensity should be the same for all exposures. This is what is meant by **exposure reproducibility**. To meet the recommendations in the code of standards for diagnostic equipment for reproducibility, the output intensity must not be greater than ±5% of the average intensities of a series of 5 exposures (Statkiewicz-Sherer et al. 7th Ed. 2015).

Exposure Linearity

The combination of different mA and time selections to produce constant mAs values should produce constant output radiation intensities (mR/mAs). This is referred to as **exposure linearity**.

For radiographic equipment, the recommendations require that the output intensities for adjacent mA selections not vary by more than 10%.

Exposure reproducibility and exposure linearity are essentials to a quality control (QC) program, and both serve to ensure optimization of radiation protection. Optimization of the dose-image quality research require that the x-ray machine be calibrated. Exposure reproducibility and linearity are part of the calibration of equipment requirements.

Fluoroscopic Equipment

Controlling the factors affecting the dose in fluoroscopy can significantly reduce the dose to both patients and operators. Although the design recommendations for fluoroscopic equipment are discussed in detail in CFR Title 21 Part 1020: Section 1020.32 (FDA 2011), this subsection of the chapter will highlight only a few important requirements. These include direct beam absorbers, output radiation intensity, filtration, collimation, SSD, exposure switch, cumulative timer, protective lead drape, and the Bucky slot shielding.

Direct Beam Absorber

All fluoroscopic units must have a **direct beam absorber**, often referred to as a **primary protective barrier**, permanently built into the unit. The purpose of this primary barrier is to limit the exposure during fluoroscopy. If this barrier is removed at anytime, the exposure will terminate. The barrier must also have a lead equivalent of 2 mm.

Output Radiation Intensity

The **exposure rate** in fluoroscopy "should not exceed 21 mGy/min (2.1 R/min) for each mA of operation at 80 kVp. If there is no optional high-level control, the intensity must not exceed 100 mGy/min (10 R/min) during fluoroscopy. If an optional high-level control is provided, the maximum table-top intensity allowed is 200 mGy/min (20 R/min)" (Bushong 2013).

Filtration

Because fluoroscopy is usually done at higher than 70 kVp, the total permanent filtration must be at least 2.5 mm Al equivalent.

Collimation

For collimation in fluoroscopy, the NCRP (1989) specifically recommends that:

> An adjustable collimator shall be provided to restrict the size of the beam to the area of interest…. The x-ray tube and collimating system shall be linked with the image receptor assembly so that the beam is centered on the image receptor assembly. The beam should be confined within the useful receptor area at all source-to-image receptor distances.

Source-to-Skin Distance (SSD)

The recommendations are such that the SSD shall not be <30 cm (12 in) for mobile fluoroscopy units and must not be <38 cm (15 in) for stationary (fixed) fluoroscopy units.

Exposure Switch

As in radiographic equipment, the exposure switch in fluoroscopy, whether it be a foot switch or a switch on the image receptor assembly (spot-film device), must be of a dead-man type.

Cumulative Timer

The NCRP's (1989) recommendation for such a timer is as follows:

> A cumulative timing device, activated by the fluoroscopy exposure switch, shall be provided. It shall indicate either by an audible or visual signal, or both, obvious to the user. The passage of a predetermined period of irradiation shall not exceed 5 minutes. The signal should last at least 15 seconds, at which time the timer must be reset manually.

Lead Protective Drape

The distribution of scattered radiation during fluoroscopy is typically 500 mR/hr, 100 mR/hr, and 50 mR/hr at 1, 2, and 3 feet from the fluoroscopy system (Bushong 2013). This scattered radiation can significantly increase the dose to personnel during the examination. To minimize the dose, a *lead protective curtain or drape* of dimensions not less than 45.7 cm × 45.7 cm (18 in × 18 in) must be attached to the image receptor assembly. For adequate protection of personnel, the drape should have at least 0.25 mm lead equivalent. In Canada, the recommendation requires a lead equivalent of not less than 0.5 mm at 100 kVp.

Bucky Slot Shielding

Another aspect of fluoroscopic equipment specifications designed to minimize scattered radiation to personnel during fluoroscopy is that of the **Bucky slot shielding**. The shielding must be a part of the equipment and should be at least 0.25 mm lead equivalent, and about 5 cm wide "at the gonadal level" (Bushong 2013).

Mobile Radiographic Equipment

Most of the general design recommendations for fixed radiographic equipment (tube shielding, focal spot location, filtration, collimation, warning signs, indicator lights, meters, and exposure timing) apply equally as well to mobile radiographic equipment. For example, NCRP's (1989) recommendation for collimation in mobile radiography is as follows:

> Mobile radiographic equipment shall be equipped with adjustable collimators containing light localizers that define the border of the entire field. The difference between the length of each x-ray beam edge and each light field edge shall not be greater than two percent of the source-to-image receptor distance at the image receptor.

One specific requirement for mobile radiographic equipment that is fundamentally different from fixed radiographic equipment is that of the *exposure switch*. The NCRP (1989) recommendation is that:

> The exposure switch on mobile radiographic units shall be so arranged that the operator can stand at least 2 m (6 feet) from the patient, the x-ray tube, and the useful beam.

Recommendations for Personnel Practices

Personnel practices simply refer to the tasks in carrying out the x-ray examination that has been prescribed by the patient's physician. These practices are intended to protect both patients and personnel from unnecessary radiation. This section addresses the more common recommendations for patient and personnel protection, as well as the general guidelines for the reduction of gonadal dose.

Protection of Personnel

In protecting personnel from unnecessary radiation, the goal is to keep exposure below the recommended dose limits by observing the ALARA philosophy. Accomplishing this goal is guided by several recommendations, not only for operating the equipment but for performing the procedure as well. The following examples are noteworthy:

Persons in the X-Ray Room

All persons whose presence is not necessary to the procedure should be excluded from the x-ray room during the radiographic/fluoroscopic exposure. Those individuals whose presence is required must be protected by some form of shielding (protective lead aprons and gloves or mobile protective barriers).

Doors to X-Ray Rooms

When rooms are occupied by patients, all doors should be kept closed. Because doors to x-ray rooms are shielded with lead, they offer some degree of protection from x-rays to individuals outside the room who may be standing or passing in the vicinity of the doors at the time of the exposure.

Distance

Personnel must remain as far away as possible from the useful beam. Personnel must not be exposed to the useful beam. During mobile radiography, the operator must stand at least 2 m (6 ft) from the x-ray machine (including the x-ray tube) and the patient. In Canada, the recommended distance is 3 m (9 ft).

Holding Patients

The NCRP (1989) specifically recommends that:

> *No person should routinely hold patients during diagnostic examinations. When a patient must be held in position for radiography, a mechanical supporting or restraining device should be used. If such use of mechanical means is not possible or human support or restraint must be used, the individual holding the patient should be chosen so that cumulative doses will be held within acceptable limits. Pregnant women or persons under the age of 18 years should not be permitted to hold patients. If a patient must be held by someone, that individual shall be protected with appropriate shielding devices such as protective gloves and aprons. Positioning should be arranged so that no part of the holder's torso, even if covered by protective clothing, will be struck by the useful beam and so that the holder's body is as far as possible from the useful beam.*

Control Booth

All operators should be remaining in the control booth during the exposure. Operators must have an unobstructed view of the patient and be able to communicate with the patient without leaving the booth. In procedures in which operators must be at the patient's side, protective clothing must be worn.

Wearing Personnel Dosimeters

Personnel dosimeters are often worn at the level of the waist or upper chest level, beside the sternum (collar level) during the procedure. In fluoroscopy, when protective aprons are worn, the dosimeter should be worn outside the apron at the level of the collar, on the front of the body. In some cases, two dosimeters may be allowed when an apron is worn. The first one is worn at the collar level outside the apron, and the second one is worn at the waist level under the apron (Bushong 2013). Furthermore, a pregnant technologist should be issued a dosimeter worn under the apron to monitor the dose to conceptors (any product of conception, e.g., fetus, placenta, umbilical cord). It is interesting to note that Health Canada recommends that the dosimeter must be worn under the apron.

In procedures in which the extremities of operators are subject to high exposures, such as in angiography, it is recommended that additional dosimeters be worn on the extremity to monitor these exposures.

Protective Clothing

Protective clothing in this context refers to lead aprons, lead gloves, and thyroid shields, which are generally made of lead-impregnated vinyl and worn during fluoroscopic and some radiographic procedures. They are available in varying sizes and shapes and different lead-equivalent thicknesses. An important characteristic is the percentage attenuation afforded by each of the lead-equivalent thicknesses at different kVp values. It is clear that as the lead-equivalent thickness increases, the percentage attenuation increases for the same kVp value. For example, the percentage attenuation afforded by an apron of 0.5 mm lead-equivalent thickness is 75%, whereas it is 94% for an apron of 1-mm lead-equivalent thickness at 100 kVp (Bushong 2013). At 75 kVp, the percentage attenuation for a 0.25-mm and 0.5-mm lead-equivalent thickness is 66% and 88% respectively (Bushong 2013).

The NCRP (1989) recommends that:

> *Protective aprons of at least 0.5 mm lead equivalent shall be worn in the fluoroscopy room by each person (except the patient). People who must move around during the procedure should wear a wraparound protective garment.*

Protective gloves are used primarily when it is likely that the hands of operators (and those holding patients) will be exposed to the useful beam, or that they are in the immediate vicinity of the primary beam. Lead gloves of at least 0.25-mm lead equivalent must be worn to provide some degree of attenuation and thus protective hand

from radiation exposure. In this regard, the NCRP (1989) recommends that:

> *The hand of the fluoroscopist shall not be placed in the useful beam unless the beam is attenuated by the patient and a protective glove of at least 0.25 mm lead equivalent.*

The recommendations for protective aprons and gloves in Canada are at least 0.5-mm and 0.25-mm lead equivalent, respectively (Health Canada, 2008).

Thyroid shields are worn by individuals performing fluoroscopy, to protect the neck and thyroid gland from radiation exposure due to scatter. These shields are available commercially and provide attenuation equivalent to at least 0.5 mm of lead.

Protection of Patients

Diagnostic radiology contributes the highest man-made radiation exposure to the population; therefore, it is absolutely necessary to reduce the dose to patients without compromising the image quality required for the examination. This goal is also guided by several regulatory and advisory recommendations directed to the technologist, the radiologist, and to the patient's physician (who prescribes the x-ray examination), in an effort to minimize the radiation exposure.

There are several general recommendations to guide technologists and radiologists in carrying out the examination, and they relate to the factors affecting dose discussed elsewhere. Examples of these are as follows:

Exposure Technique Selection

Various radiation protection agencies advocate the use of the highest kVp, since high-kVp techniques result in a lower dose to patients compared to low-kVp techniques. Additionally, the use of the automatic exposure control (AEC) timing system is recommended to ensure that exposures and repeat examinations are kept to a minimum.

Filtration

Technologists should always ensure that the proper filtration is added to the imaging system and is consistent with the requirements of the particular examination. The total permanent filtration was stated earlier.

Collimation

The purpose of collimation is to protect the patient by limiting the primary beam to the anatomical area of interest. The recommendation for collimation implies that:

1. The beam must be collimated to the smallest area of interest consistent with the goals of the examination.

2. The beam must be collimated to the size of the image receptor or smaller.

3. Evidence of collimation should be seen on the image, that is, the edges of the useful beam should be visible on the image. This requirement ensures that only the area of interest has been exposed.

Collimation is under the direct control of the operator and every effort must be made to ensure correct collimation of the primary beam for every x-ray examination.

Source-to-Skin Distance (SSD)

In carrying out the examination, the operator should use the maximum SSD consistent with the requirements of the specific examination. Furthermore, the optimum source-to-image receptor distance should be used based on the requirements of the procedure.

Image Receptor Sensitivity

The dose to the patient is inversely proportional to the sensitivity of the image receptor. If the sensitivity is increased by a factor of 2, the dose will be reduced by ½. For film-screen imaging, going from a 200-speed system to a 400-speed system, reduces the dose to the patient by 50%. For digital radiography image receptors, see Chapter 9.

Immobilization

The use of immobilization is reflected in the recommendations for holding patients stating that restraining devices should be used.

Shielding

Protection of radiosensitive organs by lead shielding is a significant task of the technologist during the examination. The NCRP (1989) specifically recommends that the eyes and gonads be shielded from exposure to the primary beam. Recommendations for doing so are:

> *Sensitive body organs (e.g., lens of the eye, gonads) should be shielded whenever they are likely to be exposed to the useful beam provided that such shielding does not eliminate useful diagnostic information or proper treatment. Shielding should never be used as a substitute for adequate collimation.*
>
> *Comment: Gonadal shielding using at least 0.5 mm lead (usual lead equivalence of aprons) should be considered whenever potentially procreative patients are likely to receive direct gonadal radiation in an examination. The lens of the eye should be shielded (2 mm lead – usual eye shield thickness) during tomographic procedures that include the eye in the useful beam.*

Fluoroscopy

The recommendations for carrying out fluoroscopy relate to the factors affecting the dose in fluoroscopy. These recommendations are highlighted in NCRP Report 102 (1989). The interested reader should refer to this report for specific details relating to requirements for ensuring that the ALARA philosophy is upheld. These requirements fall in the domain of radiologists in general.

Recommendations for Radiography in Pregnancy

Carrying out an x-ray examination on pregnant women or women of childbearing age is a topic that demands a good deal of attention because of the increased radiation risks to the embryo or fetus (Bushong 2013; Bushberg et al. 2012; McCollough et al. 2007; ICRP 2000). The decision to irradiate pregnant patients rests with the patient's physician, usually in consultation with the radiologist. The technologist carries out the examination under the direct guidance of the radiologist. As noted by Bushberg et al. (2012),

> *Professional consensus is that in no cases should medical intervention with a pregnancy be considered for estimated doses to the embryo or fetus that do not exceed 100 mSv; if the dose exceeds 100 mSv, decisions would be guided by the fetal age and individual circumstances. All x-ray imaging examinations in which the embryo or fetus is not close to the area being imaged, impart doses much less that 100 mSv to the embryo or fetus and most x-ray examinations of the abdomen and pelvis, including single phase diagnostic CT examinations, impart doses less than 100 mSv.*

For radiography of pregnant women, the more common recommendations are usually centered around informed consent and understanding, and precautions to take before irradiation, during the examination, and after irradiation (ICRP 2000). Furthermore, recommendations are also related to the 10-day rule (explained below), elective examinations, pregnancy posters, shielding, collimation, and exposure technique factors, as well as the use of diagnostic ultrasound. In addition, there are several concerns regarding the pregnant technologist. Each of these will now be briefly highlighted.

Informed Consent and Understanding

The ICRP recommendation (in Publication 84 – *Pregnancy and Radiation*) in this regard states that "the pregnant patient or worker has a right to know the magnitude and type of potential radiation effects that might result from in-utero exposure" (ICRP 2000). With regards to the examination, the ICRP (2000) states that:

> *"Almost always, if a diagnostic radiology examination is medically indicated, the risk to the mother of not doing the procedure is greater than the risk of potential*

> *harm to the fetus. Radiation doses resulting from most diagnostic procedures present no substantial risk of causing fetal death, malformation, or impairment of mental development. If the fetus is in the direct beam, the procedure often can, and should be, tailored to reduce the fetal dose"*
> **Before x-ray examination**, it should be determined whether a patient is, or may be pregnant, whether the fetus will be in the direct beam, or whether the procedure is relatively high dose… **During the examination** when an examination is indicated in which the x-ray beam irradiates the fetus, and this cannot be delayed until after pregnancy, care should be taken to minimise the dose to the fetus… **After irradiation,** for diagnostic radiology, fetal dose estimation is usually not necessary, unless the fetus is in the direct beam. Evaluation of fetal doses from pelvic fluoroscopy is subject to more uncertainty than dose from palin film radiography or CT…

The 10-Day Rule

The goal of the so-called *10-day rule* was to prevent unintentional exposure of the embryo or fetus. These recommendations were stated by the ICRP (2000) and imply that if radiography of the abdomen or pelvis on women of childbearing age is needed, then it should be done during the 10 days following the onset of menstruation, because it is highly unlikely that a woman might be pregnant during this period. Bushong (2013) pointed out that this rule is "obsolete" in present day radiology practice (in light of the current knowledge of radiobiology); however, if pregnancy is confirmed and an x ray examination is needed, every effort must be made to reduce the exposure to the embryo or fetus.

Elective Examinations

An *elective examination* is one that is not urgently needed and can be done at any time suitable to the needs and safety of the patient. The NCRP (1989) recommends that:

> *Ideally, an elective abdominal examination of a woman of childbearing age should be performed during the first few days following the onset of menses to minimize the possibility of irradiation of an embryo. In practice, the timeliness of medical needs should be the primary consideration in deciding the timing of the examination…*

Pregnancy Posters

To avoid unnecessary radiation exposure of the embryo or fetus, signs or posters that seek to obtain pregnancy information from the patient should be made available. They should appear in areas of the department where they can be clearly seen (reception areas, changing rooms, x-ray rooms) by female patients who will be undergoing a radiographic/fluoroscopic or CT examination. The ICRP suggests the following example:

> IF IT IS POSSIBLE THAT YOU MIGHT BE PREGNANT, NOTIFY THE PHYSICIAN OR RADIOGRAPHER/TECHNICIAN BEFORE YOUR X-RAY EXAMINATION.

The Pregnant Worker

Bushong (2013) presents an excellent discussion of the issues and concerns surrounding the pregnant technologist. This topic is also treated in ICRP Publication 84 under the heading of "Management of Pregnant Physicians and Other Staff." In particular, the ICRP (2000) states that:

> *Once pregnancy has been declared, and the employer notified, additional protection of the fetus should be considered. The working conditions of a pregnant worker, after the declaration of pregnancy, should be as such to make it unlikely that the additional dose to the conceptus will exceed about 1 mGy during the remainder of pregnancy. In the interpretation of this recommendation, it is important not to create unnecessary discrimination against pregnant women. There are responsibilities*

on both the worker and the employer. The first responsibility for the protection of the conceptus lies with woman herself to declare her pregnancy to the management as soon as the pregnancy is confirmed…

The recommendation from Health Canada in Safety Code 35, with regards to the pregnant worker is as follows:

> *A female operator should immediately notify her employer upon knowledge that she is pregnant, in order that appropriate steps may be taken to ensure that her work duties during the remainder of the pregnancy are compatible with the recommended dose limits as stated in Appendix I. Depending on the type of facility and on the type of work being performed by the employee, it may not be necessary to remove a pregnant staff member from their duties of operating the x-ray equipment. It is recommended that the decision to remove pregnant workers from their duties include consideration of the radiation exposure risks associated with the employees duties, as determined by a medical physicist or a radiation safety officer…*

Appendix 1 in Health Canada Safety Code 35 states that

> *…for occupationally exposed women, once pregnancy has been declared, the foetus must be protected from x-ray exposure for the remainder of the pregnancy. For women who are also occupationally exposed, an effective dose limit of 4 mSv must be applied, for the remainder of the pregnancy, from all sources of radiation…*

Shielding, Collimation, and Exposure Technique

When a medical decision has been made to irradiate a pregnant patient, it is highly recommended that the technologist:

- Use high kVp techniques

- Collimate the primary beam effectively and accurately
- Place the gonadal shield precisely on the patient so as not to compromise the quality of the examination

Use of Diagnostic Ultrasound

The ICRP (2000) and other radiation protection organizations recommend that diagnostic ultrasound be used appropriately to provide obstetrical information as well as in situations where the dose in radiography might be high.

Recommendations for Quality Assurance

A QA program is an essential subset of a radiation protection program, because it is intended to monitor appropriate activities in a department, not only in an effort to reduce costs but more importantly, to maintain system components that play a significant role in dose-image quality optimization. QA encompasses administrative, educational, and preventive maintenance as well as quality control (QC) methods. QC deals specifically with the technical aspects of ensuring optimum image quality with reduced radiation doses.

Organizations such as the ICRP, NCRP, and Health Canada recommend that depending on their size, radiology departments should have a QA program in which case QC tests are performed on all radiographic and fluoroscopic equipment (including digital instrumentation), as well as the CT scanner. Whereas some of these tests are performed on a daily basis, others are done on a weekly, monthly, semi-annually, and annually. Examples of these QC tests include film/screen contact, kVp and timer accuracy, mA linearity, radiation output reproducibility, radiation output linearity, x-ray beam filtration, automatic exposure control, x-ray field and light field alignment, x-ray beam collimation, grid performance, exposure index, dynamic range, noise, uniformity, spatial resolution, contrast detectability, image intensifier air kerma rate, maximum image intensifier air kerma rate, CT number accuracy, CT radiation dose, electronic display device performance, and the integrity of protective equipment, to mention a few.

It is not within the scope of this book to describe QA/QC in any detail, since this is a topic for an entire course on QA/QC; however, an overview of the role of QA/QC in the optimization of radiation protection is presented elsewhere.

SUMMARY OF KEY CONCEPTS

1. This chapter presented a review of mandatory requirements for the design and performance of imaging equipment as well as advisory recommendations on the safe use of the equipment and procedures used to image patients. Furthermore, these guidelines and recommendations are also focussed on how to protect personnel and members of the public from unnecessary radiation exposure.

2. Two major groups that play active roles in terms of regulation and guidance to ensure optimization of radiation protection are *regulatory agencies* and *advisory bodies*, specific to each country. Examples of two such bodies are the International Commission on Radiological Protection (ICRP) and the National Council on Radiation Protection and Measurements (NCRP – a U.S. body).

3. This chapter highlights selected regulatory and guidance recommendations, including Code of Federal Regulations Title 21: Part 1020; the NCRP Report 102; and Safety Code 35 (Health Canada).

4. For optimization of radiation protection, it is essential to pay attention to education and training of staff, equipment specifications, personnel practices, and shielding.

5. General and specific design and performance recommendations for radiographic equipment, fluoroscopic radiographic equipment and mobile radiographic equipment were identified and highlighted.

6. For personnel practices, the protection aspects of personnel and for patients were highlighted.

(Continues)

7. The recommendations for radiography in pregnancy were highlighted in terms of informed consent and understanding, elective examinations, pregnancy posters, the pregnant worker, shielding, collimation, exposure technique, and the use of diagnostic ultrasound.

8. Finally the recommendations for quality assurance in diagnostic radiography were reviewed briefly.

Discussion Questions

1. Discuss the four ways that optimization of radiation protection can be accomplished, and explain the recommendations for Quality Assurance in diagnostic radiography.

2. Discuss the general and specific design and performance recommendations for radiographic, fluoroscopic, and mobile equipment.

3. Discuss the recommendations for the protection of patients and personnel, and for radiography of the pregnant patient and pregnant worker.

References

ASRT. Code of Ethics. Albuquerque, NM: American Society of Radiologic Technologists; 2013. (Available at www.asrt.org/main/standards-regulations/ethics. Retrieved August 30 2015.)

Bushberg JT, Seibert JA, Leidholdt Jr. EM, Boone JM. *The Essential Physics of Medical Imaging* (3rd ed.). Philadelphia: Wolters Kluwer/ Lippincott Williams & Wilkins; 2012.

Bushong S. *Radiologic Science for Technologist: Physics, biology and Protection* (10th ed.) St. Louis, MO: Elsevier-Mosby; 2013.

EPA. Title 42 USC 2021 (h): *Cooperation with States-Consultative, Advisory, and Miscellaneous Functions of the Administrator of Environmental Protection Agency.* Washington, DC: Government Publishing Office; 2012a. (Available at http://www.gpo.gov/fdsys/pkg/USCODE-2011-title42/html/USCODE-2011-title42-chap55.htm; Retrieved August 30, 2015.)

EPA. EPA-402R-10003: *Federal Guidance Report No 14. Radiation Protection Guidance for Diagnostic and Interventional X-Ray Procedures.* Washington, DC: Government Publishing Office; 2012b. (Available at http://www.gpo.gov/fdsys /granule/FR-2015-01-27/2015-01468; Retrieved August 30, 2015.)

FDA. Code of Federal Regulations Title 21: Part 1020 – *Performance Standards for Ionizing Radiation Emitting Products.* Section 1020.31 Radiographic Equipment and Section 1020.32 Fluoroscopic Equipment. Silver Spring, MD: US Food and Drug Administration; 2011. (Available at http://www.gpo.gov/fdsys/pkg/CFR-2011-title21-vol8/xml/CFR-2011-title21-vol8-part1020.xml; Retrieved August 30, 2015.)

Health Canada. *Safety Code 35: Radiation Protection in Radiology – Large Facilities. Safety Procedures for the Installation, Use and Control of X-Ray Equipment in Large Medical Radiological Facilities.* Ottawa: Health Canada; 2008. (Available at http://www.hc-sc.gc.ca/ewh-semt /pubs/radiation/safety-code_35-securite/index-eng.php; Retrieved August 30, 2015.)

International Commission on Radiological Protection (ICRP). *Protection of the Patient in Diagnostic Radiology.* Elmsford, NY: Pergamon Press; 1982.

ICRP. *Pregnancy and Medical Radiation.* ICRP Publication 84. *Ann ICRP.* 2000;30(1).

ICRP. *Education and Training in Radiological Protection for Diagnostic and Interventional Procedures.* ICRP Publication 113. *Ann ICRP* 2009;39(5).

McCollough CH, Scheuler B, Atwell TD, Braun NN, Regner DM, et al. Radiation exposure and pregnancy: when should we be concerned? *Radiographics,* 2007;27:909–918.

National Council on Radiation Protection and Measurements (NCRP). *Medical X-Ray, Electron Beam and Gamma Ray Protection for Energies up to 50 MeV: Equipment Design, Performance and Use.* Report 102. Bethesda, MD: NCRP; 1989.

Statkiewicz-Sherer MA, Visconti PJ, Ritenour ER. *Radiation Protection in Medical Radiography.* (7th Ed.) Maryland Heights, MO: Mosby Elsevier; 2014.

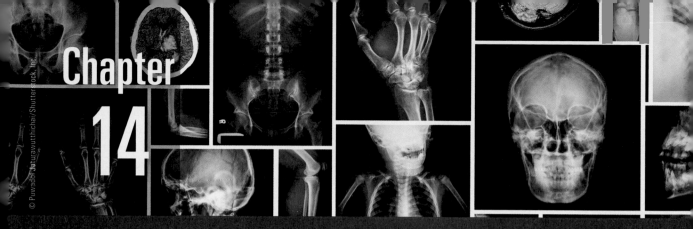

Chapter 14

Protective Shielding in Diagnostic Radiology

Outline

- Introduction
- X-ray Tube Shielding
- X-ray Room Shielding
  - Radioprotective materials
  - General principles
  - Primary and secondary barriers
- How is The Amount of Shielding Calculated?
  - Occupancy factor
  - The formulae
  - The planning process
- References

Objectives

On completion of this chapter, you should be able to:

1. Describe the nature and characteristics of x-ray tube shielding.
2. Discuss the characteristics of materials needed for shielding the x-ray room.
3. Discuss the general principles of x-ray room shielding.
4. Explain other determining features needed for x-ray room shielding.
5. Discuss the difference between primary and secondary barriers.
6. Describe how the shielding requirements for an x-ray room are calculated.
7. Discuss the requirements necessary when planning x-ray room shielding.

Introduction

Each radiation exposure in diagnostic radiology carries with it a risk of inducing a biological change that might result in a cancer. According to the Linear No-Threshold (LNT) Model, the risk is proportional to dose, and therefore, each time an exposure takes place, we attempt to keep the dose *as low as reasonably achievable* (ALARA). While the emphasis so far has been on looking at radiologic methods, technologies, and strategies that minimize dose, it is equally important that x-ray tubes and the rooms in which they are located are properly protected so that patients who are having their abdomen examined, for example, do not inadvertently have other body parts irradiated, that patients and relatives in waiting room environments are not exposed and that staff doses are kept to a minimum. All this requires appropriate radiation shielding and thoughtful room designs.

The focus of this chapter is to consider all those radiation protection structures that are required to be in place when a new x-ray room is being installed. In particular, the discussions will be around x-ray tube shielding and x-ray room shielding; radioprotective materials; primary and secondary shielding; how shielding levels are calculated, looking at both the formulae and the factors involved; and the planning process for constructing a shielded room.

There is one particular text that the authors of this book will often refer to in this chapter and recommend that anyone involved in acquiring x-ray room should access. This is NCRP *Report 147: Structural Shielding Design for Medical X-ray Facilities* (2004). It carefully examines the principles and major considerations of shielding and gives practical examples to the reader. While some of this chapter may be of most use to radiology managers planning new or altered imaging departments, the material discussed should serve as a useful reference text where some of the principles previously discussed in the book are applied in a real world situation.

X-Ray Tube Shielding

X-ray tube design is the first stage of shielding within the x-ray room. First, a reminder of the layout of an x-ray tube. In **Figure 14-1**, we can see the arrangement of the anode and the x-rays emerging from the target.

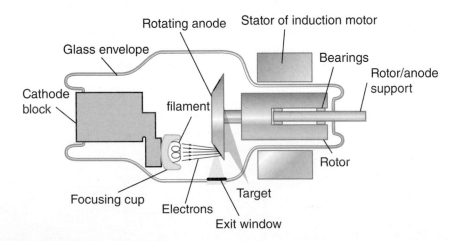

Figure 14-1 Diagram of the x-ray tube.

While a number of these x-rays are directed towards the exit window and will ultimately reach the area of interest on the patient, some x-rays could emerge from the x-ray tube and interact with the patient at some distance away from the area of interest and indeed lead to irradiation of staff and anyone who is needed to stay with the patient. Such exposures are unacceptable; therefore, the x-ray tube is designed with carefully placed shielding to ensure that x-rays only emerge from the x-ray window, otherwise known as the *x-ray tube port*.

Review (**Figure 14-2**).

In this picture, one can see that lead has now been arranged within the tube housing. This means that (in theory) the vast majority of the radiation is emitted only through the tube port while the other (misdirected) radiation is absorbed. This means that the radiographer or radiologists now can feel much more confident that the area of interest is the *only* area being irradiated.

The word *only* is italicized to bring attention to a principle regarding radiation shielding, since really my usage of the word is not strictly correct in this context. Elsewhere, we discussed the attenuation of x-rays and how materials placed in the x-ray path could reduce the intensity of x-rays being emitted, introducing the concept of the **half-value layer**. The half value layer simply is the thickness of attenuation (such as aluminum) that would reduce the original intensity of radiation by half, so for example a 5-mm-thick aluminum sheet might reduce the intensity of the radiation to a half of the original level, and an additional 5 mm would further reduce the radiation amount to one-quarter of the original (**Figure 14-3**).

However what this means is that *equal amounts of attenuating materials reduces the level of radiation by equal fractions*, thus demonstrating the exponential nature of x-ray attenuation (**Figure 14-4**). In other words, *attenuating*

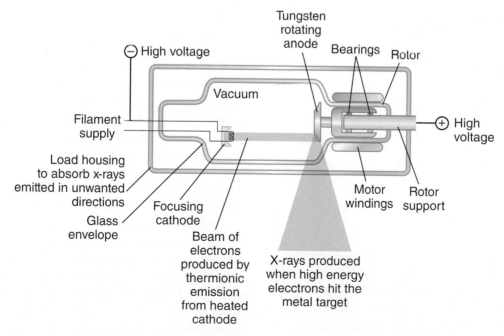

Figure 14-2 Note the lead shielding in place, making sure that the radiation is only emitted through the exit window.
Courtesy of Patrick C. Brennan.

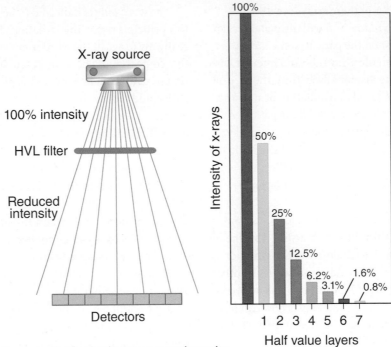

Figure 14-3 The impact of half-value layers on x-ray intensity.

Courtesy of Patrick C. Brennan.

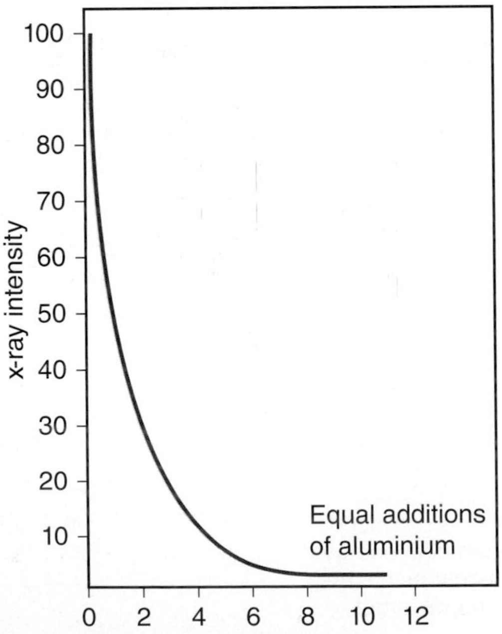

Figure 14-4 Exponential graph. Note for equal additions of aluminum (x axis), we end up with fractional reductions in x-ray intensity (y axis). Note that the x-ray intensity never reaches zero.

Courtesy of Patrick C. Brennan.

materials or shielding cannot reduce the radiation to absolutely zero, it can only reduce it to amount that is considered acceptably low.

Obviously, the more shielding we add, the lower the levels of radiation being transmitted, but ultimately there is a limit to the level of shielding that can be employed in terms of size, weight, and cost, and therefore, some level of radiation (albeit very low) is generally transmitted. This stresses the need for regular monitoring of this transmitted radiation to ensure that it does not become excessive.

This fundamental nature of x-ray shielding is relevant throughout this chapter and is demonstrated by the x-ray tube. To test this *x-ray leakage*, one can measure the level of radiation escaping through the shielding using a dosimeter placed at 1 meter from various parts of the x-ray tube housing with the collimator *closed* (indeed, there are measuring devices that allow x-ray tube leakage to be measured at 18 locations at any one time; however, most of us will have to simply repeat the experiment at several locations). Exposures are usually performed at the maximum rated continuous tube current, which according to the International Atomic Energy Agency is 3–5 mAs at 150 kVp and the radiation amount that should escape should not be any more than 1 mGy per hour (the NCRP [2004] sets it at 0.876 mGy per hour) and is usually below 0.5 mGy per hour. While this dose is very low (over a long period), it does demonstrate that shielding does not eliminate radiation transmission. It has been calculated that to achieve this level of shielding, 2.3 mm of lead is required.

Finally, with regard to tube shielding, one should consider the efficacy of the collimation device. If the aim of the shielding is that only the patient's area of interest is irradiated, accurate collimation is also fundamentally important to achieving this aim. The collimation arrangement relies on producing light that simulates the area of exposure, thus facilitating careful control of the irradiated area; however this in turn relies on the light accurately representing the radiation. If the illuminated area on the patient is smaller than the x-ray field, excessive radiation may be present. If the illuminated area on the patient is larger than the x-ray field, smaller, important body parts may be omitted from the image. There is a test whereby one can examine whether the illuminated area matches the irradiation field by irradiating a test tool (**Figure 14-5**).

In this test, one collimates the light to the rectangular perimeter (which is radio-opaque) shown in the figure and then looks at the resultant image to check the level of agreement between the light and the radiation, which should be no more than 1–2% of the source-to-receptor distance (SRD). For example, if a 100 cm SRD is being employed, the misalignment in any direction should not be greater than 1–2 cm. One additional feature of this test is that one should perform a very low exposure of the whole tool before the test exposure. This ensures that in the situation where the radiation field is smaller than the illuminated area, the radio-opaque perimeter is actually seen on the image!

X-Ray Room Shielding

Radioprotective Materials

Shortly we will discussing the construction of walls and doors, etc., and how the layout of the room is designed in such a way to minimize radiation leakage and maximize protection to patients, staff, and any other individuals in the vicinity. However, it is worth running through the type of materials that are used, which includes lead, gypsum wall board, concrete, and barium plaster (NCRP 2004; Dowsett et al. 2006).

Lead

Lead is the standard material used for x-ray walls. Its high atomic number of 82 means that it can attenuate x-rays relatively effectively compared with other materials, such as barium (atomic number: 56). This means that it can come in relatively thin sheets and therefore can offer effective protection in a non-bulky way. The cost of lead is dependent on its thickness, with a 3.17-mm thick sheet costing about 3 times more than a 0.79-mm sheet, with the latter costing roughly $200 US for a roll of 30 cm × 7.5 m at the time of writing. Weight is another consideration, since lead is heavy, and for the thicker sheet (3.17 mm) the weight is approximately 40 kg per square meter (8 pounds per square foot). Clearly, the quality of lead that can be purchased will vary, so one should be careful that the lead being acquired meets the local or national standards.

Lead is usually applied to the internal section of an x-ray room's internal walls (**Figure 14-6**). It is

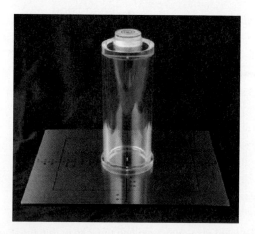

Figure 14-5 Collimator test tool.
Courtesy of Patrick C. Brennan.

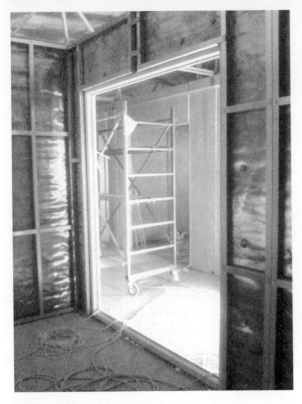

Figure 14-6 Lead being applied to the internal wall of an x-ray room.
Courtesy of Patrick C. Brennan.

either glued to a gypsum wallboard or sandwiched between pieces of wood, then nailed or screwed on (with the lead innermost if glued to gypsum). Since the nails or screws usually have at least the same level of attenuation as lead, as long as they have been introduced carefully to ensure no cracking of the lead, attenuation around these puncture holes should be minimum.

Whenever services penetrate the wall, as is needed for air conditioning and water pipes, lead will be used to baffle these penetrations to makes sure that the original protection offered by the wall is maintained. Extra attenuation must be made at junctions between lead sheets and where other joints exist with a level of overlap not be less than 1 cm. When lead is applied to doors, distinct overlap between the door, the door's frame, and the wall should be apparent (**Figure 14-7**).

Lead can also come in the form of lead glass, which is commonly used as mobile or fixed protective shielding for the radiographer or radiologist. It has the advantage of being transparent and indeed looks like normal glass (**Figure 14-8**); however, it is quite fragile and susceptible to cracking and chipping.

An alternative to lead glass is transparent lead acrylic, which, while not offering the same level of

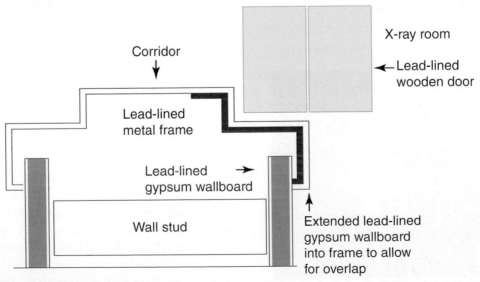

Figure 14-7 Diagrammatic illustration of lead lining. Note the level of overlap between the lead within the door, the door's frame, and the wall.
Courtesy of Patrick C. Brennan.

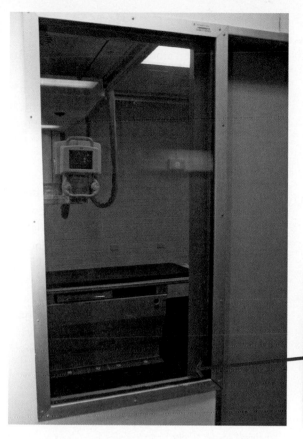
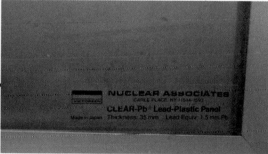

Figure 14-8 A lead glass window used in a typical x-ray room.
Courtesy of Patrick C. Brennan.

protection as glass at the same level of thickness, is lighter, stronger, and easier to install. It can be used in low-energy applications such as mammography or dental radiologic clinics.

Lead protection is quoted in *mm of lead equivalent* at specific beam energies, and for walls and glass this can vary from 1–10 mm at the type of energies used in diagnostic radiology.

Gypsum Wallboard

Gypsum wallboard, which is commonly known as plaster board, gib board, or dry wall (**Figure 14-9**), can be used in the construction of walls. It is made from calcium sulphate that has been mixed with paper fiber or fiberglass and then sandwiched between paper sheets of 1-mm thickness. It comes in thicknesses of between 9.5 mm and 15 mm, and while it has some attenuation qualities, the atomic

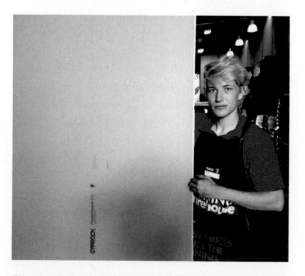

Figure 14-9 Gypsum wall boards.
Courtesy of Patrick C. Brennan.

number of its main attenuative component, calcium (20), would suggest that its main function is to absorb the lower radiation energies and therefore can be very useful in mammography.

When applied as mentioned above to the back of lead, the gypsum should be placed on the external side, since this can help absorb any of the characteristic radiation produced in lead following interactions with x-rays.

Concrete

Concrete is often used for load-bearing ceilings and floors (as well as walls) as it can offer strength as well as radioprotective properties. Its main ingredient is calcium silicate, so again, calcium is being relied on as the main attenuative feature; however, since the atomic number of calcium is much lower than lead, the thickness required of concrete to achieve the same level of attenuation as lead is much higher. For example, a layer of concrete 25-cm thick is required to achieve the same level of attenuation as 4 mm of sheet lead, and this is why a combination of lead and concrete may be required for walls if the required thickness of concrete alone is too bulky. Density of the material is also critically important, and satisfactory attenuation with concrete can be achieved at 147 pounds per cubic foot (2350 kg per cubic meter). Light-weight concrete through the introduction of an approximately 25% reduced density or empty spaces known as voids will not offer the same level of protection.

An alternative to concrete are clay bricks; however, these can have a density up to 30% less than the density on concrete stated above, which means that thicker walls will be required if bricks are being used. With all these building materials (concrete or bricks), one must take note if they have voids or empty spaces within them, as obviously this will impact importantly on radio-attenuation properties.

With all these building materials, the level of specifications can vary substantially, so full details of materials to be used such as the density and the presence of internal empty spaces must be provided by the manufacturer to ensure that the appropriate shielding calculations are made.

Barium Plaster

Barium is a useful property for attenuation purposes, having an atomic number of 56. Barium can be embedded as baryte aggregates within gypsum-based plaster. It is often used in the form of a plastering layer over the internal wall, but must be applied with great care and expertise at thicknesses of up to 25 mm.

General Principles

Before we get into the shielding calculations aimed at minimizing dose, a number of overarching principles have been made clear by the NCRP (2004), which are worth summarizing here. The author would like to stress that while regulations and arrangements may vary from country to country, it is beyond the scope of this text to summarize all arrangements, therefore the main focus here is on the information provided by the NCRP in *Report 147: Structural Shielding Design for Medical X-ray Imaging Facilities* (2004). Within that text, the shielding goal is clear and explicit. It is as follows: *That the air kerma value for a controlled and uncontrolled area is no greater than 0.1 mGy and 0.02 mGy per week respectively.*

Definitions of controlled and uncontrolled are given within the next section.

Definitions

All areas within a clinic or medical center that houses radiation-based facilities are divided into controlled or uncontrolled areas. A ***controlled area*** is where there is limited worker access to the area and only those individuals with special training, such as medical physicists, radiographers, and radiologists, are allowed to enter. These areas include the x-ray rooms and exposure selection areas. All individuals working in these areas are under the supervision of a person trained to be in charge of radiation protection and each should not receive a dose greater than 5 mGy per year. All other areas within the clinic or medical center are ***uncontrolled areas*** and are occupied by patients, non-radiologic staff, and visitors, and here the annual dose limit is 1 mGy. From these figures, we can arrive at the *weekly* shielding goal for both areas as stated at the start of this section—simply divide 5 mGy and 1 mGy by 50.

Primary radiation is that radiation that has emerged from the x-ray tube that has yet to be attenuated, thus requiring a primary barrier (**Figure 14-10**). **Secondary radiation** is scattered radiation and requires a secondary barrier.

Other factors that have impact on decision-making with respect to shielding include:

- The leakage of the x-ray tube may not exceed the regulatory limit, which as stated above for the NCRP is 0.876 mGy per hour.
- The patient attenuates x-rays between a factor of 10 and 100; however, patient attenuation is usually not used in calculations.
- Radiation interacts with walls or barriers at right angles.
- Any future changes in equipment type, radiation use, and occupancy should be considered when planning the installation, as retrospective changes to the shielding can be awkward and expensive.

Shielding calculations are conservative, meaning that resultant shielding values are on the high side. Some of the sources of such conservative calculations are:

- The field size and phantom size employed for scatter calculations are up two 4 times higher than those typically used.
- High occupancy periods are used, for example within an uncontrolled area.
- The minimum distance of a person within a shielded area to an occupied wall is 0.3 m (Figure 14-10).
- Certain materials in the x-ray room that could contribute to reducing radiation transmission such as cabinets, lead rubber aprons, etc. are not included in calculations.

Other Determining Features

There are other features determined by the varying practices and equipment used in different types of x-ray rooms that will also have a major impact on the shielding calculations. These features include:

The Output of the X-Ray Equipment Employed
The upper limit can vary from approximately 150 kVp in a general room to 35 kVp with mammography.

The Type of Exposures
In a general room, the exposures are usually very short in duration and performed at varying

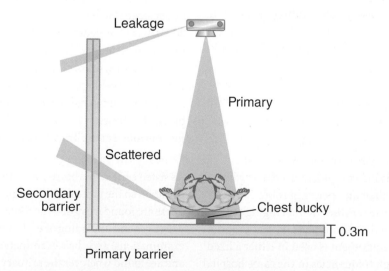

Figure 14-10 A diagram demonstrating certain principles of the shielding calculations.
Courtesy of Patrick C. Brennan.

frequencies per hour—perhaps up to 30–50 exposures per hour in a busy chest room. This is in contrast to interventional or CT facilities, where the exposures are much more prolonged and continuous with subsequently higher overall outputs.

The Movement of the X-Ray Tube

In a general or interventional room, the tube can be rotated in a number of directions—unlike a dedicated chest room, where all the radiation will be directed towards one wall via an image receptor. Whenever a wall is directly irradiated, this becomes a primary barrier.

The Relationship Between the X-Ray Source and the Receptor

In fluoroscopy, such as in the barium room, the relationship between the tube and the receptor is fixed, which means that the latter always interacts with the primary beam and serves as a primary barrier. This is also the case in modern mammography units, which means that for both fluoroscopy and mammography, only further secondary barriers are normally required, which is not the case for other x-ray facilities.

The Relationship Between the Operator of the Equipment and the Patient

In a general room, the operator is always performing the exposures behind a control booth, which thus requires a permanent structure serving as a console to operate the equipment but also as a secondary (never primary) barrier. In a fluoroscopic or interventional situation, the clinician is often positioned close to the patient.

The Mobility of the X-Ray Equipment

X-ray equipment such as that used for chest x-rays or intensifying equipment used in cardiac catheterization lab or an operating room can be brought to the patient rather than bringing the patient to protected environments with appropriate shielding. If the equipment is used in either a fixed location or in high frequencies in the same hospital environment, the need for structural shielding will need to be examined.

Primary and Secondary Barriers

Before we get into the main features used for calculating thicknesses, it is important to be clear about the two main types of barriers that are employed to protect individuals from the radiation produced within an x-ray room: primary and secondary barriers. As mentioned above very briefly, the primary barrier is aimed towards attenuating primary radiation (that is, previously unattenuated x-rays), while the secondary barrier is focused towards scattered radiation. Both barriers aim to achieve the same overall goal of protective shielding: Ensuring that the air kerma value for a controlled and uncontrolled area is no greater than 0.1 mGy and 0.02 mGy per week, respectively. As stated before this level of radiation is relevant to the nearest possible occupancy, which is assumed to be 0.3 m, 0.5 m, and 1.7 m from the shielded wall in adjacent rooms (on the same floor), above the floor for rooms above and above the floor for rooms below respectively (**Figure 14-11**).

To put the level of shielding that must be required to achieve our shielding goal (0.1 mGy/week or 0.02 mGy per week), it may be useful to consider the average value for the *unattenuated* primary beam at a distance of 1 m from the x-ray tube in a general room. Using the workload distribution figures described below, the air kerma per patient would be considered to be approximately 5.2 mGy (NCRP 2004). In a busy general room, it would be anticipated that 160 patients per week would be x-rayed, resulting in an air kerma of 832 mGy/week. Clearly, to achieve the weekly goals stated earlier, the shielding and distance must reduce this value approximately by a factor between 10,000 (controlled area) to 50,000 (uncontrolled area). This is not an insignificant task.

Primary Barrier

As stated earlier, this barrier will attenuate primary radiation so the protective shielding goal is achieved. These are found in most x-ray rooms such as those where general (including or excluding fluoroscopic examinations) and chest examinations are performed and are found wherever the primary radiation can be directed toward, such as the wall supporting an erect Bucky, the floor supporting an x-ray table, or any other

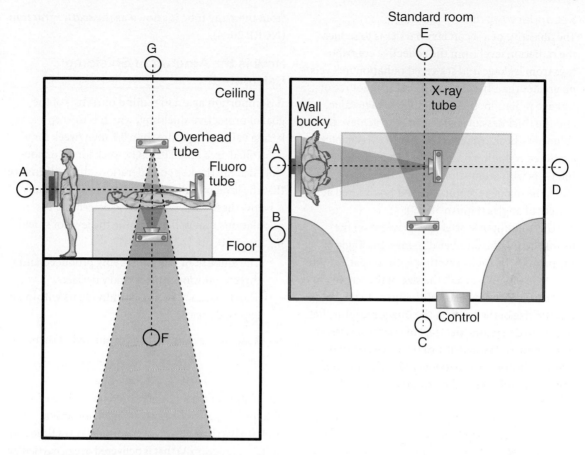

Figure 14-11 The distances from the x-ray room walls, ceiling, or floor for rooms adjacent to and on the same floor as the x-ray room (A–E), rooms on the floors immediately below (G) and rooms immediately above (F), which are used to define the shielding goals.

Courtesy of Patrick C. Brennan.

wall that may even occasionally interact with the primary beam. Since interventional facilities, dedicated fluoroscopy, and mammography units are required to have image receptors or support trays that act as attenuators for primary beams, normally only secondary barriers are required with these facilities; however, it would be prudent to check that the primary beam attenuation does actually take place effectively.

There is, however, a concept known as **preshielding** that a qualified expert can choose to include (or not) within his or her calculations. This is the level of shielding which can be stated in lead equivalent offered by the x-ray table, secondary radiation grids, x-ray receptors, and so forth; however, these may or

may not serve as effective barriers depending on the level of collimation, thus complicating the qualified expert's decision. In practice, when a table is being used for an examination where the x-rays are directed *vertically* towards the floor, preshielding may be used in the calculations; however, for lateral examinations on the table with a horizontal beam, preshielding may not be used, as the cassette is unlikely to consistently attenuate the whole beam. Obviously, one effective source of preshielding is the patient, who can reduce the radiation by a factor of 10–100; however, since the patient may not absorb the total x-ray beam, usually the safer approach of not including the patient absorption in the calculations is employed.

Secondary Barrier

The objective of a secondary barrier is to reduce the radiation level from the collective contribution from leakage *and* scattered radiation to levels no greater than the shielding goal. The source of leakage radiation, the acceptable leakage value, and the thickness of lead required to achieve these value have been discussed earlier in this chapter. Scattered radiation occurs when the primary beam interacts with attenuators such as the patient, the table, the image receptor, etc. and is scattered at a variety of angles (**Figure 14-12**).

The amount of scatter is dependent on the beam energy, the number of x-rays, the angle of the primary beam interacting with the patient, the part of the body x-rayed, the size of the patient, and the size of the x-ray field. With regard to the latter, it is the size of the beam at the image receptor that is used to determine the level of scatter. The level of scatter is measured at 1 m from the center of the primary beam at the patient, and the ratio between this value and that of the primary beam at 1 m

X-ray source

—Primary radiation

—Scatter radiation

Recording medium (digital plate or film)

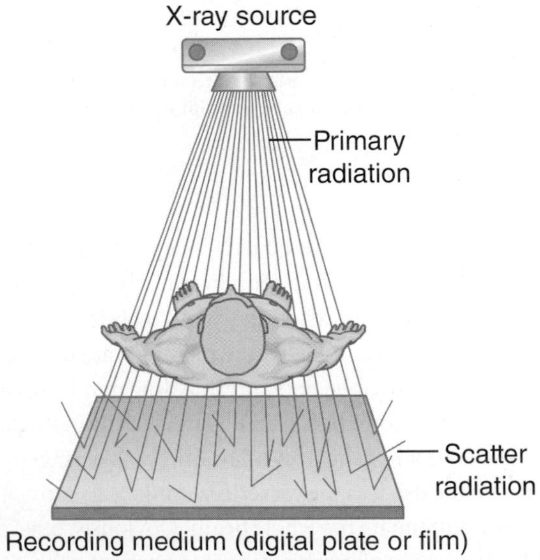

Figure 14-12 Diagram demonstrating primary and scattered radiation shown following a patient exposure.
Courtesy of Patrick C. Brennan.

from the x-ray tube is known as the *scatter fraction* (NCRP 2004).

How is the Amount of Shielding Calculated?

It is important again to remind ourselves of the goal of protective shielding, which is to keep the air kerma value to no more than 0.1 mGy/week for a controlled area and 0.02 mGy/week for an uncontrolled area. The key considerations that will ensure that the level of radiation received by individuals is below these values, and hence determine the calculations that will determine the level of shielding required, are (NCRP 2004):

- The amount of radiation being produced and directed towards the primary barriers.
- The occupancy period of individuals within an exposed area.

These two factors will be considered in turn.

The Amount of Radiation Being Produced and Directed Towards Primary Barriers

Calculation of the amount of radiation delivered by a specific piece of x-ray equipment towards a primary barrier relies on the combination of time and milliamperage (mA) that is delivered over a particular period of time, often a week, and is expressed as mA-min/week. From this value the air kerma at 1 m from the x-ray source can be calculated if the kVp is known. It can be useful to define the average workload per patient, which facilitates the following formula:

$$\text{Workload total} = \text{number of patients (e.g., per week)} \times \text{average workload per patient}$$

In the calculations demonstrated in NCRP 147 (2004) and in this chapter, this formula will be used, although this formula can be modified to suit particular circumstances such as the introduction of digital technology, which can affect, for example, the workload per patient. Also, if there are two x-ray devices in a room, say a dedicated chest unit and a general unit, and a patient is x-rayed with both, then the average workload per patient is divided appropriately across these two units.

The whole process of calculating the amount of radiation directed towards specific barriers over specific period of time is a complex one; however, here we will try to move through this in a staged approach consisting of the following main stages:

- Calculating workload per patient;
- Calculating workload per week;
- Calculating the fraction of workload per week directed towards specific barriers.

Stage 1. Calculating Average Workload Per Patient

From the above, it can be seen that the kVp selection needs to be known for the calculation of the air kerma produced at 1 m from the x-ray tube. In the past, this was based fairly conservatively at the single value of 100 kVp; however, this approach is questionable, since tube potentials vary enormously—say, for a finger versus a chest examination—and the dose behind shielding is highly dependent on beam energy. A survey performed by the American Association of Physicists in Medicine in 1996 (Simpkin 1996) showed for non-chest x-ray examinations that there was a wide distribution of kVps being employed across the varying mA-min, with the median of this distribution being well below 100 kVp (**Figure 14-13**); this type of distribution has a major impact on the radiation levels transmitted through an x-ray shield (**Figure 14-14**).

It was subsequently proposed by the NCRP to use two types of kVp distributions when performing these calculations: One for those beams directed to the chest stand and another for those directed to the floor or other structures. The varying mA-min normalized *per patient* across a variety of room types (e.g., chests, general, fluoroscopy, interventional, mammography, etc.) are tabulated in the NCRP publication (2004) for a variety of kVp settings, which is then summed to a total workload figure *per patient* that can be used for assessing shielding requirements. Examples of such workloads are 1.9 mA-min for general room (not including the chest Bucky exposures), 0.22 mA-min

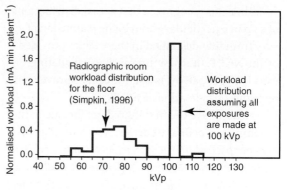

Figure 14-13 Workload distribution of examinations directed towards the floor of an x-ray room (thus not erect chests). One can see that the median value of this distribution is well below the single previously recommended value of 100 kVp.

Courtesy of Patrick C. Brennan.

for a dedicated chest room and 160 mA-min for cardiac angiography. Throughout this section of the text, we are going to use these three types of rooms to show how the calculations are performed.

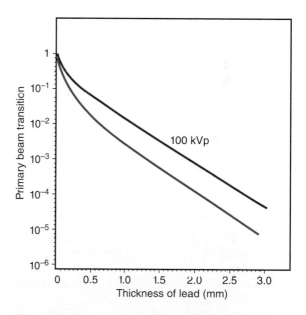

Figure 14-14 The transmitted level of primary beam transmission using varying thicknesses of lead using the 100 kVp (red curve) assumption and typical distributions of kVps (blue curve). The reduction in the level of transmission is apparent with the latter.

Courtesy of Patrick C. Brennan.

While it is recognized that actual distributions of kVp in a particular room being planned may vary from that described in these tables provided by the NCRP, this new approach to calculating workload per patient is a significant improvement on using a single value of 100 kVp.

We now have the first ingredient for calculating shielding to a primary barrier: *Normalized workload per patient in mA-min (calculated from distributions of workload across different kVps) allowing the calculation of (unshielded) air kerma per patient at 1 meter from the source.*

Stage 2. Calculating Total Workload Per Week
While we now have the workload per patient for different room situations available to us, the next stage is to get a value of workload per week, and to do this (in addition to the workload per patient), we need to know the number of patients per week. The NCRP give values for the different types of x-ray rooms ranging from 120 to 160 for a general room (not including the chest Bucky exposures), 200 to 400 for a dedicated chest room, and 20 to 30 for cardiac angiography for average and busy times respectively.

We now have the second ingredient for calculating shielding to a primary barrier: *Number of patients per week, which as you will see below can be used to arrive at workload per week.*

Now that we have these values for number of patients per week, this can for each type of x-ray activity be multiplied by the workload per patient to calculate the workload per week. These calculations are summarized in **Table 14-1**. From the table it can be seen that the workload per patient is a highly powerful factor, since for cardiac angiography while the number of patients per week is around 10% of the number in the chest room, the total workload per week (due to the high workload per patient) is around 50 times higher.

Stage 3. Calculating the Fraction of Workload Per Week Directed Towards Primary Barriers
While we now have the workload per week, it must be acknowledged that for particular activities—say, examinations in a general room or in a dedicated chest room—the fraction of the primary beam that is directed towards the primary barrier can vary. This fraction is known as the **use factor**. For example, in a dedicated chest room, the beam is always directed towards the chest Bucky, and therefore 100% of the usage is towards the primary barrier behind the chest Bucky arrangement (**Figure 14-15**) and the relevant wall.

We say here that the use factor = 1. With the general room, the x-ray tube, while a lot of the time is directed towards the floor, can be orientated in a number of different directions (**Figure 14-16**), and so the situation is more complicated.

Again the work of Simpkin (1996a), summarized in the NCRP Report No. 147 has provided these use factor values for us which for a general room (excluding the chest Bucky exposures) is 0.89 towards the floor, 0.09 towards the wall beside the table, and 0.02 to other unspecified walls.

Table 14-1

X-ray room	Workload/patient (mA-min)	Patients/ per week (a)	(b)	Workload/week (mA-min) (a)	(b)
General*	1.9	120	160	240	320
Chest	0.22	200	400	50	100
Cardiac angiography	160	20	30	3200	4800

Key: * Does not include chest Bucky exposures.

The table demonstrates the numbers required to calculate the workload per week. The final numbers are arrived at by multiplying the workload per patient by the number of patients for the average (a) and busy weeks (b). Note that while the patients per week in the cardiac angiography is much lower than in the chest room, the workload per week is much higher (NCRP 2004).

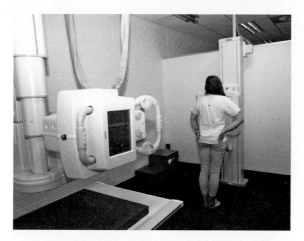

Figure 14-15 The situation presented is simulating a dedicated chest room. The x-ray tube (in theory) is directed towards the chest buck and the wall direct behind the Bucky 100% of the time—thus, a use factor of 1.

Courtesy of Patrick C. Brennan.

We now have the third ingredient for calculating shielding to a primary barrier: *The fraction of workload per week that is directed towards the primary barrier.*

Occupancy Factor

In determining the level of barrier that is required, so far we have been focusing on what has been going on within the x-ray room, i.e., the workload

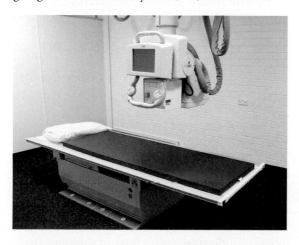

Figure 14-16 This x-ray tube, while directing x-rays toward the floor for a large part of the time, may be oriented in a number of other directions.

Courtesy of Patrick C. Brennan.

per patient, the number of patients per week, and the amount of the primary beam that is directed towards a primary barrier. However, one must also deal with what is going on in adjacent rooms, if ultimately shielding is aiming to reduce radiation dose to the shielding goal previously described. One important factor therefore is how much are these rooms occupied. This is known as the occupancy factor and is the fraction of time that the **person who will be exposed the most** is present when the x-ray beam is on. You will note that again a conservative approach is in order where the focus is on the person who is exposed the most—in other words, the person who spends the most time there. As explained by the NCRP (2004), while a waiting room may be full at all times, the occupancy factor will be low, since the people are changing all the time, in contrast with a room occupied by a single booking clerk, who might be working there up to 40 hours per week.

The NRCP has published suggested occupancy factors for a variety of locations (2004). Examples of these are shown in **Table 14-2**.

It should be stressed that occupancy factors, particularly those <1.0, are based on a number of assumptions that may change from time to time. It also stresses the importance of letting the shielding

Table 14-2 The NRCP has published suggested occupancy factors for a variety of locations (2004)

Location	Occupancy factors
Controlled area	1.0
Adjacent locations not under the control of the radiologic facility	1.0
Administrative office	1.0
Image reading office	1.0
Reception	1.0
Patient treatment room	0.5
Coffee lounges	0.2
Bathrooms	0.05
Unattended parking areas	0.025

NCRP 2004.

expert know of any future plans for the vicinity of the x-ray room that may change the occupancy calculations.

The Formulae

At this stage, the readers should be familiar with the goals of x-ray shielding along with the factors that are used to calculate the level of shielding required. Just as a reminder from the above, it is clear that of fundamental importance to these calculations are the following factors:

- Average workload per patient which will determine the average air kerma per patient
- The number of patients being x-rayed per week
- The use factor, that is the allocation of exposures in a room directed towards individual barriers
- The occupancy factor

These factors are now assembled into formulae to allow shield calculations to be for the primary and secondary barrier will be different, due to the different types of radiation directed to each of these.

Once again before the formulae are presented, let's yet again revisit our shielding goal: *That the air kerma value for a controlled and uncontrolled area is no greater that 0.1 mGy and 0.02 mGy per week, respectively.*

Therefore the aim of a barrier is to reduce the air kerma to these values, but taking into consideration factors introduced by the occupancy of the area being shielded. To achieve this we must have an appreciation of the barrier's beam transmission function [$B(x)$], which is the ratio of air kerma in a specific location behind a barrier to the air kerma in the same location if the barrier was not there. An acceptable barrier thickness achieves the following:

$$B(x_{barrier}) = (P/T) \times d^2/(K^1 \times N)$$

Where $B(x)$ is the barrier's transmission function, *barrier* is acceptable barrier thickness, P is the shielding goal, T is the occupancy factor, d is the distance between the source of radiation and person in shielded area, K is the unshielded kerma at 1 m

from the source, and N is the expected number of patients examined in the room per week.

To understand this better, lets give example values for each of the above as follows:

    P = 0.1 mGy (controlled area)
    T = 0.5 (patient treatment room)
    d = 2 meters
    K = 3 mGy
    N = 100

Using the formula: $B(x_{barrier}) = (P/T) \times d^2/(K^1 \times N)$,
$B(x_{barrier}) = (0.1/0.5) \times 4/(3 \times 100)$
$B(x_{barrier}) = 0.0026$

This means that the barrier thickness must achieve an air kerma in the shielded room that is 0.0026 that of the air kerma without the shield; in other words reduce the level of radiation by a factor of almost 385 (1/0.0026).

This is the basic formula for x-ray shielding.

This *basic* formula, however, must be adjusted for primary shielding and secondary shielding due to barrier-specific issues such as use factor and preshielding (these two factors applying solely to primary barriers and the air kerma measurement location).

Primary barrier formula (the insertion of the subscripted p represents the primary radiation; x_{pre} refers to the thickness of the preshielding); U refers to the use factor):

$$B_p(x_{barrier} + x_{pre}) = (P/T) \times d_p^2/(K_P^1 \times UN)$$

Secondary barrier formula (the insertion of the subscripted *sec* represents the secondary radiation):

$$B_{sec}(x_{barrier}) = (P/T) \times d_{sec}^2/(K_{sec}^1 \times N)$$

At this stage, the reader should have a good understanding of the shielding principles and considerations and how these contribute to the shielding formulae. In reality, the situation can be quite a bit more complicated, with several x-ray tubes in a single room and different materials used for shielding, etc. All the variations have not been addressed here, and the author encourages the reader who requires these details to access the NCRP 147 Report (2004). Within these documents, more complicated scenarios are presented, along with a chapter dedicated to providing a series of realistic examples of necessary calculations required for a variety of x-ray room types.

The Planning Process

When one is planning a new radiologic imaging center or simply a new x-ray room, or is investigating changes to the current facility, the requirements for shielding undergoes a phased project-planning process. The process requires the involvement of users of the equipment, architects, engineers, individuals with a responsibility for institutional space planning, suppliers of equipment, a person expert in radiation room shielding and a person with budget responsibilities. The NCRP (2004) describe a progressive approach to the planning, which is summarized in four key stages detailed below.

Stage 1: Strategic Planning

From time to time (often annually), the local radiologic team will consider the possibility of expanding or changing their current practice and facility and the budget implications of doing so. Compared with the price normally associated with new radiologic equipment, the shielding costs will be relatively low, but nonetheless these will need to be calculated even at this stage in a reasonably accurate way. This should provide the planning team with a good understanding of the overall effect of the change on the institution's financial situation and the feasibility of the plans.

Stage 2: Room Details

At this stage, a comprehensive description of the planned change should be provided, which should include the number and dimensions of the rooms and the use of those rooms so that the shielding expert can provide details on the shielding that may be required.

Stage 3: Designing Stage

This is where plans to scale are initially drawn up that outline the overall arrangement of the new (or changed) facility and includes details of the equipment. It is critically important that the shielding expert is involved at this stage so that cost-effective ideas to keeping shielding costs down may be presented such as the careful placement of corridors (with low occupancy) adjacent to the new facilities.

Stage 4: Refinement of the Design

After the initial design stage, the fine details of the plans are provided, such as dimensions of the room and all the associated engineering considerations around plumbing, electrical supply, and structure. Information on the surrounding areas must also be at hand so occupancy rates in adjacent locations (remembering this is a three-dimensional structure) are understood. The precise location of the x-ray equipment should be available so the shielding expert can comprehensively describe how the radiation will be delivered, attenuated and scattered and hence the type of shielding that is needed. This information will then be fed back to the engineers regarding the thicknesses of and type of materials to be used in the walls, floors, doors ceilings etc. All these details along with the shielding calculations and assumptions should be then drawn up and specified in construction and contract documents, which will be stored on a permanent basis by the person with overall responsibility for the facility.

Summary of Key Concepts

1. **Why is x-ray tube shielding needed?** While radiologic methods, technologies, and strategies that minimize dose are crucial, it is equally important that x-ray tubes and the rooms in which they are located are properly protected. All this requires appropriate radiation shielding and thoughtful room designs.

2. **Different shielding materials.** Here we discuss the construction of walls and doors etc and how the layout of the room is designed in such a way to minimize radiation leakage and maximize protection to patients, staff and any other individuals in the vicinity. However, first we run through the type of materials that are used which includes lead, gypsum wall board, concrete, and barium plaster.

(Continues)

3. **Principles behind shielding in an x-ray facility**. Before we get into the shielding calculations aimed at minimizing dose, a number of overarching principles have been made clear by the NCRP (2004), which are summarized here. The author would like to stress that while regulations and arrangements may vary from country to country, it is beyond the scope of this text to summarize all arrangements, therefore the main focus here is on the information provided by the NCRP in *Report 147: Structural Shielding Design for Medical X-ray Imaging Facilities* (2004). Within that text, the shielding goal is clear and explicit and discussed in this section.

4. **Key factors that determine the level of shielding that is required**. There are a range of features determined by the varying practices and equipment used in different types of x-ray rooms that will also have a major impact on the shielding calculations. These features include: x-ray output; exposure type; x-ray tube movement; relationship between the x-ray source and the receptor; relationship between the operator of the equipment and the patient; relationship between the operator of the equipment and the patient.

5. **Calculations that are performed to determine optimum levels of x-ray room shielding**. It is important again to restate the goal of protective shielding, which is to keep the air kerma value to no more than 0.1 mGy/week for a controlled area and 0.02 mGy/week for an uncontrolled area. The key considerations that will ensure that the level of radiation received by individuals is below these values and hence determine the calculations that will determine the level of shielding required are (NCRP 2004): the amount of radiation being produced and directed towards the primary barriers; the occupancy period of individuals within an exposed area. To determine this we must have values for average workload per patient, which will determine the average air kerma per patient; number of patients being x-rayed per week; use factor, that is, the allocation of exposures in a room directed towards individual barriers; and occupancy factor.

6. **Planning process that is needed when designing a new x-ray facility**. When one is planning a new radiologic imaging centre or simply a new x-ray room, or are investigating changes to the current facility the requirements for shielding undergoes a phased project planning process. The process requires the involvement of users of the equipment, architects, engineers, individuals with a responsibility for institutional space planning, suppliers of equipment, a person expert in radiation room shielding and a person with budget responsibilities. The NCRP describe a progressive approach to the planning, which is summarized in four key stages around: strategic planning; room details; designing stage; design refinement.

Discussion Questions

1. Discuss how an x-ray tube is shielded and how the efficacy of this shielding is tested.

2. Compare the different shielding materials that are currently available.

3. Discuss the key factors that enable an effective assessment of the level of x-ray room shielding that is required and consider the planning process that should be considered with regard to x-ray room shielding when a new installation is being planned.

References

Dowsett DJ, Kenny PA, Johnston RE. *The Physics of Diagnostic Imaging*. (2nd Ed.) New York: Hodder Arnold; 2006.

National Council on Radiation Protection and Measurement (NCRP). *Report 147: Structural Shielding Design for Medical X-ray Facilities*. Bethesda, MD: NCRP; 2004.

Simpkin DJ. Evaluation of NCRP Report No. 49: Assumptions on workloads and use factors in diagnostic radiology facilities. *Med Phys*. 1996;70:238–244.

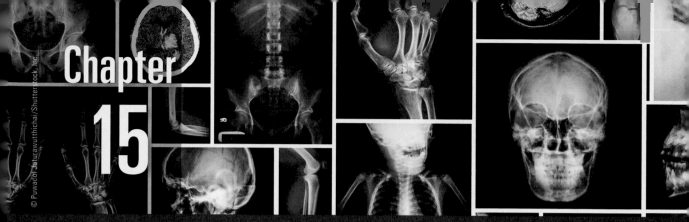

Chapter 15

Radiation Protection Through Quality Control

Outline

- Introduction
- Definitions of QA and QC
  - Quality Assurance (QA)
  - Quality Control (QC)
- Dose Optimization
  - Levels of optimization
  - QC concepts leading to dose optimization
- The Tolerance Limit in QC Testing
  - Exceeding the tolerance limit
- Dose Reduction/Optimization as a Consequence of QC
- References

Objectives

On completion of this chapter, you should be able to:

1. Define the terms *quality assurance* (*QA*) and *quality control* (*QC*).
2. Identify two levels of optimization recommended by the International Commission on Radiological Protection (ICRP) and briefly state the meaning of each level.
3. List several essential elements of a QA/QC program that play a role in dose optimization.
4. Discuss staff responsibilities in a QA/QC program.
5. Identify and explain the three major steps in a QA/QC program.
6. List several parameters in radiographic imaging subject to QC monitoring.
7. Explain the concept of the tolerance limit in QC testing.
8. State the consequence of a QA/QC program on dose reduction/optimization in diagnostic imaging.

Introduction

The activities that are characteristics of *quality assurance* (QA) and *quality control* (QC) have become increasingly important in radiation protection of the patient. It is an essential, logical step to dose optimization. The evolution of QA into other activities, such as *total quality management* (TQM) and *continuous quality improvement* (CQI) also represent integral components related to radiation protection in diagnostic x-ray imaging.

This chapter identifies and describes the essential features of QC in diagnostic x-ray imaging with the goal of emphasizing the role of QC in radiation protection of the patient. More important, the QC concepts leading to dose reduction will be highlighted. These concepts relate to responsibilities principles, test procedures, and parameters for QC monitoring. It is not within the scope of this chapter to describe QC tests, and how to conduct and interpret them; these topics are best described in texts that are devoted to comprehensive treatment of QA, QC, TQM, and CQI.

Definitions of QA and QC

The idea and concepts of QA and QC can be traced back to the early 1970s. Several definitions of QA and QC emerged in 1973, and subsequent were updated in 1979 and the 1980s to reflect advances in knowledge and technology. In 1988, the National Council on Radiation Protection and Measurements (NCRP) provided their version of these definitions, which are still current in today's practice of radiology.

Quality Assurance (QA)

The NCRP (1988) defines QA as follows:

> .... *a comprehensive concept that comprises all of the management practices instituted by the imaging physician to ensure that: (1) every imaging procedure is necessary and appropriate to the clinical problem at hand; (2) the images generated contain information critical to the solution of that problem; (3) the recorded information is correctly interpreted and made available in a timely fashion to the patient's physician; and (4) the examination results in the lowest possible radiation exposure, cost, and in convenience to the patient consistent with Objective (2) (p. 1)*

The objectives inherent in this definition identify several individuals who play significant roles in establishing a successful QA program. While Objective 1 implicates the patient's physician in the initial decision-making process, Objective 2 assigns the responsibility for making decisions about image quality to both the radiologist and technologist. Objective 3, on the other hand, narrows its focus to the radiologist, who is assumed to have a reliable degree of competency in image interpretation. Finally, Objective 4 is really the essential step of what a QA program is all about: dose reduction and hence dose optimization, since image quality is a primary concern—that is, the objective that a reduction in the dose does not compromise the image quality, needed to make a diagnosis.

In general, QA is a management concept that includes, administrative, educational, and technical measures to ensure that image quality standards are met. dose is kept to a minimum (consistent with the ALARA philosophy), and the cost of establishing and maintaining the program is low and reasonable. QA ensures efficient utilization of the resources (both human and physical) of the department.

Quality Control (QC)

QC deals with technical measures and in this respect the NCRP (1988) defined QC as:

> .... *a series of distinct technical procedures which ensure the production of a satisfaction product. Its aim is to provide quality that is not only satisfactory and diagnostic but also dependable and economic (p. 4)*

QC therefore is a major component of the QA program, since it deals with techniques and procedures for measuring image quality, as well as testing and maintaining the integrity of the components of the x-ray imaging system. In other words, QC deals with the imaging equipment. It includes several principles and concepts that ultimately lead to dose optimization as a strategy for radiation protection of patients.

Dose Optimization

The principle of dose optimization as outlined by the International Commission on Radiological Protection (ICRP) refers to keeping radiation exposures as low as reasonably achievable (ALARA) without compromising the diagnostic quality of the image. The ALARA philosophy is vital in diagnostic imaging because of the stochastic and deterministic effects of radiation exposure.

Levels of Optimization

Essentially, there are two levels of optimization addressed by the ICRP: (1) The design and function of the x-ray imaging equipment, and (2) imaging techniques and imaging protocols used during daily operation. While the former examines the design and function of the equipment to meet current radiation protection standards, the latter deals with the procedural and operational practices during the conduct of the examination.

QC involves three steps: acceptance testing, routine performance evaluation, and error correction (Bushong 2013). While acceptance testing basically examines whether the equipment meets specifications for ensuring that it operates efficiently in terms of dose output, routine performance refers to monitoring the components of the equipment that affect dose and image quality. Monitoring includes QC tests that are performed on a daily, weekly, monthly, and yearly basis. Finally, error correction deals with the evaluation of the results of the QC tests. If the machine fails to meet the tolerance limits or acceptance limits established for the particular QC test, then the machine must be serviced (or removed in some cases) to ensure that tolerance limits are met. This is the basic tenet of error correction.

QC Concepts Leading to Dose Optimization

There are several essential elements of a QA/QC program that play a role in dose optimization. These include responsibilities, QC principles and test procedures, and parameters for QC monitoring. Each of these will now be described briefly since they represent the back bone of any QA program.

Responsibilities

For a QA program to be successful, it is important that responsibilities be defined, so that individuals understand the nature of the tasks associated with a specific responsibility.

In a typical QA/QC program, the radiologist in charge of the facility or a department assumes the primary responsibility for the entire program, as identified by organizations such as The Joint Commission (TJC), the Food and Drug Administration (FDA) and Radiation Protection Bureau-Health Canada (RPB-HC), to mention only a few. As noted by RPB-HC (2008), for example:

> The owner is ultimately responsible for the radiation safety of the facility. It is the responsibility of the owner to ensure that the equipment and the facilities in which such equipment is installed and used meet all appropriate radiation safety standards, and that a radiation safety program is developed implemented, and maintained for the facility. The owner may delegate this responsibility to qualified staff. How this responsibility is delegated will depend upon the number of staff members, the nature of the operation and on the number of x-ray equipment owned. In any event, the owner must ensure that one or more qualified persons are designated to carry out the roles ... (p. 7)

The responsibility for QC is a group effort. Everyone in the department, from radiologists, medical physicists, biomedical engineers, QC technologists, and all technologists, should play a role, no matter how small, to maintain the integrity and success of the program. Since medical physicists and biomedical engineers are educated and trained at a higher level than technologists, they play major roles in the more sophisticated and advanced QC tests. The engineer's role may relate to repair and general servicing of the equipment. In general, there are a wide variety of QC tests that may fall within the domain of the technologist.

QC Principles and Test Procedures

As noted earlier in the chapter, the principles of QC are related to three major steps: (1) Acceptance testing, in which equipment is tested to verify that it functions according to the manufacturer's specifications; (2) routine performance and evaluation, and (3) error correction (Bushong 2013). Conducting performance evaluation tests requires the use of a set of rules for solving a problem. Included in these rules are the test procedures, image quality standards, and performance criteria or tolerance limit.

The *test procedure* outlines the steps taken in performing the QC test. These steps should be clear and precise and should be based on a format that is easy to follow. One such format may be as follows:

1. The name and purpose of the test
2. The equipment needed to perform the test
3. How often the test should be conducted; in other words, the testing frequency
4. Equipment set-up and measurements to be recorded
5. Documentation of the test results
6. Measures to correct unsatisfactory results

The notion of image quality standards is vital to a QC program. Such standards must be established by the department and are usually based on subjective and objective criteria. While subjective standards are related to feelings and opinions of observers (radiologists and technologists) in evaluating images, objective standards are based on the results of scientific research. In QA/QC programs, objective standards should prevail.

Standards should have certain defined limits, referred to as *acceptance limits* or *tolerance limits*. Equipment performance is deemed acceptable when the results of the QC test fall within these limits. In this situation, a patient will not be subjected to unnecessary radiation exposures due to faulty equipment.

The principles of QC include other considerations that affect the integrity of the program. These include preventive and corrective maintenance measures, record keeping, and a QC policy and procedural manual.

Elements and Parameters for QC Monitoring

In terms of dose optimization via QC, there are several elements and parameters in the imaging chains for radiography, fluoroscopy, mammography, and computed tomography (CT) that vary in time. Therefore, all parameters that affect dose and image quality must be subject to QC monitoring.

It is not within the scope of this chapter to list all of the elements or to describe how the parameters are tested. QC tests for all major components of the imaging systems listed above are described in detail by Bushong (2013) and Papp (2011). It is important, however, to identify those elements common to x-ray imaging systems, and provide examples of tolerance limits for a few representative parameters. Common elements for film-screen and digital radiography, fluoroscopy, mammography, and CT systems include the x-ray generator, x-ray tubes, collimation, filtration, anti-scatter devices, image detectors, and image processing. X-ray generator parameters subject to QC monitoring are the radiation output, exposure reproducibility, linearity, kVp and exposure timer accuracy, and automatic exposure control (Bushong 2013; Papp 2011).

Parameters for x-ray tubes and collimators are filtration, alignment of the light field and radiation field defined by the collimator, focal spot size, off-focus radiation, and several others. Because filtration and collimation are intended to protect the patient from unnecessary radiation, they are extremely important to QC monitoring.

The Tolerance Limit in QC Testing

Each of the QC tests for different parameters has an associated tolerance limit, previously established by various radiology and medical physics organizations such as the American College of Radiology (ACR) and the American Association of Physicists in Medicine (AAPM) respectively. The results of QC tests during routine performance evaluations are subsequently matched against the established tolerance limits. As mentioned earlier, these limits can be expressed qualitatively (pass-fail or no significant areas of poor contact seen) or quantitatively (±0.5 or $\pm3\%$ or ≤1.3 mC-kg^{-1}/mm). The tolerance limit usually has a $\pm$ value.

Exceeding the Tolerance Limit

Papp (2011) states that the tolerance limit for the kVp accuracy QC test should be within $\pm5\%$. Suppose a test was conducted for the 80 kVp setting on the control panel; the acceptable limits would be $\pm5\%$ of 80, which equals ±4. The tolerance limits for this test would then be 76–84 kVp. Any value >84 or <76 would render the test results unacceptable and would suggest the need for repairs or recalibration. It is clear, then, that the machine must function correctly in order to optimize the dose-image quality relationship. The tolerance limits for a wide variety of QC tests for film-screen radiography, fluoroscopy, mammography, digital radiography, and CT are provided by Bushong (2013) and Papp (2011).

Dose Reduction/ Optimization as a Consequence of QC

It is logical that an effective QA/QC program will result in dose reduction as well as dose optimization. Maintaining the proper functioning of those technical factors that affect dose and image quality will clearly demonstrate the ultimate value of radiation protection through QC.

A dose optimization study requires several important elements, such as ensuring that the system components affecting dose and image quality be calibrated before the study begins. This means that the parameters affecting dose confirm to the established tolerance limits that indicate the machine performance is acceptable. Thus, the first thing that should be done is QC testing of these components. For example, the generator parameters, such as radiation output exposure reproducibility, linearity, kVp, and timer accuracy, must be within established tolerance limits. Other elements such as filtration, collimation, x-ray tube focal spot size, and the image receptors (deflectors) meet acceptable QC tolerance limits.

Another important consideration in dose optimization studies relates to the dose measurement. It is vital that a calibrated dosimeter be used to record dose measurements. In addition, if observers are used to evaluate images in a dose optimization study, they should be instructed in procedures for evaluate images. These are all elements of QC that play an important role in dose optimization (Seeram 2013).

Summary of Key Concepts

1. This chapter presented a review of the general ideas concerning QA and QC in diagnostic radiography.

2. QA is a management concept that includes, administrative, educational, and technical measures to ensure that image quality standards are met; dose is kept to a minimum (consistent with the ALARA philosophy) and the cost of establishing and maintaining the program is low and reasonable. QA ensures efficient utilization of the resources (both human and physical) of the department.

3. QC deals with techniques and procedures for measuring image quality, as well as testing and maintaining the integrity of the components of the x-ray imaging systems. QC deals with the imaging equipment, and includes several principles and concepts that ultimately lead to dose optimization as a strategy for radiation protection of patients.

(Continues)

4. Two levels of optimization addressed by the ICRP relate to the design and function of the x-ray imaging equipment, and imaging techniques and imaging protocols used during daily operation.

5. The essential elements of a QA/QC program that play a role in dose optimization include responsibilities, QC principles and test procedures, and parameters for QC monitoring.

6. In a typical QA/QC program, the radiologist in charge of the facility or a department assumes the primary responsibility for the entire program as identified by organizations such as The Joint Commission (TJC), the Food and Drug Administration (FDA) and Radiation Protection Bureau-Health Canada (RPB-HC).

7. Three major steps of QC are acceptance testing, in which equipment is tested to verify that it functions according to the manufacturer's specifications; routine performance and evaluation, and error correction.

8. In terms of dose optimization via QC there are several elements and parameters in the imaging chains for radiography, fluoroscopy, mammography, and computed tomography (CT) that vary in time. Therefore, all parameters that affect dose and image quality must be subject to QC monitoring. Common elements for film-screen and digital radiography, fluoroscopy, mammography, and CT systems include, for example, the x-ray generator, x-ray tubes, collimation, filtration, antiscatter devices, image detectors, and image processing.

9. Parameters for x-ray tubes and collimators are filtration, alignment of the light field and radiation field defined by the collimator, focal spot size, off-focus radiation, and several others. Because filtration and collimation are intended to protect the patient from unnecessary radiation, they are extremely important to QC monitoring.

10. QC tests for different parameters are in general assigned a tolerance limit. The results of QC tests during routine performance evaluations are subsequently matched against the established tolerance limits that can be expressed qualitatively (pass-fail or no significant areas of poor contact seen) or quantitatively (±0.5 or $\pm3\%$ or ≤1.3 mC.kg^{-1}/mm). The tolerance limit usually has a $\pm$ value.

11. An effective QA/QC program will result in dose reduction as well as dose optimization. Maintaining the proper functioning of those technical factors that affect dose and image quality will clearly demonstrate the ultimate value of radiation protection through QC.

Discussion Questions

1. Discuss staff responsibilities in a QA/QC program, and explain the three major steps in a QA/QC program.

2. Identify several parameters in radiographic imaging subject to QC monitoring, and explain the concept of the tolerance limit in QC testing.

3. Outline the consequence of a QA/QC program on dose reduction/optimization in diagnostic imaging.

References

Bushong S. *Radiologic Science for Technologist: Physics, Biology and Protection*. St. Louis, MO: Elsevier-Mosby; 2013.

Papp J. *Quality Management in the Imaging Sciences*. (4th ed.). St. Louis, MO: Mosby-Elsevier; 2011.

Seeram E. Optimization of the exposure index of a CR system as a radiation dose management strategy. *Scientific abstract - quality, safety & radiation dose – part 1*. Society for Imaging Informatics in Medicine (SIIM). Dallas, Texas; 2013.

Appendix A

Mapping the ARRT Exam Specifications for Radiation Protection to this Text*

ARRT Radiation Protection Examination Specifications	Relevant Chapters in *Radiation Protection in Diagnostic Imaging*
1. Biological Aspects of Radiation Protection A. Radiosensitivity B. Somatic Effects C. Acute Radiation Syndromes D. Embryonic and Fetal Effects E. Genetic Impact F. Photon Interaction with Matter	Chapter 1 (A, including all subtopics) Chapter 2 (F, including all subtopics) Chapter 4 (A–E, including all subtopics)
2. Minimizing Patient Exposure A. Exposure Factors B. Shielding C. Beam Restriction D. Filtration E. Exposure Reduction F. Image Receptors G. Grids H. Fluoroscopy	Chapter 7 (A–F, including all subtopics) Chapter 8 (H, including all subtopics) Chapter 9 (A–H for digital radiography) Chapter 10 (All topics relating to CT) Chapter 15 (Quality control in minimizing radiation exposure to patients and personnel)
3. Personnel Protection A. Sources of Radiation Exposure B. Basic Methods of Protection C. Protective Devices D. Special Considerations (Portable and Fluoroscopy) E. Guidelines for Portable and Fluoroscopy Units (NCRP #102 and 21 CFR)	Chapter 1 (A) Chapter 3 (A) Chapter 6 (B) Chapter 14 (B and C) Chapter 13 (D and E)

ARRT Radiation Protection Examination Specifications	Relevant Chapters in *Radiation Protection in Diagnostic Imaging*
4. Radiation Exposure and Monitoring	Chapter 3 (A)
A. Units of Measurement	Chapter 13 (B)
B. Dosimeters	Chapter 5 (B)
C. NCRP Recommendations for Personnel Monitoring (NCRP # 116)	Chapter 12 (A) Chapter 13 (C)

*The textbook **Radiation Protection in Diagnostic X-Ray Imaging** includes several chapters covering topics beyond those prescribed by the ARRT Radiation Protection Examination Specifications. These chapters (and associated topics) include more recent topics on radiation protection that should be a part of a Radiation Protection course of study, as follows:

- Chapter 6: Radiation Protection Organizations
- Chapter 9: Dose in Digital Radiography
- Chapter 10: Radiation Dose in Computed Tomography (CT)
- Chapter 11: Image Quality Assessment Tools for Dose Optimization in Digital Radiography
- Chapter 12: Diagnostic Reference Levels
- Chapter 15: Radiation Protection through Quality Control

Appendix B

Mapping the ASRT Objectives for Radiation Protection (47 Objectives) and Radiation Biology (21 Objectives) to this Text

ASRT Radiation Protection Objectives	Content Addressed in the Text
1. Identify and justify the need to minimize unnecessary radiation exposure of humans.	Chapter 1 Radiation Protection Overview Chapter 4 The Radiobiology of Low-Dose Radiation Chapter 5 Radiation Protection Practice
2. Distinguish between somatic and genetic radiation effects.	Chapter 1 Radiation Protection Overview Chapter 4 The Radiobiology of Low-Dose Radiation
3. Differentiate between the stochastic (probabilistic) and nonstochastic (deterministic) effects of radiation exposure.	Chapter 1 Radiation Protection Overview Chapter 4 The Radiobiology of Low-Dose Radiation
4. Explain the objectives of a radiation protection program.	Chapter 1 Radiation Protection Overview Chapter 5 Radiation Protection Practice
5. Define radiation and radioactivity units of measurement.	Chapter 2 Basic Physics for Radiation Protection: An Overview Chapter 3 Radiation Exposure and Dose Units
6. Identify effective dose limits (EDL) for occupational and non-occupational radiation exposure.	Chapter 5 Radiation Protection Practice
7. Describe the ALARA concept.	Chapter 1 Radiation Protection Overview Chapter 3 Radiation Exposure and Dose Units Chapter 5 Radiation Protection Practice
8. Identify the basis for occupational exposure limits.	Chapter 5 Radiation Protection Practice
9. Distinguish between perceived risk and comparable risk.	Chapter 1 Radiation Protection Overview Chapter 4 The Radiobiology of Low-Dose Radiation Chapter 5 Radiation Protection Practice

ASRT Radiation Protection Objectives	Content Addressed in the Text
10. Describe the concept of the negligible individual dose (NID).	
11. Identify ionizing radiation sources from natural and man-made sources.	Chapter 2 Basic Physics for Radiation Protection: An Overview
12. Comply with legal and ethical radiation protection responsibilities of radiation workers.	Chapter 6 Radiation Protection Organizations Chapter 13 Optimization of Radiation Protection: Regulatory and Guidance Recommendations
13. Describe the relationship between irradiated area and effective dose.	Chapter 3 Radiation Exposure and Dose Units Chapter 5 Radiation Protection Practice Chapter 7 Factors Affecting Dose in Radiographic Imaging
14. Describe the theory and operation of radiation detection devices.	Chapter 5 Radiation Protection Practice
15. Identify appropriate applications and limitations for each radiation detection device.	Chapter 5 Radiation Protection Practice
16. Describe how isoexposure curves are used for radiation protection.	Chapter 5 Radiation Protection Practice
17. Identify performance standards for beam limiting devices.	Chapter 7 Factors Affecting Dose in Radiographic Imaging Chapter 15 Radiation Protection through Quality Control
18. Describe procedures used to verify performance standards for equipment and indicate the potential consequences if the performance standards fail.	Chapter 15 Radiation Protection through Quality Control
19. Describe the operation of various interlocking systems for equipment and indicate potential consequences of interlock system failure.	Chapter 7 Factors Affecting Dose in Radiographic Imaging Chapter 8 Factors Affecting Dose in Fluoroscopy
20. Identify conditions and locations evaluated in an area survey for radiation protection.	
21. Distinguish between controlled and non-controlled areas and list acceptable exposure levels.	Chapter 14 Protective Shielding in Diagnostic Radiology
22. Describe "Radiation Area" signs and identify appropriate placement sites.	Chapter 13 Optimization of Radiation Protection: Regulatory and Guidance Recommendations Chapter 14- Protective Shielding in Diagnostic Radiology
23. Describe the function of federal, state and local regulations governing radiation protection practices.	Chapter 6 Radiation Protection Organizations Chapter 13 Optimization of Radiation Protection: Regulatory and Guidance Recommendations
24. Describe the requirements for and responsibilities of a radiation safety officer.	Chapter 6 Radiation Protection Organizations

ASRT Radiation Protection Objectives	Content Addressed in the Text
25. Express the need and importance of personnel monitoring for radiation workers.	Chapter 5 Radiation Protection Practice
26. Describe personnel monitoring devices, including applications, advantages and limitations for each device.	Chapter 5 Radiation Protection Practice
27. Interpret personnel monitoring reports.	Chapter 5 Radiation Protection Practice
28. Compare values for individual effective dose limits for occupational radiation exposures (annual and lifetime).	Chapter 5 Radiation Protection Practice
29. Identify anatomical structures that are considered critical for potential late effects of whole body irradiation exposure.	Chapter 4 The Radiobiology of Low-Dose Radiation
30. Identify effective dose limits for the embryo and fetus in occupationally exposed women.	Chapter 5 Radiation Protection Practice
31. Distinguish between primary and secondary radiation barriers.	Chapter 14 Protective Shielding in Diagnostic Radiology
32. Demonstrate how the operation of various x-ray and ancillary equipment influences radiation safety and describe the potential consequences of equipment failure.	Chapter 7 Factors Affecting Dose in Radiographic Imaging Chapter 8 Factors Affecting Dose in Fluoroscopy Chapter 15 Radiation Protection through Quality Control
33. Perform calculations of exposure with varying time, distance and shielding.	Chapter 7 Factors Affecting Dose in Radiographic Imaging
34. Discuss the relationship between workload, energy, half-value layer (HVL), tenth-value layer (TVL), use factor, and shielding design.	Chapter 14 Protective Shielding in Diagnostic Radiology
35. Identify emergency procedures to be followed during failures of x-ray equipment.	Chapter 6 Radiation Protection Organizations Chapter 15 Radiation Protection through Quality Control
36. Demonstrate how time, distance and shielding can be manipulated to keep radiation exposures to a minimum.	Chapter 14 Protective Shielding in Diagnostic Radiology
37. Explain the relationship of beam-limiting devices to patient radiation protection.	Chapter 7 Factors Affecting Dose in Radiographic Imaging

ASRT Radiation Protection Objectives	Content Addressed in the Text
38. Discuss added and inherent filtration in terms of the effect on patient dosage.	Chapter 7 Factors Affecting Dose in Radiographic Imaging
39. Explain the purpose and importance of patient shielding.	Chapter 6 Radiation Protection Organizations Chapter 7 Factors Affecting Dose in Radiographic Imaging Chapter 13 Optimization of Radiation Protection: Regulatory and Guidance Recommendations
40. Identify various types of patient shielding and state the advantages and disadvantages of each type.	Chapter 7 Factors Affecting Dose in Radiographic Imaging Chapter 13 Optimization of Radiation Protection: Regulatory and Guidance Recommendations
41. Use the appropriate method of shielding for a given radiographic procedure.	Chapter 7 Factors Affecting Dose in Radiographic Imaging Chapter 13 Optimization of Radiation Protection: Regulatory and Guidance Recommendations
42. Explain the relationship of exposure factors to patient dosage.	Chapter 7 Factors Affecting Dose in Radiographic Imaging Chapter 8 Factors Affecting Dose in Fluoroscopy Chapter 9 Dose in Digital Radiography Chapter 10 Radiation Dose in Computed Tomography
43. Explain how patient position affects dose to radiosensitive organs.	Chapter 7 Factors Affecting Dose in Radiographic Imaging Chapter 8 Factors Affecting Dose in Fluoroscopy
44. Identify the appropriate image receptor that will result in an optimum diagnostic image with the minimum radiation exposure to the patient.	Chapter 7 Factors Affecting Dose in Radiographic Imaging Chapter 8 Factors Affecting Dose in Fluoroscopy Chapter 9 Dose in Digital Radiography Chapter 10 Radiation Dose in Computed Tomography
45. Select the immobilization techniques used to eliminate voluntary motion.	Chapter 7 Factors Affecting Dose in Radiographic Imaging Chapter 13 Optimization of Radiation Protection: Regulatory and Guidance Recommendations
46. Describe the minimum source-to-tabletop distances for fixed and mobile fluoroscopic devices.	Chapter 13 Optimization of Radiation Protection: Regulatory and Guidance Recommendations
47. Apply safety factors for the patient, health care personnel and family members in the room during radiographic procedures.	Chapter 13 Optimization of Radiation Protection: Regulatory and Guidance Recommendations

ASRT Radiation Biology Objectives	Content Addressed in the Text
1. Describe principles of cellular biology.	Chapter 4 The Radiobiology of Low-Dose Radiation
2. Identify sources of electromagnetic and particulate ionizing radiations.	Chapter 3 Radiation Exposure and Dose Units
3. Differentiate between ionic and covalent molecular bonds.	
4. Discriminate between direct and indirect ionizing radiation.	Chapter 2 Basic Physics for Radiation Protection: An Overview Chapter 4 The Radiobiology of Low-Dose Radiation
5. Discriminate between the direct and indirect effects of radiation.	Chapter 2 Basic Physics for Radiation Protection: An Overview Chapter 4 The Radiobiology of Low-Dose Radiation
6. Identify sources of radiation exposure.	Chapter 1 Radiation Protection Overview Chapter 3 Radiation Exposure and Dose Units
7. Describe radiation-induced chemical reactions and potential biologic damage.	Chapter 4 The Radiobiology of Low-Dose Radiation
8. Evaluate factors influencing radiobiologic/biophysical events at the cellular and subcellular level.	Chapter 4 The Radiobiology of Low-Dose Radiation
9. Identify methods to measure radiation response.	Chapter 4 The Radiobiology of Low-Dose Radiation
10. Describe physical, chemical and biologic factors influencing radiation response of cells and tissues.	Chapter 4 The Radiobiology of Low-Dose Radiation
11. Explain factors influencing radiosensitivity.	Chapter 4 The Radiobiology of Low-Dose Radiation
12. Recognize the clinical significance of lethal dose (LD).	
13. Identify specific cells from most radiosensitive to least radiosensitive.	Chapter 4 The Radiobiology of Low-Dose Radiation
14. Employ dose response curves to study the relationship between radiation dose levels and the degree of biologic response.	Chapter 1 Radiation Protection Overview Chapter 4 The Radiobiology of Low-Dose Radiation
15. Examine effects of limited vs. total body exposure	Chapter 4 The Radiobiology of Low-Dose Radiation Chapter 5 Radiation Protection Practice
16. Relate short-term and long-term effects as a consequence of high and low radiation doses.	Chapter 4 The Radiobiology of Low-Dose Radiation
17. Differentiate between somatic and genetic radiation effects and discuss specific diseases or syndromes associated with them.	Chapter 4 The Radiobiology of Low-Dose Radiation
18. Discuss stochastic (probabilistic) and nonstochastic (deterministic) effects.	Chapter 1 Radiation Protection Overview Chapter 4 The Radiobiology of Low-Dose Radiation
19. Discuss embryo and fetal effects of radiation exposure.	Chapter 4 The Radiobiology of Low-Dose Radiation

ASRT Radiation Biology Objectives	Content Addressed in the Text
20. Discuss risk estimates for radiation-induced malignancies.	Chapter 4 The Radiobiology of Low-Dose Radiation
21. Discuss acute radiation syndromes.	

This text also provides knowledge beyond what is required in the above objectives in current topics on Radiation Protection including:

Chapter 10: Radiation Dose in Computed Tomography

Chapter 11: Image Quality Assessment Tools for Dose Optimization in Digital Radiography

Chapter 12: Diagnostic Reference Levels

Index

A

AAPM TG. *See* American Association of Physicists in Medicine Task Group

abdomen AP
    cancer risks for, 103*f*
    diagnostic reference levels for, 101*f*
    effective doses for, 102*f*
    patient radiation doses for, 64*t*

abdomen CT, 53*t*, 55*t*
    cancer risks for, 105*f*
    effective doses for, 104*f*

abdomen x-ray exam, 55*t*

abdominal angiography, 54*t*, 55*t*

absorbed dose, 9, 14, 57–58
    calculation for, 9
    female phantom, 60*f*
    male phantom, 60*f*
    sex-averaged, 60*f*

acceptance limits, 282

added filtration, 153

AEC. *See* automatic exposure control

AERC. *See* automatic exposure rate control

ALARA. *See* as low as reasonably achievable

alpha particles, 21, 23, 23*f*, 24*f*
    weighting factors for, 58*t*

American Association of Physicists in Medicine Task Group (AAPM TG), 179
    exposure indicator report, 180*f*
    116 solution, 185–190, 186*f*, 187*f*, 188*f*, 197

angiocardiography, 54*t*, 55*t*

angiography, 53*t*
    radiation exposure with, 53–54, 54*t*

angstrom, 20

anti-scatter grids
    fluoroscopy with, 171
    radiographic imaging with, 156–157, 162

anti-scatter radiation grid, 171

aortography, 54*t*, 55*t*

apoptosis, 77, 80, 81*f*

as low as reasonably achievable (ALARA), 5, 12
    computed tomography with, 204
    diagnostic reference levels with, 222
    digital radiography with, 176
    film-screen technology with, 176
    protective shielding with, 262
    radiation protection practice with, 100
    stochastic effects and risk with, 68

a-Se TFT direct detector, 168

ATCM. *See* automatic tube current modulation

atmospheric nuclear testing, 49*f*

atomic mass, 21

atomic number
    defined, 20
    effective, 20–21, 21*f*
    examples of, 21*f*

atomic structure
    atom in, 19–20, 20*f*, 44
    electrons in, 20–22, 22*f*, 22*t*
    element in, 19, 19*t*
    isotope with, 21
    neutrons in, 20
    nucleus in, 20–21
    protons in, 20
    quarks in, 20

attenuation, 9

Auger electron, 35

automatic exposure control (AEC), 152, 161, 203

automatic exposure rate control (AERC), 171, 174

automatic tube current modulation (ATCM), 206, 208

B

B. *See* Bucky factors

beam alignment, 155, 161

beam geometry, 204

BEIR. *See* Biological Effects of Ionizing Radiation
beta particles, 21, 23–24, 24*f*
β⁻ decay, 23
β⁺ decay, 23
biliary and urinary interventional x-ray exam, 55*t*, 231*t*, 232*t*
biliary system x-ray exam, 55*t*, 231*t*, 232*t*
binding energy, 22, 22*t*
biological effects, 3, 4. *See also* relative biological effectiveness
    deterministic effects with, 4, 14, 18, 87–89, 88*f*, 89*t*
    low-dose radiation, 67–96
    stochastic effects, 4, 14, 18, 68–87, 69*f*–71*f*, 73*f*, 75*f*–79*f*, 81*f*, 82*f*, 84*t*–88*t*
Biological Effects of Ionizing Radiation (BEIR), 3, 139, 143–144
bladder
    nominal risk coefficient associated with, 85*t*
    radiation weighting factors for, 59*t*
    x-ray exam, 55*t*
bone
    mineral densitometry CT, 53*t*
    nominal risk coefficient associated with, 85*t*
    surface, radiation weighting factors for, 59*t*
bone marrow
    nominal risk coefficient associated with, 85*t*
    radiation weighting factors for, 59*t*
brain, radiation weighting factors for, 59*t*
breast
    nominal risk coefficient associated with, 85*t*
    tissue, radiation weighting factors for, 59*t*
bremsstrahlung radiation, 28*f*, 29, 29*f*
Bucky factors (B), 157, 162
Bucky slot shielding, 253
bystander effect, 95

C

cancer
    conversion of, 83–84, 84*t*, 85*t*
    detriment-adjusted nominal risk coefficient for, 83, 84*t*, 87
    initiation of, 82–83
    nominal risk coefficient associated with, 83, 85*t*–86*t*
    progression of, 83

    risks for fluoroscopic and CT exams, 105*f*
    risks for non-fluoroscopic and non-CT exams, 103*f*
    stages of, 82
    stochastic detriment-adjusted nominal risk coefficient for, 87, 88*f*
cardiovascular interventional x-ray exam, 55*t*
Carestream Health (Kodak), 183–184, 184*f*
C-arm computed tomography fluoroscopy (C-arm CT), 173, 174
C-arm fluoroscopy, 172
CC images. *See* cranio-caudal images
CDRH. *See* Center for Devices and Radiological Health
cell cycle arrest, 77–79, 78f, 79f, 80
cell membranes, free radicals effects on, 77
cell repair mechanisms
    adaptation in, 81
    apoptosis, 77, 80, 81*f*
    cell cycle arrest, 77–79, 78*f*, 79*f*
    DNA repair mechanism, 77, 79–80
Center for Devices and Radiological Health (CDRH), 140–141, 144
cerebral angiography, 54*t*, 55*t*
cervical spine AP
    cancer risks for, 103*f*
    effective doses for, 102*f*
    patient radiation doses for, 64*t*
cervical spine Lat
    cancer risks for, 103*f*
    effective doses for, 102*f*
    patient radiation doses for, 64*t*
cervical spine x-ray exam, 55*t*
characteristic radiation, 27–29, 28*f*, 29*f*
charged pions, weighting factors for, 58*t*
Chernobyl accident, 49*f*
chest AP, patient radiation doses for, 64*t*
chest CT, 53*t*, 55*t*
    cancer risks for, 105*f*
    effective doses for, 104*f*
chest Lat, effective doses for, 102*f*
chest PA
    cancer risks for, 103*f*
    diagnostic reference levels for, 101*f*

effective doses for, 102*f*

   patient radiation doses for, 64*t*

chest x-ray exam, 55*t*

children

   pediatric values for DRLs, 241, 242*t*

   radiation's effects on, 95–96

chromosomal aberrations, 82, 82*f*

coherent scattering. *See* elastic scattering

collective effective dose, 61

collimation, 10

   computed tomography, 206, 208

   deviation index with, 195

   electronic, 155

   fluoroscopic equipment, 253

   patients protection with, 256

   pregnancy radiation protection with, 258–260

   radiography and, 154–155, 161

   total, 203

colon

   nominal risk coefficient associated with, 85*t*

   radiation weighting factors for, 59*t*

   x-ray exam, 55*t*

Compton scattering, 33, 36–40, 37*f*, 38*f*, 39*f*, 41*f*

computed tomography (CT)

   ALARA principle in, 204

   C-arm, 173, 174

   deterministic effects in, 204

   diagnostic reference levels for, 236

   dose descriptors for, 204–206

      CTDI, 204

      DLP, 205, 208

      effective dose, 204

   dose optimization study example for, 208

   dose-image quality optimization research in, 208

   dose-image quality optimization with, 10

   effective doses for, 104*f*

   factors affecting dose in

      ATCM, 207, 209

      collimation, 206, 209

      exposure technique factors, 206

      iterative image reconstruction, 207

      patient centering, 207, 209

      pitch, 206, 209

human risk with exposure to, 72

Nobel prize work for development of, 200, 208

principles and components of, 200–203, 201*f*, 202*f*

   data flow in, 202–203, 202*f*, 208

   image quality characteristics, 203, 208

   multislice technology, 202, 208

radiation dose in, 199–209

radiation exposure with, 52–53, 53*t*

risks of, 204

stochastic effects in, 204

computed tomography dose index (CTDI), 204

contact shields, 159

continuous fluoroscopy mode, 170

continuous quality improvement (CQI), 9, 280

contrast resolution, 203, 209, 214, 218

controlled area, 268

coronary angiography

   cancer risks for, 105*f*

   effective doses for, 104*f*

cosmic radiation from space, 49*f*, 50

coulomb per kilogram, 10, 15, 57

CQI. *See* continuous quality improvement

cranio-caudal (CC) images, 106, 107*f*

CsI a-Si TFT indirect detector, 168

CT. *See* computed tomography

CT numbers, 201, 208

CTDI. *See* computed tomography dose index

cumulative timer, 170

D

DAPs. *See* dose-area product meters

data acquisition, 200, 208

DBT. *See* digital breast tomosynthesis

DDREF. *See* dose and dose rate effectiveness factor

dental examinations

   diagnostic reference levels for, 236, 236*f*

   radiation exposure with, 54

   teeth x-ray exam, 55*t*

detective quantum efficiency (DQE), 157, 214, 218

deterministic effects, 4, 14, 18, 87–89

   computed tomography with, 204

   early effects, 89

   example of, 88*f*

deterministic effects (*Cont.*)
 factors influencing low-dose radiation with
  cell radiosensitivity, 89–92, 90*f*, 91*f*, 92*f*, 96
  dose rate, 93
  kinetics, 92–93
  oxygen presence, 93, 94*f*
  radioprotectants and radiosensitizers, 93–94
 late effects, 89
 three main principles applied to, 88
 with threshold doses, 89*t*
detriment-adjusted nominal risk coefficient,
  83, 84*t*, 87
deviation index
 action levels, 190–191, 190*t*
 attenuating materials within x-ray beam with,
  195–196, 195*f*
 audits of exposure index opportunity, 191–195,
  192*f*, 193*t*, 194*t*
 beam energy in, 196
 caution with, 196
 collimation with, 195
 exposure index importance, 190
 IEC publication, 191
diagnostic efficacy, 116
diagnostic exposures, 52–54, 55*t*
 angiographic examinations in, 53–54, 54*t*
 CT in, 52–53, 53*t*
 dental examinations in, 54
 doses from medical x-ray, 52*t*
diagnostic imaging
 dose risks in, 100–104, 102*t*, 103*t*,
  104*t*, 105*t*, 131
 patient doses in, 63, 64*t*
 staff doses in, 63–65
diagnostic reference levels (DRLs), 11, 15, 101*f*, 110,
  221–245
 ALARA principle with, 222
 CT examinations with, 236
 defined, 224–227, 227*f*
 dental examinations with, 236, 236*f*
 establishment of
  calculation for, 237–241, 240*f*, 245
  data gathering practical for, 243–245
  global activity in, 241–243

 pediatric values in, 241, 242*t*
 survey for, 230–237, 231*t*, 232*t*, 234*f*, 235*f*,
  236*f*, 238*f*, 239*f*
 importance of, 229
 improved awareness of radiation doses with,
  229–230
 mammography with, 236–237
 methods of dose measurement in, 233–236
  DAP measurement, 234–235, 234*f*
  entrance surface doses, 222, 224*t*, 234, 244
  free-in-air measurements, 235–236, 235*f*
 reduced doses with, 229
 regulatory requirement with, 229
 societal benefits with, 229
 what DRL is not, 228, 244
digital breast tomosynthesis (DBT), 106–107
digital radiography
 ALARA principle in, 176
 assessment tools for dose optimization in, 211–218
 deviation index
  action levels, 190–191, 190*t*
  attenuating materials within x-ray beam with,
   195–196, 195*f*
  audits of exposure index opportunity, 191–195,
   192*f*, 193*t*, 194*t*
  beam energy in, 196
  caution with, 196
  collimation with, 195
  exposure index importance, 190
  IEC publication, 191
 dose in, 175–197
 exposure creep in, 179
 exposure indices establishment in
  AAPM TG 116 solution, 185–190, 186*f*,
   187*f*, 188*f*, 197
  exposure represented by, 183
  options for, 183, 183*f*
  previous manufacturers solutions, 183–185, 184*f*
 exposure indices principles of
  practical criteria for, 181, 181*f*, 182*f*
  scientific criteria for, 179–180, 180*f*
 film-screen technology before, 176–177,
  176*f*, 177*f*, 197
 highlighting inappropriate exposures in, 179

image quality in, 212–215
    assessment of, 214–215
    defined, 213–214, 213f
LNT model with, 176
manufacturers of previous solutions to exposure in
    Carestream Health, 183–184, 184f
    Philips Healthcare, 185
    Siemens, 184–185
new paradigm using, 177–179, 178f, 179f
protective shielding in, 261–278
    ALARA principle for, 262
    calculating shielding amount for, 272–278, 273f,
        274t, 275f, 275t
    x-ray room shielding, 265–272, 266f, 267f, 269f,
        271f, 272f, 277–278
    x-ray tube shielding, 262–265, 262f, 263f,
        264f, 265f, 277
radiation dose quantities in, 212
saturation in, 177
visual grading of normal anatomy in
    dose optimization research, 216–217
    dose optimization study example, 217–219
    visual grading analysis, 215–216, 218–219
direct beam absorber, 252
direct ionization, 32
DLP. See dose length product
DNA
    cell repair mechanisms following irradiation and,
        77–81, 78f, 79f, 81f
    defined, 74, 75f
    double strand of, 75f
    double-strand breaks with, 76f
    free-radical damage on, 77
    nitrogen bases of, 75f
    nucleotide base damage with, 76f
    radiation causing change within, 73–74, 73f
    single-strand breaks with, 76f
    time to manifest for damaged, 81–87,
        81f, 82f, 84t–88t
        chromosomal aberrations, 82, 82f
        genetic mutations, 82
        hereditary effects, 84–87, 85t, 86t, 87t
        induction of cancer, 82–84, 84t
    x-ray interaction with, 74–76, 76f

DNA repair mechanism, 77, 79–80
    cell repair mechanisms following irradiation,
        77–81, 78f, 79f, 81f
    homologous recombination in, 79–80
    non-homologous end joining in, 79–80
    single-strand annealing in, 80
dosage
    computed tomography, 199–209
        dose descriptors for, 204–206, 209
        factors affecting dose in, 206–207
        image quality optimization research for, 208
        optimization study example for, 208
        rationale for dose optimization in, 203
    deterministic effects with threshold doses, 89t
    digital radiography, 175–197
        assessment tools for optimization in, 211–218
        deviation index in, 190 196, 192f, 193t, 194t, 195f
        exposure creep in, 179
        exposure indices establishment in, 183–190,
            183f, 184f, 186f, 187f, 188f, 197
        exposure indices principles of, 179–181, 180f,
            181f, 182f
        highlighting inappropriate exposures in, 179
        image quality in, 212–215, 213f, 218
        new paradigm using, 177–179, 178f, 179f
        saturation in, 177
        visual grading of normal anatomy in, 215–219
    factors in fluoroscopy affecting, 165–174
    factors in radiographic imaging affecting, 147–162
        anti-scatter grids in, 156–157, 162
        automatic exposure control in, 152, 161, 203
        beam alignment in, 155, 161
        clinical factors in, 149–151, 161
        collimation in, 154–155, 161
        components of radiographic systems affecting,
            148–149, 149f
        density in, 156, 161
        exposure technique factors in, 151–152
        field size in, 154–155, 161
        film processing in, 157–158
        filtration in, 153–154, 161
        patient thickness in, 156, 161
        patient's responsibility in, 150
        radiography technical factors in, 151–162, 156f

dosage (*Cont.*)
  radiologist's role in, 150
  referring physician's responsibility in, 149–150
  repeat radiographic examinations in, 158–159
  repeat rates in digital radiography in, 159, 162
  responsibilities and radiation protection in, 150–151
  sensitivity of image receptor in, 157, 162
  shielding radio-sensitive organs in, 159–160, 162
  source-to-image receptor distance in, 155–156, 156*f*, 161
  source-to-skin distance in, 155–156, 156*f*, 161
  system components affecting, 148–149, 149*f*
  technologist' role in, 150
  x-ray generator waveform in, 152–153
  fixed fluoroscopy factors in, 169–172
    fluoroscopic exposure factors, 170
    fluoroscopic instrumentation factors, 170–172
  mobile fluoroscopy factors in, 172
  optimization, quality control with, 281–282, 284
  patient dose variations
    historical perspective for, 222, 222*t*, 223*f*
    today, 222–224, 224*t*, 225*t*
  patient doses in diagnostic imaging, 63, 64*t*
  staff doses in diagnostic imaging, 63–65
dose and dose rate effectiveness factor (DDREF), 83
dose creep, 179
dose equivalent limit, 7
dose length product (DLP), 205
dose limitation, 212
dose optimization, quality control with, 281–282, 284
dose settings, 170–171
dose units
  absorbed dose, 57–58
  collective effective dose, 61
  dosimetric quantities and units, 57–63, 65
  effective dose, 58–61
  equivalent dose, 58–59
  kinetic energy released per unit mass, 61–63, 62*f*
  quantities of radiation dose, 57
  units of exposure, 57
dose-area product meters (DAPs), 131
  function of, 122–124, 124*f*
  ionization chamber location with, 124–126, 125*f*

limitations with, 126–127
measurements, 234–235, 234*f*
overview, 122, 123*f*, 124*f*
readout unit, 123*f*, 124*f*
uncertainty in measurements with, 127
dose-image quality optimization, 10–11
dose-response models, 3–4, 14
down quarks, 20
DQE. *See* detective quantum efficiency
DRLs. *See* diagnostic reference levels
duodenum x-ray exam, 55*t*

E
effective atomic number, 20–21, 21*f*
effective dose, 9, 14, 58–61
  calculation of, 10, 60–61, 60*f*
  computed tomography, 204
  formula for, 59
  summary for non-fluoroscopic and non-CT exams, 102*t*
effective dosimetry, 100
elastic scattering, 34–35, 34*f*
elective examination, 257–258
electromagnetic radiation, 24–27, 25*f*, 44
  dual characteristics of, 25–27
  particles of, 25
  properties of, 25, 26*f*
electromagnetic spectrum, 25, 25*f*
electron optical magnification, 171
electronic collimation, 155
electronic magnification, 172
electronic noise, 214
electrons, 20–22
  binding energy of, 22, 22*t*
  orbit of, 22, 22*f*
  shells of, 22, 22*t*
  valence, 22
  weighting factors for, 58*t*
electrostatic lenses, 171
element, 19, 19*t*
embryos, radiation's effects on, 95–96
entrance surface air kerma (ESAK), 235
entrance surface doses (ESD), 222, 224*t*, 234, 244
epidemiologic studies, 3

equivalent dose, 7, 14, 58–59
  calculation for, 9
  deriving, 59–60
ESAK. *See* entrance surface air kerma
ESD. *See* entrance surface doses
esophagus x-ray exam, 55*t*
excitation, 33
exposure, 9, 14. *See also* diagnostic exposures;
      medical exposures; radiation exposure
  automatic exposure control, 152, 161, 203
  automatic exposure rate control, 171, 174
  coulomb per kilogram, 10, 15, 57
  dose units of, 57
  fluoroscopic exposure factors, 170
  highlighting inappropriate, 179
  human risk with, 72
  low-dose, risk debate with, 68–69, 69*f*, 70*f*
  radiation effects from x-ray, 166
exposure control, 251
exposure creep, 179
exposure index
  establishment of
    AAPM TG 116 solution, 185–190, 186*f*,
      187*f*, 188*f*, 197
    exposure represented by, 183
    options for, 183, 183*f*
    previous manufacturers solutions, 183–185, 184*f*
  importance of, 190
  opportunity in audits of, 191–195, 192*f*, 193*t*, 194*t*
  principles of
    practical criteria for, 181, 181*f*, 182*f*
    scientific criteria for, 179–180, 180*f*
exposure linearity, 252
exposure rate, 252
exposure reproducibility, 252
exposure switch, 253
exposure technique, pregnancy radiation protection
    with, 258–260
exposure technique factors
  exposure time, 152
  radiation quantity, 152
  tube current, 152
  tube potential energy, 151–152
exposure time, 152
extremity CT, 53*t*

F
FBP algorithm. *See* filtered back projection algorithm
female phantom absorbed doses, 60*f*
femoral angiography
  cancer risks for, 105*f*
  effective doses for, 104*f*
femur AP, effective doses for, 102*f*
femur Lat, effective doses for, 102*f*
fetuses, radiation's effects on, 95–96
field size, 154–155, 161
field-of-view (FOV), 148
  fluoroscopy, 167, 170, 174
film processing, 157–158
film-screen technology, 176–177, 176*f*, 177*f*, 197
  ALARA principle in, 176
filtered back projection (FBP) algorithm, 201
filters, 153
filtration
  added, 153
  fluoroscopy with, 171, 252
  inherent, 153
  patients protection with, 255–256
  radiographic equipment, 251–252
  radiographic imaging with, 153–154, 161
  total, 153
fission fragments, weighting factors for, 58*t*
fixed fluoroscopy, 169
  major dose factors in, 169–172
    exposure factors, 170
    instrumentation factors, 170–172
flat-panel digital detector-based fluoroscopy system
    (FPDD), 168–169, 168*f*, 169*f*
fluoroscopic exposure factors, 170
fluoroscopic instrumentation factors, 170–172
  anti-scatter radiation grid, 171
  automatic exposure rate control, 171, 174
  dose level settings, 170–171
  filtration, 171
  image magnification, 171–172
  image recording techniques, 172
  last frame hold, 172
  modes of operation, 170
fluoroscopy
  cancer risks with, 105*f*
  C-arm, 172

fluoroscopy (*Cont.*)
   C-arm CT, 173, 174
   dosage affected by, 165–174
   dose-image quality optimization with, 10
   equipment, 252–253
   fixed, 169
      fluoroscopic exposure factors in
         dosage, 170
      fluoroscopic instrumentation factors in dosage,
         170–172
      major dose factors in, 169–172
   high-level control, 171, 174
   intermittent, 170
   mobile, 169
      major dose factors in, 172
   patients protection with, 256
   pulse-progressive, 169
   radiation effects from x-ray exposure in, 166
   system types and components in, 166–169
      flat-panel digital detector-based system,
         168–169, 168*f*, 169*f*
      image intensifier-based system, 167, 167*f*
   variable frame-rate pulsed, 170
foot exam
   cancer risks for, 103*f*
   effective doses for, 102*f*
for-presentation image, 186
FOV. *See* field-of-view
FPDD. *See* flat-panel digital detector-based
        fluoroscopy system
frames per second (FPS), 170
free radicals, 74
   DNA with damage from, 77
free-in-air measurements, 235–236, 235*f*
Fukushima Daiichi nuclear disaster, 50, 70*f*

G
gamma radiation, 21
gamma rays radiation
   internal conversion with, 31–32
   production of, 30–31, 31*f*, 32*f*
   x-rays radiation Interactions with, 33–42
      Compton scattering, 36–40, 37*f*,
         38*f*, 39*f*, 41*f*
      elastic scattering, 34–35, 34*f*

      pair production, 40–42, 42*f*
      photoelectric absorption, 35–36, 35*f*
genetic effects, 4
genetic mutations, 82
genomic instability, 95
geometric magnification, 172
gonads
   nominal risk coefficient associated with, 85*t*
   radiation weighting factors for, 59*t*
gray (Gy), 57, 65
grid frequency, 157
grid ratio, 157
Gy. *See* gray

H
hadron, 20
half-life, 47
half-value layer, 263
head AP
   cancer risks for, 103*f*
   effective doses for, 102*f*
head CT, 53*t*, 55*t*
   cancer risks for, 105*f*
head Lat
   cancer risks for, 103*f*
   effective doses for, 102*f*
head PA
   cancer risks for, 103*f*
   effective doses for, 102*f*
heavy ions, weighting factors for, 58*t*
hereditary effects, 84–87, 85*t*, 86*t*
   detriment-adjusted nominal risk
      coefficient for, 87, 87*f*
   stochastic detriment-adjusted nominal risk
      coefficient for, 87, 88*f*
high-level control (HLC), 171, 174
highlighting inappropriate exposures, 179
hip AP, effective doses for, 102*f*
hip x-ray exam, 55*t*
Hiroshima nuclear explosion, 69*f*
historical perspectives, 6–7
HLC. *See* high-level control
homologous recombination, 79–80
hydrogen free radical, 74
hydroxy free radical, 74

I

IAEA. *See* International Atomic Energy Agency
ICRP. *See* International Commission on
    Radiological Protection
ICRU. *See* International Commission on Radiological
    Units and Measurements
IEC. *See* International Electrotechnical Commission
image detector, 157, 162
image intensification, 167
image intensifier-based fluoroscopy system,
    167, 167*f*
image magnification, 171–172
image quality, 116
    assessment of, 214–215
    computed tomography, 203, 208
    contrast resolution in, 214, 218
    detective quantum efficiency in, 214, 218
    digital radiography, 212–215, 213*f*, 218
    dose for optimization of, 10–11, 15
    fluoroscopy dose optimization for, 10
    noise in, 214, 218
    objective physical measures in, 214–215, 218
    radiation dose optimization for, 9
    spatial resolution in, 213, 218
    subjective observer performance in, 214, 218
image quality quartet, 213
image receptor, 157, 162
image receptor sensitivity, 157, 162
image receptor speed, 157, 162
image reconstruction, 200
image recording techniques, 172
indirect ionization, 33
inherent filtration, 153
intensity, 205
intermittent fluoroscopy, 170
internal conversion, 31–32
International Atomic Energy Agency (IAEA), 11
International Commission on Radiological Protection
    (ICRP), 11, 136–138, 143, 248
    definition of terms used in reports by,
        142, 142*t*, 144
    framework, 5, 14
    radiation protection guidance by, 248, 249
International Commission on Radiological Units and
    Measurements (ICRU), 11, 138, 143

International Electrotechnical Commission (IEC),
    191, 197
interspace material, 157
interventional CT, 53*t*, 55*t*
intravenous urogram x-ray exam, 55*t*
inverse square law, 8, 43–44, 43*f*
ionizing radiation, 32–33, 33*f*
    benefits and hazards from, 2, 14
    biological effects of, 3
isomeric transition, 31
isotope, 21

J

joule (J), 57
justification, 131, 212
    broad implementation of, 106–108,
        106*f*, 107*f*
    defined, 104–106
    individual implementation of, 108–109

K

kerma. *See* kinetic energy released per unit mass
kinetic energy, 29
kinetic energy released per unit mass (kerma),
    61–63, 62*f*
kinetics, 92–93
knee AP
    cancer risks for, 103*f*
    effective doses for, 102*f*
knee Lat
    cancer risks for, 103*f*
    effective doses for, 102*f*
Kodak. *See* Carestream Health
kVp. *See* tube potential energy

L

Lambert-Beer's law, 201
last frame hold, 172
lead protective curtain or drape, 253
LET. *See* linear energy transfer
Life Span Study, 69
ligation, 80
line spectra, 31
linear attenuation coefficient, 42
linear energy transfer (LET), 23, 42

Linear No-Threshold Model (LNT model), 262
  application of, 72
  debate over, 71–72, 71f
  digital radiography with, 176
  "linear" part of, 69–70, 70f
  "no-threshold" part of, 70–71
  three alternative models to, 71f
lithophiles, 47
liver
  nominal risk coefficient associated with, 85t
  radiation weighting factors for, 59t
LNT model. See Linear No-Threshold Model
low-dose radiation
  biological effects of, 67–96
  factors influencing effects at
    cell radiosensitivity, 89–92, 90f, 91f, 92f, 96
    dose rate, 93
    kinetics, 92–93
    oxygen presence, 93, 94f
    radioprotectants and radiosensitizers, 93–94
lumbar sacral joint x-ray exam, 55t
lumbar spine AP
  cancer risks for, 103f
  diagnostic reference levels for, 101f
  effective doses for, 102f
  patient radiation doses for, 64t
lumbar spine Lat
  cancer risks for, 103f
  effective doses for, 102f
  patient radiation doses for, 64t
lumbar spine x-ray exam, 55t
lumbo-sacral joint Lat, effective doses for, 102f
lung
  nominal risk coefficient associated with, 85t
  tissue, radiation weighting factors for, 59t

M
mA. See tube current
male phantom absorbed doses, 60f
mammography
  diagnostic reference levels for, 236–237
  dose-image quality optimization with, 10
  x-ray exam, 55t
mAs. See radiation quantity

mass attenuation coefficient, 42–43
maximum permissible dose (MPD), 7
mean glandular dose (MGD), 110, 236
medical exposures, 51–56
  diagnostic, 52–54, 52t, 53t, 54t, 55t
  doses, 56
  nuclear medicine, 48f, 51f, 52, 54, 56t
  radiation therapy, 54–56, 56t
medical radiodiagnostic practices, 226
mediolateral oblique (MLO) images, 106, 107f
metastable state, 31
MGD. See mean glandular dose
millisievert (mSv), 58
mitochondria, free radicals effects on, 77
MLO images. See mediolateral oblique images
mm of lead equivalent, 267
mobile fluoroscopy, 169
  major dose factors in, 172
MPD. See maximum permissible dose
MSCT. See multislice CT scanners
mSv. See millisievert
multislice CT scanners (MSCT), 202, 208
muons, weighting factors for, 58t

N
Nagasaki nuclear explosion, 69f
National Council on Radiation Protection and
    Measurements (NCRP), 5, 140, 144, 248
  definition of terms used in reports by,
      142, 142t, 144
  radiation protection guidance by, 248, 259
National Institute for Health and Care Excellence
    (NICE), 108
National Radiological Protection Board-United
    Kingdom (NRPB-UK), 141, 144
natural background radiation, 47–50, 48f, 49t
NCRP. See National Council on Radiation Protection
    and Measurements
neck CT, 53t, 55t
neutron radiation, 24
neutrons, 20
  weighting factors for, 58t
NICE. See National Institute for Health and
    Care Excellence

noise, 203, 208
  electronic, 214
  image quality and, 214, 218
  quantum, 214, 218
nominal risk coefficient, 83, 85t–86t
non-homologous end joining, 79–80
non-stochastic effects, 4
NRPB-UK. *See* National Radiological Protection Board-United Kingdom
nuclear medicine, 48f, 51f, 52, 54, 56t
nucleons, 20
nucleus, 20–21

O

objective physical measures, 214–215, 218
OER. *See* oxygen enhancement ratio
oesophagus
  nominal risk coefficient associated with, 85t–86t
  radiation weighting factors for, 59t
116 solution, 185–190, 186f, 187f, 188f, 197
optically stimulated luminescent dosimetry (OSL), 122, 122f, 123f
optimization, 109–116, 131, 212
  assessment tools for digital radiography dose, 211–218
  cost of, 116
  defined, 109–111
  dose for of image quality, 10–11, 15
  dose optimization research, 216–217
  dose optimization study example, 217–219
  fluoroscopy dose for image quality, 10
  image quality research for CT, 207
  image quality *versus* diagnostic efficacy with, 116
  initiatives for, 115–116
  non-optimization evident instead of literature on, 115
    new technologies in, 113–115, 113f, 114f
    reliance on traditionally procedures with, 111–113, 111f, 112f
  personnel practices recommendations for
    pregnancy, 256–260
    protection of patients, 255–256, 259
    protection of personnel, 254–255, 259
  quality control with dose, 281–282, 284

radiation dose for image quality, 9
radiation protection, 247–260
  education and training in, 249–250, 259
  equipment specifications in, 250
  personnel practices in, 250
  shielding in, 250
  radiation protection practice and, 109–116, 111f, 112f, 113f, 114f, 131
  rationale for dose in CT, 203
OSL. *See* optically stimulated luminescent dosimetry
ovary, nominal risk coefficient associated with, 85t–86t
oxygen enhancement ratio (OER), 93, 94f

P

P. *See* pitch
PACS. *See* picture archiving and communications system
pair production, 33, 40–42, 42f
particle beam, 23
particulate radiation, 22–24, 44
  alpha particles, 23, 23f, 24f
  beta particles, 23–24, 24f
  neutrons, 24
patient entrance dose (PED), 236
patient thickness and density, 156, 161
patient-image intensifier distance (P-IID), 172, 174
PBL. *See* positive beam limitation
PED. *See* patient entrance dose
pediatric values, DRLs establishment for, 241, 242t
pelvimetry CT, 53t
pelvis AP
  cancer risks for, 103f
  diagnostic reference levels for, 101f
  effective doses for, 102f
  patient radiation doses for, 64t
pelvis CT, 53t, 55t
pelvis x-ray exam, 55t
penetrating ability, 23
penumbra, 111, 112f
periodic table, 19t
peripheral angiography, 54t
  x-ray exam, 55t
peroxyl free radical, 74

personnel dosimeters, 254

personnel practices

pregnancy, 256–260

protection of patients, 255–256, 259

protection of personnel, 254–255, 259

Philips Healthcare, 185

photoelectric absorption, 33, 35–36, 35*f*

photons, weighting factors for, 58*t*

picture archiving and communications system (PACS), 202

P-IID. *See* patient-image intensifier distance

pitch (P), 203, 206, 209

pitch ratio, 203

positive beam limitation (PBL), 154, 251

potential energy, 30

pregnancy

children, embryos, and fetuses, radiation's effects on, 95–96

radiation protection recommendations for, 256–260

diagnostic ultrasound use, 259

elective examination, 257–258

informed consent and understanding, 257

pregnant worker, 258

shielding, collimation, and exposure technique, 258–260

signs or posters, 258

10-day rule, 257

preshielding, 271

primary protective barrier, 252

primary radiation, 268

protective clothing, 255

protective gloves, 255

protective shielding, 250

ALARA principle in, 262

calculating shielding amount for

amount of radiation being produced in, 272–275, 273*f*, 274*t*, 275*f*

formulae in, 276

occupancy factor in, 275, 275*t*

planning process in, 277, 278

in digital radiography, 261–278

shielding radio-sensitive organs, 159–160, 162

x-ray room

general principles for, 268–270, 269*f*, 278

primary and secondary barriers for, 270–272, 271*f*, 272*f*

radioprotective materials in, 265–268, 266*f*, 267*f*, 277

x-ray tube, 262–265, 262*f*, 263*f*, 264*f*, 265*f*, 277

proteins, free radicals effects on, 77

protons, 20

weighting factors for, 58*t*

pulmonary angiography, 54*t*

pulse-progressive fluoroscopy, 169

Q

QC. *See* quality control

quality assurance (QA)

defined, 280

radiation protection, 8–9, 256–260

quality control (QC)

defined, 280–281

dose optimization in, 281–284

radiation protection through, 279–284

tolerance limits in, 282–284

quantum mottle, 179

quantum noise, 214, 218

quarks, 20

R

R. *See* roentgen

rad, 57, 65

radiation

bremsstrahlung, 28*f*, 29, 29*f*

characteristic, 27–29, 28*f*, 29*f*

children effected by, 95–96

cosmic, 49*f*, 50

defined, 22

effects of, 18

electromagnetic, 24–27, 25*f*, 26*f*, 44

embryos effected by, 95–96

fetuses effected by, 95–96

gamma rays, 27–42, 31*f*, 32*f*, 35*f*, 37*f*, 38*f*, 39*f*, 41*f*, 42

ionizing, 2, 3, 14, 32–33, 33*f*

linear attenuation coefficient with, 42

linear energy transfer with, 23, 42
mass attenuation coefficient with, 42–43
natural background, 47–50, 48f, 49t
natural history of, 46–47, 46f, 65
neutron, 24
particulate, 22–24, 23f, 24f, 44
terrestrial, 50
types of, 22–33
UV, 47
x-rays, 27–32, 28f, 29f, 33–42, 35f, 37f, 38f, 39f, 41f, 42f, 43
radiation detection and measurement
DAPs in, 122–127, 123f, 124f, 125f, 131
radiochromic film in, 129–131, 129f, 130f
solid-state meters in, 127–129, 128f, 131
TLDs in, 118–122, 118f, 119f, 120f, 121f, 122f, 123f, 131
radiation dose
quantities of, 57
radiation exposure, difference from, 57, 65
radiation dose limits, 5–6, 6t, 116–118, 117t, 131
radiation dose-image quality optimization, 9
Radiation Effects Research Foundation (RERF), 3, 139, 143–144
Life Span Study undertaken by, 69
radiation exposure
biological effects of, 3, 4
bystander effect with, 95
diagnostic exposures, 52–54, 52t, 53t, 54t, 55t
genomic instability with, 95
non-irradiated cells changes with, 94–95
radiation dose, difference from, 57, 65
sources of, 65
man-made, 48f, 50–51
medical, 48f, 51–56, 51f, 52f, 52t, 53t, 54t, 55t, 56t
natural, 47–50, 48f, 49t
radiation protection
concepts, 6–11
diagnostic reference levels with, 11
dose-image quality optimization with, 10–11, 15
dose-response models for, 3–4, 14
equipment design and performance for
fluoroscopic equipment, 252–253
mobile radiographic equipment, 253
radiographic equipment, general, 250–251
radiographic equipment, specific, 251–252
four areas of responsibility in, 12–14
four quartets of, 7–9, 7f, 14
historical perspectives for, 6–7
ICRP framework for, 5
optimization of, 247–260
education and training in, 249–250, 259
equipment specifications in, 250
personnel practices in, 250
shielding in, 250
organizations for, 11, 15
personal actions in, 7, 7f, 14
personnel practices recommendations for
pregnancy, 256–260
protection of patients, 255–256, 259
protection of personnel, 254–255, 259
philosophy of, 4–6, 7f, 9
quality assurance with, 8–9, 256–260
quality control for, 279–284
dose optimization in, 281–284
tolerance limits in, 282–284
rationale for, 3–4
reports and publications for, 11–12, 248–249
technologist and, 12–15
x-ray dosimetry with, 9–10, 14
Radiation Protection Bureau-Health Canada (RPB-HC), 141, 144
definition of terms used in reports by, 142, 142t, 144
radiation protection organizations, 135–144
common elements in recommendations by, 142, 144
definition of terms used in reports by, 141–142, 142t, 144
international
BEIR, 3, 139, 143–144
ICRP, 5, 11, 14, 136–138, 142, 142t, 143
ICRU, 11, 138, 143
RERF, 3, 69, 139, 143–144
UNSCEAR, 11, 51, 138–139, 143
national
CDRH, 140–141, 144
NCRP, 5, 140, 142, 142t, 144
NRPB-UK, 141, 144
RPB-HC, 141, 142, 142t, 144

radiation protection practice, 99–131
  ALARA principle with, 100
  DAPs in, 122–127, 123f, 124f, 125f, 131
  diagnostic reference levels for, 101f
  dose risks in diagnostic imaging with, 100–104, 102t, 103t, 104t, 105t, 131
  justification in, 104–109, 106f, 107f, 131
  optimization in, 109–116, 111f, 112f, 113f, 114f, 131
  radiation detection and measurement in, 118–131, 118f–125f, 128f, 129f, 130f
  radiation dose limits in, 116–118, 117t, 131
  radiochromic film in, 129–131, 129f, 130f
  solid-state meters in, 127–129, 128f, 131
  three main systems in, 100
  TLDs in, 118–122, 118f, 119f, 120f, 121f, 122f, 123f, 131
radiation quantity (mAs), 152
radiation safety officer (RSO), 12
radiation therapy, 54–56, 56t
radio sensitivities, 58
radioactive decay, 21
radiobiology, 2
  bystander effect with, 95
  children, embryos, and fetuses in, 95–96
  deterministic effects with, 4, 14, 18, 87–89, 88f, 89t
  epigenetics with, 95
  genomic instability with, 95
  low-dose radiation of, 67–96
  non-irradiated cells changes with, 94–95
  stochastic effects with, 4, 14, 18, 68–87, 69f–71f, 73f, 75f–79f, 81f, 82f, 84t–88t
radiochromic film, 129–131, 129f, 130f
radiography
  anti-scatter grids in, 156–157, 162
  automatic exposure control in, 152, 161, 203
  beam alignment in, 155, 161
  collimation in, 154–155, 161
  exposure technique factors in
    exposure time, 152
    radiation quantity, 152
    tube current, 152
    tube potential energy, 151–152
  field size in, 154–155, 161
  film processing in, 157–158

  filtration in, 153–154, 161
  patient thickness and density in, 156, 161
  repeat radiographic examinations in, 158–159
  repeat rates in, 159, 162
  sensitivity of image receptor in, 157, 162
  shielding radio-sensitive organs in, 159–160, 162
  source-to-image receptor distance in, 155–156, 156f, 161
  source-to-skin distance in, 155–156, 156f, 161
  technical factors in, 151–162, 156f
  x-ray generator waveform in, 152–153
radiologist, 149, 150
radioprotectants, 93–94
radiosensitivity of cell, 89–92, 90f, 91f, 92f, 96
radiosensitizers, 93–94
radon, 48, 48f
Rayleigh scattering. See elastic scattering
RBE. See relative biological effectiveness
receiver operating characteristics (ROC), 10, 214
recoil, 35
referring physician, 149–150
reject analysis, 159, 162
relative biological effectiveness (RBE), 7
rem, 58, 65
repeat radiographic examinations, 158–159
repeat rates, 159, 162
RERF. See Radiation Effects Research Foundation
resection, 80
RNA, free radicals effects on, 77
ROC. See receiver operating characteristics
roentgen (R), 57, 65
RPB-HC. See Radiation Protection Bureau-Health Canada
RSO. See radiation safety officer

S
salivary glands, radiation weighting factors for, 59t
saturation, 177
scatter fraction, 272
secondary radiation, 268
sex-averaged absorbed dose, 60f
shadow shields, 159
shells, 22, 22t
shielding radio-sensitive organs, 159–160, 162

shoulder AP, effective doses for, 102*f*

SID. *See* source-to image receptor distance

Siemens, 184–185

sievert (Sv), 58, 65

signal-to-noise ratio (SNR), 214

single-slice CT (SSCT), 202

single-strand annealing, 80

skin. *See also* source-to-skin in distance

    nominal risk coefficient associated with, 85*t*–86*t*

    radiation weighting factors for, 59*t*

slice thickness, 203

small intestine x-ray exam, 55*t*

SNR. *See* signal-to-noise ratio

solid-state meters, 127–129, 128*f*, 131

somatic effects, 4

source-to image receptor distance (SID)

    fluoroscopy, 170, 174

    radiographic imaging, 148, 155–156, 156*f*, 161

source-to-skin in distance (SSD), 148, 155–156, 156*f*, 161

    patients protection with, 256

    radiation protection guidance with, 252, 253

spatial resolution, 203, 209, 213, 218

specific-area shielding, 250

spine CT, 53*t*, 55*t*

spine x-ray exam, 55*t*

SSCT. *See* single-slice CT

SSD. *See* source-to-skin in distance

stochastic effects, 4, 14, 18

    ALARA relevant to, 68

    background of, 68

    computed tomography with, 204

    detriment-adjusted nominal risk coefficient with, 87, 88*f*

    DNA in, 73–87, 73*f*, 75*f*–79*f*, 81*f*, 82*f*, 84*t*–88*t*

    human risk of x-ray exposures with, 72

    LNT model with, 69–72, 70*f*, 71*f*

    low-dose exposure risk debate with, 68–69, 69*f*, 70*f*

    principles of, 68–69, 69*f*, 70*f*

    radiation-induced change responsible for, 73–77, 73*f*, 75*f*, 76*f*, 77*f*

stomach

    nominal risk coefficient associated with, 85*t*–86*t*

    tissue, radiation weighting factors for, 59*t*

    x-ray exam, 55*t*

strand invasion, 80

subatomic entities, 44

subjective observer performance, 214, 218

Sv. *See* sievert

T

technical factors, 151–162, 156*f*

technologist, 149, 150

teeth x-ray exam, 55*t*

terrestrial radiation, 50

test procedure, 282

thermoluminescent dosimetry (TLDs), 131, 234, 234*f*

    calibration for, 120

    function of, 119

    OSL with, 122, 122*f*, 123*f*

    overview, 118–119

    patient dose measurements with, 119–120, 119*f*

    reading, 120–121, 121*f*

    staff dose measurements with, 120, 120*f*

    uncertainty in measurements with, 121–122, 122*f*, 123*f*

thoracic spine AP

    cancer risks for, 103*f*

    effective doses for, 102*f*

    patient radiation doses for, 64*t*

thoracic spine Lat

    cancer risks for, 103*f*

    effective doses for, 102*f*

    patient radiation doses for, 64*t*

thoracic spine x-ray exam, 55*t*

thyroid

    nominal risk coefficient associated with, 85*t*–86*t*

    radiation weighting factors for, 59*t*

thyroid shields, 255

TIPSS. *See* transjugular intrahepatic portosystemic stent shunting

tissue weighting factors (W_T), 7

TLDs. *See* thermoluminescent dosimetry

tolerance limits, 282–284

total collimation, 203

total filtration, 153

total quality management (TQM), 9, 280

transaxial images, 200

transjugular intrahepatic portosystemic stent
  shunting (TIPSS), 88
troposphere, 50
tube current (mA), 152
tube potential energy (kVp), 151–152
typical examinations, 226

U
ultraviolet (UV) radiation, 47
United Nations Scientific Committee on the Effects
  of Atomic Radiation (UNSCEAR), 11, 51,
  138–139, 143
up quarks, 20
urethra x-ray exam, 55t
UV radiation. *See* ultraviolet radiation

V
valence electrons, 22
variable frame-rate pulsed fluoroscopy, 170
visual grading analysis (VGA), 10, 214–216,
  218–219

W
W_T. *See* tissue weighting factors

X
x-ray dosimetry, 9–10, 14
x-ray generator waveform, 152–153
x-ray room shielding
  calculating shielding amount for
    amount of radiation being produced in, 272–275,
      273f, 274t, 275f
    formulae in, 276

occupancy factor in, 275, 275t
planning process in, 277, 278
general principles for, 268–270, 269f, 278
primary and secondary barriers for, 270–272,
  271f, 272f
radioprotective materials in
  barium plaster, 268, 277
  concrete, 268, 277
  gypsum wallboard, 267–268, 267f, 277
  lead, 265–268, 266f, 267f, 277
x-ray table top, 156, 161
x-ray tube port, 263
x-rays
  attenuating materials within beam of,
    195–196, 195f
  DNA interaction with, 74–76, 76f
  exam using, 55t, 231t, 232t
  first known image using, 18f
  human risk with exposure to, 72
  radiation effects from, 166
x-rays radiation, 27–32, 28f, 29f
  bremsstrahlung radiation with, 28f, 29, 29f
  characteristic radiation with, 27–29, 28f, 29f
  efficiency of, 30
  gamma rays radiation Interactions with, 33–42
    Compton scattering, 36–40, 37f, 38f, 39f, 41f
    elastic scattering, 34–35, 34f
    pair production, 40–42, 42f
    photoelectric absorption, 35–36, 35f
  interactions with biological tissue, 44
  properties of, 27, 44
  types of, 27–30, 28f, 29f